FIRST AID FOR THE®

Emergency Medicine Clerkship

Third Edition

D1240972

LATHA GANTI STEAD, MD, MS, FACEP
Chief, Division of Clinical Research
Professor of Emergency Medicine
University of Florida College of Medicine at Gainesville
Gainesville, Florida
Adjunct Professor of Emergency Medicine
Mayo Clinic, College of Medicine
Rochester, Minnesota
Executive Committee, Clerkship Directors in Emergency
    Medicine (CDEM)
Editor-in-Chief, *International Journal of Emergency
    Medicine*

MATTHEW S. KAUFMAN, MD
Assistant Professor of Medicine
Department of Hematology-Oncology
Albert Einstein College of Medicine
Bronx, New York
Resident, Emergency Medicine
Long Island Jewish Medical Center
New Hyde Park, New York

TORREY A. LAACK, MD, FACEP
Assistant Professor of Emergency Medicine
Emergency Medicine Clerkship Director
Mayo Clinic, College of Medicine
Rochester, Minnesota

JONATHAN FISHER, MD, MPH, FACEP
Assistant Professor of Medicine
Harvard Medical School
Director of Undergraduate Education
Harvard Affiliated Emergency Medicine Residency
Beth Israel Deaconess Medical Center
Boston, Massachusetts
Founding Member and Chair 2010–2011, Clerkship
    Directors in Emergency Medicine (CDEM)

ANUNAYA JAIN, MBBS, MCEM (UK)
Stroke Research Fellow
Department of Neurosurgery
University of Rochester Medical Center
Rochester, New York

MINAL JAIN, MBBS
Stroke Research Fellow
Department of Neurosurgery
University of Rochester Medical Center
Rochester, New York

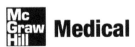 **Medical**

New York / Chicago / San Francisco / Lisbon / London / Madrid / Mexico City
Milan / New Delhi / San Juan / Seoul / Singapore / Sydney / Toronto

First Aid for the® Emergency Medicine Clerkship, Third Edition

1 2 3 4 5 6 7 8 9 0 QDB/QDB 14 13 12 11

ISBN 978-0-07-173906-1
MHID 0-07-173906-8

This book was set in Electra LH by Rainbow Graphics.
The editors were Catherine A. Johnson and Christine Diedrich.
The production supervisor was Catherine Saggese.
Project management was provided by Rainbow Graphics.
Quad/Graphics was the printer and binder.

Library of Congress Cataloging-in-Publication Data
Stead, Latha G.
    First aid for the emergency medicine clerkship / Latha Ganti Stead,
[et al.]. — 3rd ed.
        p. ; cm.
    Rev. ed. of: First aid for the emergency medicine clerkship : the
student to student guide / Latha G. Stead, S. Matthew Stead, Matthew S.
Kaufman. 2nd ed. 2005.
    Includes index.
    ISBN-13: 978-0-07-173906-1 (pbk.)
    ISBN-10: 0-07-173906-8 (pbk.)
    1. Emergency medicine—Outlines, syllabi, etc. 2. Clinical
clerkship—Outlines, syllabi, etc. I. Stead, Latha G. II. Stead, Latha
G. the student to student guide. First aid for the emergency medicine
clerkship :
    [DNLM: 1. Emergencies. 2. Clinical Clerkship. WB 105]
    RC86.92.S74 2011
    616.02′5—dc22

                                                    2011004090

To my parents, Ganti and Prabha Rao, for selflessly giving their time and encouragement so that I may continue to write; and to my four gifted sons, Thor, Tej, Trilok, and Karthik, for showing me by example how to enjoy life to its fullest.

—Latha

To my energy-packed nephews, Noah and Leo, providers of extra epinephrine.

—Matt

To my mom and dad for their support and encouragement; my wife, who is the love of my life; and all of the doctors and nurses who took care of me as a child and continue to teach me every day.

—Jonathan

We dedicate this book to our families for their love and support.

—Torrey, Anunaya, and Minal

CONTENTS

SECTION III: CLASSIFIED   515

SERIES EDITORS

LATHA GANTI STEAD, MD, MS, FACEP
Chief, Division of Clinical Research
Professor of Emergency Medicine
University of Florida College of Medicine at
    Gainesville
Gainesville, Florida
Adjunct Professor of Emergency Medicine
Mayo Clinic, College of Medicine
Rochester, Minnesota
Executive Committee, Clerkship Directors in
    Emergency Medicine (CDEM)
Editor-in-Chief, *International Journal of Emergency
    Medicine*

MATTHEW S. KAUFMAN, MD
Assistant Professor of Medicine
Department of Hematology-Oncology
Albert Einstein College of Medicine
Bronx, New York
Resident, Emergency Medicine
Long Island Jewish Medical Center
New Hyde Park, New York

TITLE EDITORS

TORREY A. LAACK, MD, FACEP
Assistant Professor of Emergency Medicine
Emergency Medicine Clerkship Director
Mayo Clinic, College of Medicine
Rochester, Minnesota

JONATHAN FISHER, MD, MPH, FACEP
Assistant Professor of Medicine
Harvard Medical School
Director of Undergraduate Education
Harvard Affiliated Emergency Medicine Residency
Beth Israel Deaconess Medical Center
Boston, Massachusetts
Founding Member and Chair 2010–2011, Clerkship
    Directors in Emergency Medicine (CDEM)

ANUNAYA JAIN, MBBS, MCEM (UK)
Stroke Research Fellow
Department of Neurosurgery
University of Rochester Medical Center
Rochester, New York

MINAL JAIN, MBBS
Stroke Research Fellow
Department of Neurosurgery
University of Rochester Medical Center
Rochester, New York

FACULTY CONTRIBUTORS

FALK EIKE FLACH, MD
Co-Director, Ultrasound Education
Assistant Professor
Department of Emergency Medicine
University of Florida College of Medicine
Gainesville, Florida

MATTHEW F. RYAN, MD, PHD
Medical Student Clerkship Director
Assistant Professor
Department of Emergency Medicine
University of Florida College of Medicine
Gainesville, Florida

LESLIE CONNOR NICKELS, MD, RDMS
Co-Director, Ultrasound Education
Assistant Professor
Department of Emergency Medicine
University of Florida College of Medicine
Gainesville, Florida

STUDENT REVIEWERS

The authors would like to thank the following student reviewers from the University of Rochester School of Medicine & Dentistry (URSMD) who carefully reviewed and made valuable improvements to the text. We would also like to thank Dr. David Lambert, Senior Associate Dean, Medical Student Education, and Dr. David Guzick, Former Dean of URSMD, for helping us to recruit these stellar students. Dr. Guzick is now Senior Vice President for Health Affairs and President, UF & Shands Health System.

SAMUEL HORR, CLASS OF 2010

KATHRYN KELLOGG, CLASS OF 2011

AJAY KURIYAN, CLASS OF 2010

EMILY MCQUAID, CLASS OF 2011

TARA WEISELBERG, CLASS OF 2010

The authors would also like to thank:

JOSHUA J. LYNCH, DO
Class of 2008
Lake Erie College of Osteopathic Medicine

FOREWORD

Emergency medicine has become one of the most popular and satisfying clinical clerkships in undergraduate medical education. The busy emergency department (ED) is one of the few places left in a student's experience where they can grapple with the difficulty and challenges of managing patients who are truly undifferentiated. The challenge to a student's success in the ED is to combine all the elements of punctuality, dedication, superior communication skills, empathy, procedural dexterity, efficient time management, and mastery of an essential knowledge base. All of these skills have to be used to manage the care of patients under as challenging a circumstance as any in the undergraduate medical education experience. The crutch of having teams of physicians who have already exercised diagnostic routines and have implemented treatment and management protocols are no longer available to the student in the ED. The student is expected to quickly master a broad base of knowledge that is essential to the specialty of emergency medicine, while at the same time focusing on specific areas of interest that would allow enough depth of knowledge to result in a comprehensive experience. This is particularly difficult to achieve in 4 weeks, but the exhilaration of the challenge and the sense of accomplishment after a successful rotation is the inspiration behind the third edition of *First Aid for the Emergency Medicine Clerkship*. This "how to succeed" guide for students who intend to complete a clerkship in emergency medicine is a comprehensive yet concise outline of core knowledge and concepts. The pages and margins of the guide are filled with absolutely relevant and clearly highlighted factoids and practical tips that supervising residents or faculty will be bound to ask about or will be found as questions in clerkship examinations. The "typical scenarios" highlights are tips in management and diagnostics that are case based and complaint driven. These scenarios guide the student to consider very specific common diagnoses based on common presentations they may encounter. The guide is organized in a format that allows for both quick reference and a comprehensive preview by students in preparation for their clerkship experience and their clerkship exam. Medical students who are transitioning from their preclinical years or intend to do a fourth-year elective should find this book an essential and extremely practical resource that will optimize the value of their experience in emergency medicine and should result in a true sense of accomplishment at the end of a 4-week rotation. The *First Aid* concept is superb and highly relevant. No student in emergency medicine should leave home without it.

Joseph A. Tyndall, MD, MPH
Associate Professor & Chairman
Department of Emergency Medicine
University of Florida College of Medicine
Gainesville, Florida

INTRODUCTION

This clinical study aid was designed in the tradition of the *First Aid* series of books. It is formatted in the same way as the other books in the series; however, a stronger clinical emphasis was placed on its content. You will find that rather than simply preparing you for success on an exam, this resource will also help guide you in the clinical diagnosis and treatment of many of the problems seen by emergency physicians.

The content of the book is based on the American College of Emergency Physicians (ACEP) and Society of Academic Emergency Medicine (SAEM) recommendations for the Emergency Medicine curriculum for fourth-year medical students. It also contains information derived from the Core Curriculum, an outline developed by the Residency Review Committee, which details the information that EM residents are expected to learn and will ultimately be responsible for on their oral and written board exams. Each of the chapters contains the major topics central to the practice of EM and has been specifically designed for the medical student learning level. In addition, special chapters such as Diagnostics and Procedures have been included to emphasize the more clinical nature of EM.

The content of the text is organized in the format similar to other texts in the *First Aid* series. Topics are listed by bold headings, and the "meat" of the topic provides essential information. The outside margins contain mnemonics, diagrams, exam and ward tips, summary or warning statements, and other memory aids. Exam tips are marked by ✎, ED tips by the symbol ⚕, and typical scenarios by the symbol 👤.

ABOUT THE CLERKSHIP DIRECTORS IN EMERGENCY MEDICINE

Clerkship Directors in Emergency Medicine (CDEM) is dedicated to promoting excellence in medical student education in emergency medicine. CDEM was founded as an Academy within the Society for Academic Emergency Medicine (SAEM) to represent medical student educators. Members of CDEM are medical student educators who are committed to enhancing medical student education within our specialty. CDEM provides an opportunity for EM clerkship directors and medical student educators to join forces, collaborate, and become a unified voice at the national level. CDEM serves as forum to establish guidelines, curricula and methods of evaluation. CDEM seeks to develop and disseminate these and other resources for medical student educators. CDEM is committed to promoting and supporting educational research and providing career development for its members.

Jonathan Fisher, MD, MPH
Founding Member and Chair 2010–2011, CDEM

HOW TO CONTRIBUTE

To continue to produce a high-yield review source for the radiology clerkship, you are invited to submit any suggestions or correction. Please send us your suggestions for:

- New facts, mnemonics, diagrams, and illustrations
- Low-yield facts to remove

For each entry incorporated into the next edition, you will receive personal acknowledgment. Diagrams, tables, partial entries, updates, corrections, and study hints are also appreciated, and significant contributions will be compensated at the discretion of the authors. Also let us know about material in this edition that you feel is low yield and should be deleted. You are also welcome to send general comments and feedback, although due to the volume of e-mails, we may not be able to respond to each of these.

The **preferred way** to submit entries, suggestions, or corrections is via **electronic mail**. Please include name, address, school affiliation, phone number, and e-mail address (if different from the address of origin). If there are multiple entries, please consolidate into a single e-mail or file attachment. Please send submissions to:

firstaidclerkships@gmail.com

Otherwise, please send entries, neatly written or typed or on disk (Microsoft Word), to:

Latha Ganti Stead, MD
c/o Catherine A. Johnson
Executive Editor
McGraw-Hill Medical
1221 Avenue of Americas, 45th Floor
New York, NY 10020

All entries become property of the authors and are subject to editing and reviewing. Please verify all data and spellings carefully. In the event that similar or duplicate entries are received, only the first entry received will be used. Include a reference to a standard textbook to facilitate verification of the fact. Please follow the style, punctuation, and format of this edition if possible.

INTERNSHIP OPPORTUNITIES

The author team is pleased to offer part-time and full-time internships in medical education and publishing to motivated physicians. Internships may range from three months (eg, a summer) up to a full year. Participants will have an opportunity to author, edit, and earn academic credit on a wide variety of projects, including the popular *First Aid* series. Writing/editing experience, familiarity with Microsoft Word, and Internet access are desired. For more information, e-mail a résumé or a short description of your experience along with a cover letter to **lathagantimd@gmail.com.**

NOTE TO CONTRIBUTORS

All entries become properties of the authors and are subject to review and edits. Please verify all data and spelling carefully. In the event that similar or duplicate entries are received, only the first entry received will be used. Include a reference to a standard textbook to facilitate verification of the fact. Please follow the style, punctuation, and format of this edition if possible.

CONTRIBUTION FORM

Contributor Name: _____

School/Affiliation: _____

Address: _____

Telephone: _____

E-mail: _____

Topic:

Location:

Cause:

Image findings:

Notes, Diagrams, Tables, and Mnemonics:

Reference:

You will receive personal acknowledgment for each entry that is used in future editions.

How to Succeed in the Emergency Medicine Clerkship

- What to Expect
- What to Bring
- How to Dress
- What to Do (How to Behave)
- What Not to Do
- What to Read
- Exam
- Specific Advice for Emergency Medicine Applicants

Emergency medicine (EM) takes a slightly different approach to patients from other specialties. The focus of emergency medicine is on acute stabilization; as such, we first look to rule out emergent, life-threatening causes of each patient's presentation rather than focusing on the most likely diagnoses.

Emergency medicine is a specialty with many unique and challenging aspects for medical students. These include:

- A large variety of presenting complaints over the entire range of ages.
- Being the first one to see a patient, which means being the first one to come up with a diagnosis.
- Opportunity to do a number of procedures.
- Opportunity to function as a real member of the resuscitation teams (eg, performing chest compressions).
- Opportunity for close interaction with attendings.
- Constant ongoing teaching, with the opportunity to pick up many "pearls."
- The emergency department (ED) can be a crazy place. You will undoubtedly have many very memorable cases and experiences during your rotation.

Many of the things that make EM so enjoyable may also pose a challenge at times:

- For many, the ED is the only place to obtain care; what a patient perceives as an emergency may not be what you perceive as one. Often, eliciting the underlying issue requires a little finesse and remaining nonjudgmental. For example, the patient who presents with a rash of 3 weeks' duration at 4 AM may actually be a victim of domestic violence. Since many patients who present to the ED have underlying social, psychological, and substance abuse issues, history taking can be quite challenging. It is important to remain nonjudgmental and provide the best possible care under sometimes less-than-optimal circumstances.
- The 24-hour open door policy of the ED, long waiting times, and uncomfortable waiting environment combined with the stress of high-acuity complaints, predispose to violence in the ED. Students should be aware of their environment and practice personal safety behavior as they would in any other potentially dangerous environment.
- While resuscitations are an exciting opportunity for students to learn and practice procedures, students often forget about universal precautions because of all the excitement, putting themselves at risk for needle-stick injuries. Remember, ALWAYS wear gloves and other personal protective equipment and NEVER recap needles. Report any exposure to body fluids to the EM attending immediately.

WHAT TO BRING

There is very little you will need to have on your person while working in the department. A basic list of equipment to carry with you includes:

1. Several black pens.
2. Stethoscope.
3. Trauma shears.
4. Small notepad to track patients and record important teaching points.
5. Penlight.
6. A pocket-sized or PDA/smartphone drug reference (eg, Tarascon's *Pharmacopeia*).
7. EMRA's *Guide to Antibiotic Use in the Emergency Department* or Sanford's *Guide to Antimicrobial Therapy*.
8. A good attitude!

HOW TO DRESS

Every ED will have a dress code. It is in your best interest to find out prior to your first shift what you are expected to wear. If you are unsure what to wear, you should dress in professional attire on the first day of the rotation with a white coat. Although most people wear scrubs, it is not a universal rule that one can wear scrubs in the ED. The ED can be a messy environment; while appropriate dress is required, very expensive clothes should be avoided (nice shoes seem to attract the most blood). You will be on your feet most of the day, so comfortable shoes are a must.

WHAT TO DO (HOW TO BEHAVE)

There are a few things we can say about what makes a medical student look good. Generally, a medical student who can function with some level of independence and stay on top of his or her patients is well received. For example, if a test is ordered for your patient, you should either know the result or what the delay is to getting the result.

- It is best to try to emulate an efficient and thorough resident that you may work beside. Every institution has its particular procedures for assigning patients, charting, "starting up" patients, admitting and discharging patients, and ordering labs or radiologic studies. Your efficiency in the department will be markedly improved if you can familiarize yourself with these administrative hurdles early on.
- A few general pointers:
  - Punctuality speaks for itself. Be the first one to arrive for sign-out rounds, codes, lectures, and grand rounds. Sign-out at the beginning of a shift is often one of the best learning opportunities and should not be missed.
  - Know all the important numbers for the department (door and copier codes, pager numbers, etc).
  - Ask the nurses for their help should you need it. They can be valuable allies and generally have the ear of the attendings.

3

- Treat everyone with respect; this includes nurses, ancillary staff, and even the hospital resident trying to "block" an admission at 3 AM.
- Be thorough but focused in your history and physical. Presentations should include only the essentials of relevant pertinent positives and negatives.
- Be brave: Avoid the temptation to present the history and wait for the attending or resident to come up with a plan of action. Try to present an action plan for each patient you see, even if you are unsure (this will help guide the attending or resident to teach you what you need to learn).
- Show an interest in what you are doing (fecal disimpactions can be fun!).
- Charting—essential components below:
  - Times of initial evaluation, all orders, repeat exams, radiology/lab results, discharge instructions.
  - Chief complaint and a good history *with review of systems*.
  - Exam (don't forget the neurologic, mental status, pelvic exams, etc) and *repeat* exam data as things change.
  - Orders must be countersigned by a resident or attending.
  - *Document* the lab, radiology, and electrocardiogram results on the chart.
  - Discharge instructions should be specific: Who to follow up with and when, as well as specific symptoms that warrant an immediate return to the ED (eg, fever, chest pain, shortness of breath, etc).
- If a patient wants to sign out against medical advice, notify the attending.
- Avoid being the rate-limiting step in a patient's care (eg, *you* forget to order the x-ray).
- Always sign out your patients at the end of the shift—this is essential.

WHAT NOT TO DO

- Be late.
- Make up an answer to a question you might not know (just say you don't know or didn't check that), particularly a fact about the patient or a test result.
- Look sloppy.
- Delay your patient's care.
- Seem uninterested.
- Be a "gunner." You are not competing against your peers, but should instead be helping each other along. If you are not perceived as a "team player," it will reflect negatively on you.
- Turn down the opportunity to do a procedure (even if you have done it before).
- Leave a shift prior to signing over care of your patients to another student or resident.

WHAT TO READ

Most EDs have a small collection of texts (usually locked up in a rack). There are, of course, almost limitless online resources as well (UpToDate, eMedicine, eMedHome, MDConsult, etc). If you have time to read during a shift, try to review topics related to each patient you see. You may find some specific information so you look sharp when presenting the patient and have a clear plan of action. Remember, patient care is an "open-book" endeavor, so utilize whatever resources are available to you.

As far as general reading for the clerkship, *this book* alone will likely provide enough reading material and information. The Academy of Clerkship Directors in Emergency Medicine published "Emergency Medicine Clerkship Primer: A Manual for Medical Students," which is available for free from: www.saem.org/saemdnn/Portals/0/NTForums_Attach/ED%20Primer.pdf.

The primer serves as guidebook with valuable advice for students rotating in emergency medicine and is a nice complement to the content of this book. If you desire to learn a topic in more detail, we advise that you jot down notes about each patient you see during your shift, and then read up about them when you get home.

Textbooks in emergency medicine that can be used as a reference include:

- *Emergency Medicine (A Comprehensive Study Guide)* by Judith Tintinalli: Designed as board review for residents.
- *Harwood-Nuss' Clinical Practice of Emergency Medicine*: Used by many residencies as the core textbook.
- *Rosen's Emergency Medicine (Concepts and Clinical Practice)*: The definitive text in emergency medicine and a good resource for reading on the pathophysiology as well as clinical aspects of disease.
- *Clinical Procedures in Emergency Medicine* by James R. Roberts and Jerris R. Hedges: A how-to for nearly all procedures you might be doing within the department.

EXAM

Some departments will have their own exam designed for the fourth-year medical student rotator (almost always multiple guess). There is no standardized shelf exam for EM. Some programs have an oral exam. This is a lot like taking the oral board exam as a graduating resident, only less strenuous and with less at stake. Others will use an Objective Structured Clinical Examination (OSCE), medical simulation cases, or other practical type exams. Clerkships may also use an online testing site known as SAEMTESTS.org.

The best strategy for doing well on a written, multiple-choice exam is to do practice questions beforehand. *PEER VIII* is a collection of questions put out by the American College of Emergency Physicians (ACEP) as an EM board preparation. These questions are often beyond what is expected of a medical student, but they contain extensive explanations for each question. Your best bet to obtain a copy of *PEER VIII* is to ask the residents in the program for a copy to borrow. There are a number of other commercially published question-and-answer texts that are available but not as good. However, going through this many resources is probably overkill, as this book, *First Aid for the Clinical Clerkship in Emergency Medicine*, will have the facts you need for both the test and the clerkship (ie, if you know what is in this book, you will do well).

Seeing as many patients as possible and presenting cases to the attendings and senior residents is the best form of preparation for the oral exam.

First- to Third-Year Students

- This is a time of exploration:
  - Be open to all specialties—ask yourself, "Could I see myself doing this as a career?"
  - Remember, EM is not the best choice for everyone.
- Seek mentorship from EM attendings or residents. Consult the Society for Academic Emergency Medicine (SAEM) web site for the "virtual advisors" program if you do not have an EM residency at your school.
- Seek out opportunities for clinical experience in EM (shadowing shifts, electives).
- Look for research opportunities within EM. This is also a great way to make connections with EM faculty.
- Become active in your school's emergency medicine interest group (EMIG). If you do not have an EMIG at your school, seek a faculty mentor to help start one.

Fourth-Year Planning

- EM clerkships:
  - In general, 2 months of EM early in the fourth year is adequate.
  - Ideally, 1 month will be at your home institution and 1 month will be away.
- Away EM rotations:
  - Consider an institution that is different than your own (eg, county hospital, inter-city, academic university hospital, etc).
  - Preferably will be done early in the year to allow you to obtain a standardized letter of recommendation (SLOR).
  - It need not be at your top choice, but it should be at a residency you would consider joining.
  - ED attendings, residency directors, and department chairpersons will be observing you as a potential resident. You are, in a sense, auditioning for a position in the match. Residents can be your allies and help you "look good" to the attendings; they may also have a role in the rank list decision making.
  - Have a good attitude and have fun; attendings are not going to want to work with a bunch of negative residents.
- Take advantages of unique learning opportunities:
  - Avoid turning your fourth year into a pre-residency.
  - Try electives you may not get to do again as a resident.
  - Program directors (PD) want well-rounded individuals with a breadth of experience.

HOW DO I KNOW IF I AM COMPETITIVE?

- Solicit feedback from EM faculty with whom you have worked.
- Try to find a mentor who will be honest with you (attending or resident).
- Be realistic: If you are not very competitive, you must be willing to apply very broadly.

WHAT ARE PDS LOOKING FOR?

- Honest, intelligent, hardworking residents who are teachable (nobody wants to work with an overconfident, difficult resident).
- USMLE scores:
  - Important in that they may be used to screen out applicants, especially at highly competitive programs (they cannot interview everyone).
  - Once you secure an interview, these scores become much less important.
  - Poor performance or failure in USMLE may predict later difficulties on written board exam.
- Timing of Step 2:
  - Generally can be taken whenever it is convenient for you.
  - Consider taking early if you think you can significantly improve upon your performance from Step 1.
- Non-EM clinical rotations:
  - Even if you know you want to do EM, performance on core clinical rotations is important.
  - May be viewed by PDs as a reflection of how you will perform clinically as a resident.
- Personal statement (PS):
  - Occasionally can help you stand out.
  - Opportunity to address any red flags (explanation of past failures, discipline, etc).
  - A very odd or negative PS can hurt you.
- SLORs (standardized letters of recommendation):
  - Very important, especially for programs where you have not rotated (no firsthand exposure).
  - Try to choose faculty with whom you have had good rapport or clinical experience to complete the SLOR.
  - Some departments may provide a joint letter from the PD and/or clerkship director with input from faculty and residents.
  - Ask if the individual can provide you with a "strong letter of recommendation." Be receptive for any hesitation, as you don't want to pressure someone to write you a letter if they are not comfortable or enthusiastic.
  - It is OK to follow up with faculty on the status of SLORs, but try to avoid being demanding or unrealistic, as this may negatively affect the letter.

Interviews

- Be realistic about the number of interviews you can accept (don't accept too few or too many).
- Avoid restricting your interviews to only highly competitive programs.
  - You may be competitive enough to get interviews at these programs, but not quite make the rank list. "Almost matching" doesn't help you.
  - Have a balanced number of highly competitive, midrange, and less competitive programs (keeping in mind that there are no "safety schools" and all programs are quite competitive).
  - There is no formal rating for EM programs—primarily based on word of mouth and reputation (ask around, use online resources).

- Be nice to everyone; the PD is likely to find out if you are rude to the residency coordinator.
- Cancel any interviews you do not intend to keep as soon as you know your plans. Last minute cancellations or "no shows" reflect poorly on you as well as fellow students from your school.

Rank List

- Consider discussion with all those affected by the decision (spouse, family, etc).
- Remember, there is no harm in putting your "dream program" number one, even if you do not think you will match there.
- Finally, rank every program unless you would rather scramble for a slot than match to that program.

OK, good luck . . . enjoy the book.

The following material will be useful to keep on hand during rounds. We have arranged it so that you can Xerox the pages, cut them out, and carry them in your pocket on the wards.

Trauma Card

Primary Survey

- **Airway:** Secure airway while maintaining C-spine immobilization. Verify endotracheal tube placement if patient arrives intubated.
- **Breathing:** Assist breathing if needed. Excessive positive pressure ventilation may reduce venous return to the heart.
- **Circulation:** Verify adequate circulation. Do chest compressions if pulseless, open cardiac massage for patients with penetrating chest trauma who initially had a pulse but lost it within 5 minutes or less of arrival.
- **Disability:** Deformity: GCS, wiggle toes. Identify and stabilize (splint) life threatening deformity.
- **Exposure:** Remove all clothing.
- **Flip:** While maintaining spine immobilization, log roll patient to examine back, rectal exam, between extremities. Concurrent with ABCDEF by other staff; secure two IVs, draw bloods, place Foley.

Secondary Survey

"AMPLE" history; obtain from patient, witnesses and paramedics.

- **A** Allergies
- **M** Medications
- **P** Past medical history
- **L** Last meal
- **E** Events

Physical Examination

- **Head:** Lacerations, depressions
- **Eyes:** Trauma, bulging
- **Ears:** Lacerations, blood or CSF in canal
- **Nose:** Blood or CSF
- **Mouth:** Missing teeth, gum fractures, maxillary instability
- **Jaw:** Mandible instability
- **Neck:** Posterior C-spine tenderness, anterior swelling or impending airway compromise, jugular venous distention. Record NEXUS criteria.
- **Chest:** Observe chest rise, auscultate, look for penetrating trauma
- **Abdomen:** Distention, tenderness, FAST exam (ultrasound)
- **Pelvis:** Instability, blood at urethral meatus
- **Rectal:** Sphincter tone, blood, position of prostate
- **Extremities:** Tenderness, deformity, pulses
- **Neuro:** Focal deficits

- Concurrent with secondary survey: portable films if needed: C-spine, chest, pelvis, and unstable extremity fractures. Give tetanus and antibiotics as needed. Record second GCS.

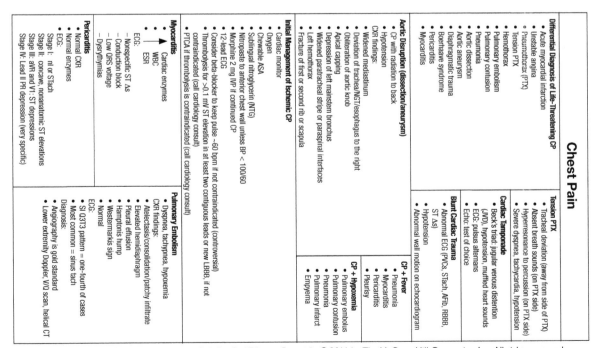

Chest Pain

Differential Diagnosis of Life-Threatening CP

- Acute myocardial infarction
- Unstable angina
- Pneumothorax (PTX)
- Tension PTX
- Hemothorax
- Pulmonary embolism
- Pulmonary contusion
- Pneumonia
- Aortic dissection
- Aortic aneurysm
- Diaphragmatic trauma
- Boerhaave syndrome
- Pericarditis
- Myocarditis

Tension PTX
- Tracheal deviation (away from side of PTX)
- Absent breath sounds (on PTX side)
- Hyperresonance to percussion (on PTX side)
- Severe dyspnea, tachycardia, hypotension

Cardiac Tamponade
- Beck's triad: jugular venous distention (JVD), hypotension, muffled heart sounds
- ECG: pulsus alternans
- Echo: test of choice

Blunt Cardiac Trauma
- Abnormal ECG (PVCs, STach, AFib, RBBB, ST ΔAs)
- Hypotension
- Abnormal wall motion on echocardiogram

Aortic Disruption (dissection/aneurysm)
- CP with radiation to back
- Hypotension
- CXR findings:
  - Widened mediastinum
  - Deviation of trachea/NGT/esophagus to the right
  - Obliteration of aortic knob
  - Apical capping
  - Depression of left mainstem bronchus
  - Widened paratracheal stripe or paraspinal interfaces
  - Left hemothorax
  - Fracture of first or second rib or scapula

CP + Fever
- Pneumonia
- Myocarditis
- Pericarditis
- Pleurisy

CP + Hypoxemia
- Pulmonary embolus
- Myocarditis
- Pulmonary contusion
- Pneumonia
- Pulmonary infarct
- Empyema

Initial Management of Ischemic CP
- Cardiac monitor
- Oxygen
- Chewable ASA
- Sublingual nitroglycerin (NTG)
- Nitroglycerin to anterior chest wall unless BP < 100/60
- Morphine 2 mg IVP if continued CP
- Consider beta-blocker to keep pulse ~60 bpm if not contraindicated (controversial)
- Thrombolysis for >0.1 mV ST elevation in at least two contiguous leads or new LBBB, if not contraindicated (call cardiology consult)
- PTCA if thrombolysis is contraindicated (call cardiology consult)

Pulmonary Embolism
- Dyspnea, tachypnea, hypoxemia
- CXR findings:
  - Atelectasis/consolidation/patchy infiltrate
  - Elevated hemidiaphragm
  - Pleural effusion
  - Hampton's hump
  - Westermark's sign
  - Normal
- ECG:
  - S1 Q3T3 pattern = one-fourth of cases
  - Most common = sinus tach
- Diagnosis:
  - Angiography is gold standard
  - Lower extremity Doppler V/Q scan, helical CT

Myocarditis
- ECG:
  - Cardiac enzymes
  - WBC
  - ESR
  → 12-lead ECG
  - Nonspecific ST Δs
  - Conduction block
  - Low QRS voltage
  - Dysrhythmias

Pericarditis
- Normal CXR
- Normal enzymes
- ECG:
  - Stage I: ↑I or STach
  - Stage II: concave, nonanatomic ST elevations
  - Stage III: aVR and V1: ST depressions
  - Stage IV: Lead II PR depression (very specific)

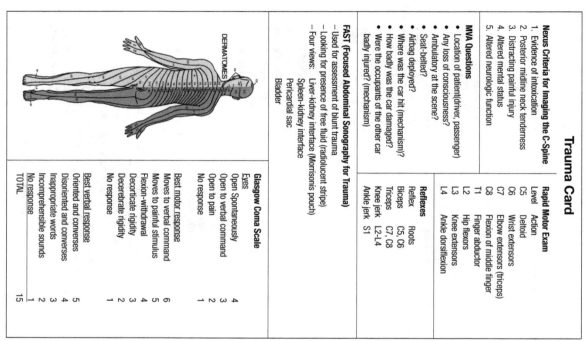

Trauma Card

Nexus Criteria for Imaging the C-Spine
1. Evidence of intoxication
2. Posterior midline neck tenderness
3. Distracting painful injury
4. Altered mental status
5. Altered neurologic function

MVA Questions
- Location of patient(driver, passenger)
- Any loss of consciousness?
- Ambulatory at the scene?
- Seat-belted?
- Airbag deployed?
- Where was the car hit (mechanism)?
- How badly was the car damaged?
- Were the occupants of the other car badly injured? (mechanism)

FAST (Focused Abdominal Sonography for Trauma)
— Used for assessment of blunt trauma
— Looking for presence of free fluid (radiolucent stripe)
— Four views:　Liver-kidney interface (Morrison's pouch)
　Spleen-kidney interface
　Pericardial sac
　Bladder

DERMATOMES

Rapid Motor Exam

Level	Action
C5	Deltoid
C6	Wrist extensors
C7	Elbow extensors (triceps)
C8	Flexion of middle finger
T1	Finger abductor
L2	Hip flexors
L3	Knee extensors
L4	Ankle dorsiflexion

Reflexes

Reflex	Roots
Biceps	C5, C6
Triceps	C7, C8
Knee jerk	L2-L4
Ankle jerk	S1

Glasgow Coma Scale

Eyes	
Open Spontaneously	4
Open to verbal command	3
Open to pain	2
No response	1
Best motor response	
Moves to verbal command	6
Moves to painful stimulus	5
Flexion-withdrawal	4
Decorticate rigidity	3
Decerebrate rigidity	2
No response	1
Best verbal response	
Oriented and converses	5
Disoriented and converses	4
Inappropriate words	3
Incomprehensible sounds	2
No response	1
TOTAL	15

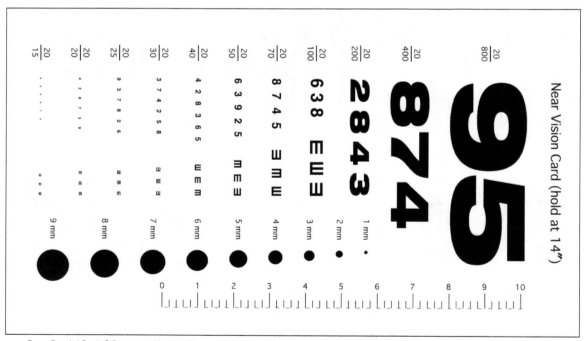

Near Vision Card (hold at 14")

High-Yield Facts

Resuscitation

Based on 2010 American Heart Association Guidelines for CPR and Emergency Cardiovascular Care

- Goals of BLS:
  - Recognition of sudden cardiac arrest
  - Activation of Emergency Response System
  - Early performance of high-quality cardiopulmonary resuscitation (CPR)
  - Rapid defibrillation when appropriate
- **BLS Protocol (3 A's plus CAB)**
  - Assessment: Determine unresponsiveness of the patient.
  - Activate the EMS system immediately by calling 9-1-1.
  - AED activation if available
  - CABs of CPR (chest compressions, airway, breathing)

Circulation

- Chest compressions should be continuous, over the middle of the chest.
- Proper hand position is on the lower half of the sternum, with one hand on top of the other.
- **Push hard, push fast. Allow the chest to recoil after each compression.**
- Compression depth should be at least 2 inches.
- Rate of chest compressions should be at least 100 per minute.
- A compression-ventilation ratio of 30:2 is recommended.

Airway with C-Spine Control

- Position the patient supine on a flat surface using "logroll" technique.
- Open the airway using head tilt–chin lift maneuver or the jaw thrust maneuver if cspine injury possible.

Breathing

- Perform **rescue breathing** after 30 chest compressions.
- Give two initial breath over 1 second each.
- Give enough tidal volume to produce a visible chest rise (equivalent to 500-600 mL).
- When an advanced airway is in place, during 2 person CPR, give 1 breath every 6–8 seconds without attempting to synchronize between compressions for delivery of ventilations.

Risk Factors

- Large, poorly chewed pieces of food.
- Excessive alcohol intake.
- Dentures.
- Children swallowing small objects (toys, beads, marbles, thumbtacks).

The most common cause of sudden cardiac death in adults is ventricular fibrillation (V-fib).

The most significant change in the 2010 AHA guidelines for CPR and ECC is the change of order, with chest compressions being first.

Survival rates from cardiac arrest are highest when BLS is initiated within 4 minutes and advanced cardiac life support (ACLS) is initiated within 8 minutes.

The 2010 AHA guidelines for CPR and ECC have removed the "look, listen, and feel" from the algorithm and have deemphasized the check for breathing and look for pulse.

The **tongue** is the most common cause of airway obstruction in the unconscious victim.

HIGH-YIELD FACTS

Resuscitation

Foreign body airway obstruction should be considered in any victim who suddenly becomes cyanotic and stops breathing, especially children.

In adults, poorly chewed meat is the most common cause of foreign body obstruction.

The **Heimlich maneuver** is the recommended method of expelling a foreign object from the airway.

- Children eating foods that require adequate chewing (hot dogs, peanuts, popcorn, candy).
- Children running/playing while eating.

Management of Partial Airway Obstruction

Do not interfere with any choking victim who is able to cough or speak. Coughing is the most effective way to clear a foreign body from the airway, and the ability to speak indicates that adequate ventilation is still occurring.

Signs of Complete Airway Obstruction

- High-pitched, stridorous sounds during inhalation
- Weak and ineffective coughing
- Respiratory distress
- Inability to speak
- Cyanosis

Heimlich Maneuver (Abdominal Thrusts)

 You are at dinner with friends when the woman at the next table and stands up and starts screaming that she is choking and cannot breathe. Her color is pink, and she coughing forcefully. What should you do?

The person in question has a partial airway obstruction indicated by the fact that she is able to speak and has a strong cough. At this point, you should monitor the situation until she clears the obstruction on her own or develops a complete obstruction. Signs of complete obstruction include inability to speak, weak cough, and cyanosis.

In a Standing (Conscious) Victim
- Stand behind victim and wrap arms around waist.
- Make fist and place thumb of fist slightly above the navel of the victim's abdomen.
- Grasp fist with the other hand and quickly thrust inward and upward into victim's abdomen.
- Repeat until object is dislodged or patient becomes unconscious.

In an Unconscious Victim
- Lay victim supine.
- Straddle victim, place heel of palm just above navel (well below the xiphoid), and deliver quick inward and upward abdominal thrusts (up to five).
- Open the mouth of the unconscious victim to look for foreign body and remove if present.
- Reposition the head and attempt rescue breathing.
- Repeat the sequence of the Heimlich maneuver, finger sweep, and rescue breathing attempts until victim resumes breathing or definitive help arrives.

Goals

To provide rapid assessment and definitive management of the cardiac arrest situation using cardiac monitoring equipment, advanced airway management, as well as electrical and pharmacologic therapy.

Primary Survey

Focus on the CABs of CPR and keep in mind defibrillation.

Secondary Survey

Secondary survey of ACLS focuses on establishing a definitive airway, establishing access to the circulation, assessing cardiac rhythms, pharmacologic interventions, etc.

Secondary survey "A-B-C-D"
- Airway—laryngeal mask airway (LMA) or endotracheal intubation.
- Breathing—assess bilateral chest rise and bilateral breath sounds.
- Circulation—establish intravenous (IV) access, determine the cardiac rhythm, and give the appropriate medication for that rhythm.
- Differential diagnosis—why did the arrest occur? Are there any causes that are reversible and have a specific therapy?

Airway

- **Nasal airway:** Rubber nasal trumpet inserted into the nostril and passed into the posterior pharynx keeps the tongue from falling back and obstructing the airway.
- **Oral airway:** Curved rigid airway, inserted using a tongue blade so that the distal edge prevents the tongue from falling backward. Often *incorrectly* used as a "bite block." Should be used only in unconscious patients with absent gag reflexes (ie, it will cause gagging if any gag reflex remains).
- **Laryngeal mask airway:** A supraglottic airway management device. Distal tip of LMA cuff presses against upper esophageal sphincter, upper border rests against tongue (see Figure 1-1). Cuff is then inflated, forming a seal over the larynx and permiting positive pressure ventilation.
- **Endotracheal intubation:** Establishes a definitive airway that also protects against aspiration of blood, vomit, and pharyngeal secretions.

ACLS is a continuum of BLS.

Remember your **CAB**s:
- **C**irculation
- **A**irway with C-spine control
- **B**reathing
Don't forget to **D**efibrillate.

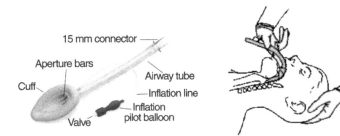

FIGURE 1-1. Laryngeal mask airway (LMA).

Several cardiac medications can be given directly through the endotracheal tube (ETT). Usual ETT dose is 2–2.5 times the IV dose followed by 10 mL of normal saline flush and several ventilations by bag-valve ventilation. Intravenous and intraosseous routes are preferred for administration of resuscitation medications.

Breathing

- Assess the status of ventilations after intubation (listen for equal breath sounds over both lung fields and make sure there are no sounds of gastric insufflation) and adjust the tube as necessary.
- Assess the movement of the chest wall with ventilations.
- If in a hospital setting, obtain a stat portable chest x-ray (CXR).
- Confirm ETT placement with a continuous wave capnography. If not available, can use exhaled end-tidal CO_2 detector, but remember this is not any better than visualization or auscultation.
- If there is any doubt of placement, consider extubation and reintubation under direct visualization with a laryngoscope.

Circulation

- Establish IV access (easiest access is usually the antecubital vein).
- *Normal saline* is the fluid of choice in the resuscitation setting.
- Determine cardiac rhythm.

Differential Diagnosis

- Continually ask yourself, "What caused this arrest?"
- Examine the rhythm and consider all the possible causes.
- Treat each of those possible causes that are reversible and/or have a specific therapy.

New 2010 ACLS Cardiac Arrest Algorithm

1. Activate emergency response.
2. Start CPR (CABs, 2 minutes of continuous compressions).
3. O_2, monitor, intravenous (IV) or intraosseous (IO) access.
4. Check rhythm.
5. If return of spontaneous circulation (ROSC), proceed to post–cardiac arrest care (PCAC).
6. If rhythm is ventricular fibrillation (VF)/ventricular tachycardia (VT), shock and check rhythm.
7. If at any time there is ROSC, proceed to PCAC.
8. If not, continue CPR for 2 minutes before doing another rhythm check.
9. Drug therapy (IV or IO):
   - Epinephrine 1 mg every 3–5 minutes.
   - Vasopressin 40 mg can be used in lieu of first or second dose of epinephrine.
   - Amiodarone for refractory VF/VT (first dose = 300 mg bolus; second dose = 150 mg).
10. Consider advanced airway (see section on page 25).
11. Treat reversible causes.

RETURN OF SPONTANEOUS CIRCULATION (ROSC)

Characterized by:

- Presence of spontaneous pulse and blood pressure.
- Abrupt and sustained ↑ in pressure of end-tidal carbon dioxide ($PETCO_2$) typically > 40 mm Hg.

MARKERS OF HIGH-QUALITY CPR

- Compression depth > 2 inches
- Compression rate > 100/minute
- Complete recoil between compressions
- Minimal interruptions between compressions
- No excessive ventilation
- Chest compressor rotated every 2 minutes
- 30:2 compression ventilation ratio when no advanced airway present

MARKERS OF COMPROMISED-QUALITY CPR

- $PETCO_2$ < 10 mm Hg
- Intra-arterial relaxation phase (diastolic) pressure < 20 mm Hg

VENTRICULAR FIBRILLATION OR PULSELESS VENTRICULAR TACHYCARDIA (VF/VT)

VF and Pulseless VT Algorithm

- It is essential to remember that early defibrillation is the most important therapy for this rhythm. (See Figures 1-2 and 1-3.)
- Defibrillation should take precedence over establishing IV access, intubation, or the administration of any drug.
- Initiate and continue CPR until defibrillator is attached.
- Defibrillate (shock), 360J (monophasic) or 150 to 200J (biphasic).
- Perform 2 minutes of CPR in between each shock.
- **Epinephrine** 1 mg IV q 3–5 minutes or **vasopressin** 40 U IV × 1.
- **Amiodarone** 300 mg IV for VF/pulseless VT, then infusion.
- **Lidocaine** if amiodarone not available: 1–1.5 mg/kg IV; can repeat once.
- **Magnesium sulfate** 1–2 g IV, then infusion if torsades de pointes present.

> Magnesium sulfate is especially useful in *torsades de pointes* and suspected hypomagnesemia; it should be given whenever these etiologies are suspected.

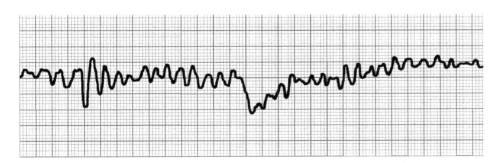

FIGURE 1-2. Ventricular fibrillation.

Causes of PEA:
Remember that cute lab partner in gross anatomy?
HOT MATCH MD
- **H**ypovolemia (volume — normal saline infusion)
- Hyp**O**xia (oxygen, intubation, ventilation)
- Hypo**T**hermia (warmed normal saline infusion)
- **M**assive pulmonary embolism (thrombolytics)
- **A**cidosis (sodium bicarbonate)
- **T**ension pneumothorax (needle decompression)
- **C**ardiac tamponade (pericardiocentesis)
- **H**yperkalemia (calcium, sodium bicarbonate)
- Massive acute **M**yocardial infarction
- **D**rug overdose from TCAs, digoxin, beta blockers, calcium channel blockers

Asystole = no pulse + no electrical activity. Always confirm flatline in more than one lead. Never shock asystole.

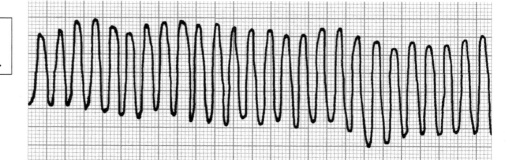

FIGURE 1-3. Ventricular tachycardia.

PULSELESS ELECTRICAL ACTIVITY (PEA)

Definition

- Any normally perfusing rhythm in which there is no detectable pulse.
- The differential diagnosis for PEA is key because certain etiologies of PEA have specific treatments and therefore the arrhythmia may be easly reversible.
- CPR and ACLS should be continued until correctable causes of PEA have been addressed.

ASYSTOLE

 You are walking through the airport when a fellow passenger grabs his chest and drops to the ground. You run over to discover he is cyanotic and does not have a pulse. What do you do?

The passenger is suffering sudden cardiac arrest. You should identify a particular person to call 911, and should begin CPR. Given that this is a stranger, you can consider doing compression-only CPR, and skip providing rescue breast via mouth to mouth. There is good evidence that compression-only CPR is as effective as traditional CPR. Many airports have automated external defibrillators (AED). The AED is a device that can be attached to a patient suffering from cardiac arrest via two pads. The device will analyze the patient's rhythm and recommend a shock if the patient is in ventricular fibrillation or tachycardia. If an AED is available, you should apply it to victim and follow the instructions. Early defibrillation is the key to survival from sudden cardiac arrest.

Definition

- A "flatline" rhythm is indicative of the absence of any electrical activity of the heart.
- The most common cause of a flatline tracing on electrocardiogram (ECG) is a detached lead or malfunctioning equipment, not asystole; therefore, always confirm asystole in more than one lead!
- Asystole is always pulseless.
- Asystole will not respond to shocking (no matter what you see on TV).

Definition

- Defined as heart rate < 60 beats per minute.
- It is considered symptomatic or "unstable" when accompanied by hypotension, shock, congestive heart failure (CHF), pulmonary edema, shortness of breath, cyanosis, lethargy, or chest pain.

Bradycardia Algorithm

- ABCs, O_2, IV access, cardiac monitor, pulse oximetry, ECG, portable CXR.
- Call for transcutaneous pacer to bedside earlier rather than later.

Treatment of Unstable Bradycardia

1. **Atropine** 0.5 mg IV bolus q 3–5 minutes, max dose 3 mg (remember that transplanted hearts are *denervated* and will not respond to atropine, go straight to pacing).
2. **Transcutaneous pacing (TCP)** (this is *painful*, use sedation and/or analgesia as needed) verifying electrical capture and mechanical contractions.
3. **Dopamine** 5–20 µg/kg/min—titrate to acceptable heart rate (HR) and blood pressure (BP).
4. **Epinephrine** 2–10 µg/min—titrate to acceptable HR and BP.
5. Prepare for **transvenous pacing.**

"Unstable bradycardia" = ↓ LOC, ↓ BP, CHF, ischemic chest pain.

Atropine may convert Type II second-degree block into complete heart block; thus, TCP is indicated.

Definition

- Any rhythm in which the heart is beating faster than 100 times per minute.
- As with bradycardia, treatment of tachydysrhythmia is largely dictated by the severity of the signs and symptoms.
- If serious signs and symptoms are present, you should ask whether the tachycardia is causing the symptoms or an underlying symptom is causing the tachycardia.
- "Unstable" refers to the presence of:
  - Hypotension
  - Acute altered mental status
  - Signs of shock
  - Ischemic chest discomfort
  - Acute heart failure

Tachycardia Algorithm

1. ABCs, O$_2$, IV access, cardiac monitor, pulse oximetry, ECG, portable CXR.
2. If unstable: Synchronized cardioversion.
   a. Narrow regular: 50–100J
   b. Narrow irregular: 120–200J biphasic; 200J monophasic
   c. Wide regular: 100J
   d. Wide irregular; Unsynchronized cardioversion
3. If stable: vagal menuevers, adenosine if regular, expert consultation

ATRIAL FIBRILLATION AND ATRIAL FLUTTER

A 55-year-old male presents with palpitations. His heart rate is 155 with a blood pressure of 160/92. The monitor shows a narrow complex tachycardia that is irregular. What are the treatment options?
The rhythm represent atrial fibrillation with rapid ventricular response. The first question is whether the patient is stable or unstable. The patient appears stable. The goal of therapy should be rate control. An IV beta blocker or calcium channel blocker is a reasonable choice. If the patient becomes unstable, synchronized cardioversion should be performed.

See Figures 7-13 and 7-14 (Cardiovascular Emergencies chapter) for ECGs of atrial fibrillation and atrial flutter.

Atrial Fibrillation/Flutter Algorithm

1. ABCs, O$_2$, IV access, cardiac monitor, pulse oximetry, ECG, portable CXR.
2. Decide if *stable* or *unstable*.
3. If unstable, administer **synchronized cardioversion** (120–200J biphasic or 200J monophasic).
4. If stable, pharmacologic interventions for rate control include:
   - **Diltiazem** 0.25 mg/kg IV slowly over 2 minutes. Wait 15 minutes. If no response, then increase diltiazem dose to 0.35 mg/kg IV slowly over 2 minutes, then infusion at 5 to 15 mg/h IV. Wait 15 minutes.
   - If no result, consider short-acting beta blocker (cautiously use beta blockers only after enough time has passed since last dose of calcium channel blockers; many prefer to stick with either a calcium channel blocker or a beta blocker to avoid blocking both channels):
     - **Metoprolol** 5 mg IV q 5 minutes × 3.
     - **Esmolol** 500 μg/kg IV over 1 minute (loading dose), then 50–200 μg/kg/min infusion.
     - **Attenolol** 2.5–5.0 mg IV over 2 minutes.
5. Agents for rhythm control are rarely used in the acute setting. When used, these are usually done with expert cardiology consultation.
6. Anticoagulation.

Awake patients should be sedated prior to synchronized cardioversion.

Definition

- Heart rate usually > 160 beats per minute.
- Usually demonstrates a narrow regular QRS complex (< 0.10 second) on ECG (see Figure 1-4).

PSVT Algorithm

1. ABCs, O_2, IV access, cardiac monitor, pulse oximetry, ECG, portable CXR.
2. Decide if *stable* or *unstable*.
3. If unstable, synchronized cardioversion (50–100J).
4. If stable, proceed as follows:
   - **Vagal maneuvers:** Valsalva; carotid massage (listen first for bruits); ice water bath (not if history of myocardial infarction [MI]).
   - **Adenosine** 6 mg *rapid* IV push.
   - Important: Wait 1–2 minutes.
   - **Adenosine** 12 mg rapid IV push, repeat after 1 to 2 minutes.
5. If tachycardia persists, analyze QRS complex on ECG and rhythm strip:
   - If **wide complex tachycardia** (and patient remains stable), treat as ventricular tachycardia.
   - If **narrow complex tachycardia** (and patient remains stable), several agents can be used for cardioversion:
     - Diltiazem 20 mg or verapamil 3–10 mg over 2 minutes; can repeat in 30 minutes. Hypotension from these calcium channel blockers can be treated with IV calcium chloride 35 mg.
     - Esmolol followed by infusion, or metoprolol 5–10 mg IV.
     - Digoxin 5 mg IV.
6. If at any time the patient becomes unstable, proceed directly to synchronized cardioversion.

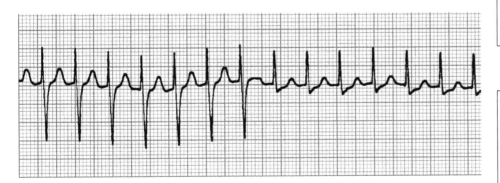

FIGURE 1-4. Paroxysmal supraventricular tachycardia.

PSVT = narrow regular QRS and rate > 160

Avoid *carotid massage* if bruits present. Avoid ice bath if history of myocardial infarction (MI). Push adenosine *rapidly* with an immediate saline flush. The biggest mistake when using adenosine is it is not *pushed rapidly enough.*

Adenosine feels like a *mule kick* to the chest—warn patients prior to giving it.

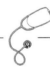

Adenosine is contraindicated in patients with asthma.

Reduce adenosine dose in patients with heart transplants, and those taking dipyramidole or carbemazepine.

HIGH-YIELD FACTS

Resuscitation

Definition

- Rate > 100 **beats per minute.**
- **Wide QRS** complexes that are **regular.**
- Constant QRS axis.
- Readily converts to ventricular fibrillation (**BAD!**).
- If pulseless VT, proceed immediately with defibrillation (remember VF/pulseless VT algorithm).
- Some wide complex tachycardias are not VT, but when in doubt treat as VT.

VT = wide QRS + rate > 100 msec

VT with Pulse Algorithm

1. ABCs, O_2, IV access, cardiac monitor, pulse oximetry, ECG, portable CXR.
2. Decide if stable or unstable.
3. If unstable, immediate synchronized cardioversion (100J).
4. If stable:
   - Procainamide 20–50 mg/min IV until arrhythmia suppressed, hypotension ensues, QRS duration ↑ > 50%, or maximum dose (17 mg/kg) reached. Avoid in patients with CHF.
   - Amiodarone 150 mg IV bolus over 10 minutes. Can repeat once, then follow with maintenance infusion of 1 mg/min for 6 hours.
   - Sotalol 100 mg IV (1.5 mg/kg) over 5 minutes. Avoid if prolonged QT.
   - Sedation and synchronized cardioversion.

Shock = inadequate tissue perfusion

Definitions

- **Hypotension** is generally defined as an SBP < 90 and a DBP < 60.
- **Shock** is defined as inadequate tissue perfusion.

These topics will be covered elsewhere, but they are included in the ACLS course and will therefore be discussed (briefly).

Causes

In order to rapidly assess a hypotensive patient, it is often helpful to divide the causes of shock into three etiologies.

Rate Problems
- Bradyarrhythmias:
  - Sinus bradycardia
  - Second- and third-degree heart block
  - Pacemaker failures
- Tachyarrhythmias:
  - Sinus tachycardia
  - Atrial flutter
  - Atrial fibrillation
  - PSVT
  - Ventricular tachycardia

Pump Problems
- Primary pump failure:
  - Myocardial infarction
  - Myocarditis
  - Cardiomyopathies
  - Ruptured chordae or papillary muscle damage
  - Aortic or mitral regurgitation/failure
  - Septal defect/damage
- Secondary pump failure:
  - Cardiac tamponade
  - Tension pneumothorax
  - Pulmonary embolism
  - Superior vena cava syndrome
  - Cardiodepressant drugs

Volume Problems
- Volume loss:
  - Blood loss
  - Gastrointestinal (GI) losses (vomiting, diarrhea, etc)
  - Urine output
  - Third-space losses
- ↓ vascular resistance:
  - Central nervous system (CNS) or spinal injury
  - Sepsis
  - Vasodilatory drugs
  - Adrenal insufficiency

ADVANCED AIRWAY MANAGEMENT

The 2010 AHA guidelines for CPR and ECC do not recommend the persistent use of cricoid pressure in cardiac arrest. This is because cricoid pressure can prevent gastric inflation, which can impede ventilation in addition to the benefits of decreasing regurgitation and aspiration.

Rapid Sequence Intubation Algorithm

1. Prepare the necessary equipment:
   - IV access, cardiac monitor, pulse oximetry.
   - Bag-valve mask (Ambu bag).
   - Suction equipment (make sure it works!).
   - Laryngoscope with blade (check lightbulb!).
   - ETT (7.0 adult female/8.0 adult male).
   - Insert ETT stylet (if desired).
   - Medications.
   - Prepare adjunct airway (fiberoptic scope, cricothyroidotomy tray, etc) in case ETT is unsuccessful.
2. Pretreat:
   - Lidocaine for head injury patients (↓ intracranial pressure).
   - Atropine for children (prevents bradycardia).
3. Position the patient:
   - Raise bed to height appropriate for intubation.
   - Place head in "sniffing position" with neck extended (except when C-spine injury suspected).

4. Preoxygenate the patient:
   - Bag-valve mask with 100% oxygen.
   - Pulse oximetry should read 100%.
   - Hyperventilate patient to accomplish nitrogen washout.
6. Sedation: Many agents are available, including:
   - Etomidate (does not cause hypotension).
   - Ketamine (does not cause hypotension, used in pediatric patients).
   - Midazolam (short acting benzodiazepine).
   - Propofol (nonbarbiturate hypnotic, can cause hypotension).
7. Paralyze the patient:
   - Succinylcholine (1.5 mg/kg IVP) onset 45–60 seconds, duration 5–10 minutes. Do not use in hyperkalemia, crush injuries, or history of neuromuscular diseases.
   - Rocuronium (1.2 mg/kg IVP) onset 1–2 minutes, duration 25–30 minutes.
   - Vecuronium (0.1 mg/kg IVP) onset 2–3 minutes, duration 25–30 minutes.
8. Place the tube:
   - Open the mouth and displace the jaw inferiorly.
   - Holding the laryngoscope in the left hand, insert the blade along the right side of the tongue, and the tongue is swept toward the left.
   - If using a curved (Macintosh) blade, the tip should be inserted to the vallecula (the space between the base of the tongue and the epiglottis).
   - If using a straight (Miller) blade, the tip is inserted beneath the epiglottis.
   - The laryngoscope is the used to *lift* the tongue, soft tissues, and epiglottis to reveal the vocal cords (remember, it is a *lifting* motion, not a *rocking* motion).
   - Upon direct visualization of the cords, the tube is directed through the cords, the stylet (if used) is removed, the tube is connected to an oxygen source, and it is secured after proper placement is confirmed.
9. Confirm position of the tube by two methods:
   - Bilateral breath sounds (check both apical lung fields!)
   - Absence of breath sounds in abdomen
   - End-tidal carbon dioxide detection
   - Portable CXR
   - Condensation in ETT corresponding to bag-valve mask breaths

Prepare = equipment
Pretreat = drugs
Position = sniffing position
Preoxygenate = pulse oximetry of 100%
Paralyze = drugs
Placement of the tube
Position of tube = confirm by two methods

NEEDLE CRICOTHYROIDOTOMY

Definition

- Temporizing measure to provide oxygen to a patient emergently after a failed or impossible endotracheal intubation.
- The procedure entails inserting a large-bore angiocatheter through the cricothyroid membrane (see Figure 1-5) and providing oxygen through the catheter.
- It is important to note that while oxygen delivery can be established with this procedure, adequate elimination of carbon dioxide is not achieved.

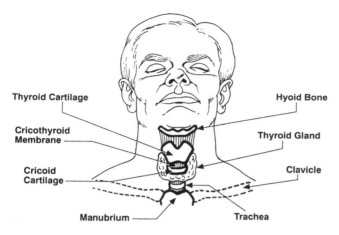

Thyroid Cartilage

Hyoid Bone

Cricothyroid Membrane

Thyroid Gland

Cricoid Cartilage

Clavicle

Manubrium

Trachea

FIGURE 1-5. Anatomical landmarks for needle and surgical cricothyroidotomy.

Needle Cricothyroidotomy Algorithm

1. Prep area with alcohol and povidone-iodine (Betadine).
2. Hyperextend neck (if no C-spine injury is suspected).
3. Identify cricothyroid membrane.
4. Insert 14G angiocatheter on a syringe at a 45-degree angle (toward feet) through cricothyroid membrane.
5. Advance with negative pressure until air is freely aspirated.
6. Remove needle and advance angiocatheter.
7. Use a syringe to verify placement in trachea.
8. Attach adapter from 3.0 ETT and ventilate with bag-valve delivery system or use transtracheal jet ventilation system.

SURGICAL CRICOTHYROIDOTOMY

Definition

- Allows for rapid establishment of an airway when endotracheal intubation has failed or is impossible (eg, severe facial trauma, burns, impacted obstruction).
- Permits both oxygen delivery and ventilation for elimination of carbon dioxide.

Indications and Contraindications

Indications
- Inability to obtain an airway by orotracheal or nasotracheal intubation due to anatomic distortion, massive hemorrhage, or severe aspiration.
- Presence of severe maxillofacial trauma renders other airways impossible.
- Upper airway obstruction due to foreign body.
- Massive upper airway edema.

Contraindications
- Age under 5–10 years, depending on child's size.
- Significant injury to larynx or cricoid.
- Tracheal transection.
- Expanding hematoma over the cricothyroid membrane.
- Preexisting laryngeal pathology.

Procedure

1. Prep area with alcohol and povidone-iodine (Betadine).
2. Hyperextend neck (if no C-spine injury is suspected).
3. Identify cricothyroid membrane.
4. Holding a #10 scalpel at the hub of the blade, make an incision through the skin and cricoid membrane (hold at the hub to ensure the stab incision does not go too deep!).
5. Enlarge the stab incision to approximately 1.5–2.0 cm with a horizontal motion of the scalpel.
6. Keeping the scalpel in place, insert a tracheal hook next to the scalpel and retract the larynx.
7. Remove the scalpel.
8. Using the scalpel handle, or a dilator, dilate the surgical opening.
9. Place a tracheostomy tube into the opening, secure the airway, and ventilate with bag-valve oxygen delivery system.

Complications

Esophageal perforation, hemorrhage, subcutaneous emphysema, vocal cord injury.

Diagnostics

- Laboratory examinations are one of the most variable aspects of emergency medicine practice.
- Diagnostic tests ordered differ greatly from one physician to another.
- In general, a test should not be ordered unless it could → change in the management of a patient.

ELECTROLYTES

Calcium

- Parathyroid hormone (PTH) and calcitonin are counterregulatory hormones that respond to levels of ionized Ca. Remember, PTH ↑ serum Ca.
- Vitamin D metabolites (calcitriol) are synthesized in liver/kidney in response to ↓ calcium levels.

IONIZED CALCIUM

- Ionized calcium is most important physiologically. Approximately 50% of total body calcium is in this form.
- Hypoalbuminemia (40–45% of calcium is bound to albumin) will ↓ total calcium, but ionized calcium is unaffected.
- Acid-base disorders will affect ionized calcium levels (↓ with alkalosis, ↑ with acidosis).
- Blood transfusion will also ↓ ionized calcium (because of citrate ions; other ions that reduce ionized calcium include phosphate, bicarbonate, and calcium chelators in radiographic contrast media).
- **Critical value:** Life threatening if values < 2 mg/dL or 0.5 mmol/L.

HYPERCALCEMIA

CAUSES

Malignancy (lung, breast, kidney, leukemia, myeloma) and hyperparathyroidism are most common causes.

SIGNS AND SYMPTOMS

- Neurologic: Weakness, fatigue, ataxia, altered mental status, seizures (rare).
- Gastrointestinal (GI): ↓ motility (constipation), vomiting.
- Renal: Osmotic diuresis (polyuria), polydipsia, nephrolithiasis, potassium/magnesium losses.
- Cardiovascular: ECG changes, potentiates digoxin toxicity.

ECG

May reveal shortened QT interval, bradycardia, or heart blocks.

TREATMENT

Aimed at correcting dehydration and promoting urinary excretion of calcium:

- Rehydrate with large amounts of intravenous (IV) saline (0.9% preferred) until volume status is restored.

Most accurate calcium level:
4 − serum albumin (g/dL) × 0.8 + serum calcium

Rough correction for total body calcium in hypoalbuminemia: Add 1 mg/dL to serum calcium for every 1 mg/dL reduction in albumin below 4 mg/dL.

Signs of hypercalcemia:
- Bones (bony pain)
- Stones (kidney stones)
- Groans (abdominal pain)
- Psychiatric overtones (change in mental status)

Caveats of hypercalcemia:
- ↑ serum chloride, low serum bicarbonate in a ratio > 33:1 is suggestive of primary hypothyroidism.
- High total protein with reversed albumin-to-globulin (A/G) ratio suggestive of multiple myeloma.

HIGH-YIELD FACTS

Diagnostics

31

Causes of hypercalcemia—SPLITTing HEADACHE
Sarcoid
Pheochromocytoma
Lithium
Immobilization
Tuberculosis
Thiazides
1° **H**yperparathyroidism
Estrogens
Vitamin **A** excess
Vitamin **D** excess
Adrenal insufficiency
Cancers (lung, breast, kidney, leukemia, myeloma)
Hyperthyroidism
Estrogen antagonists (therapy for breast cancer)

Chvostek's sign: Tapping facial nerve below zygomatic arch induces tetany of facial muscles.

Trousseau's sign: Inflating blood pressure (BP) cuff above systolic BP for 3 minutes induces carpal spasm.

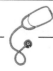

Ca gluconate is less irritating than Ca chloride when given via peripheral IV (rather than central line).

- Furosemide (loop diuretic) may be added to promote diuresis once volume status is restored.
- Thiazide diuretics must be avoided as they ↓ urinary calcium excretion.
- Electrolytes must be monitored carefully (hypokalemia/hypomagnesemia).
- Dialysis in the setting of renal failure.

HYPOCALCEMIA

CAUSES

- Hypoalbuminemia (cirrhosis, nephrotic syndrome); does not lower the ionized Ca^{2+}.
- Hypoparathyroidism (intrinsic or post-thyroid surgery).
- Malnutrition/malabsorption.
- Renal failure.
- Pancreatitis (saponification).
- Medications (cimetidine, proton pump inhibitors, selective serotonin reuptake inhibitors [SSRIs], etc).

PATHOPHYSIOLOGY

Neuronal membranes become more excitable secondary to ↑ sodium permeability.

SIGNS AND SYMPTOMS

- Perioral and digital paresthesias.
- ↓ myocardial contractility (relaxation is inhibited) can predispose to congestive heart failure (CHF). Severe hypocalcemia can also cause laryngeal spasm and seizures.

ECG

ECG characteristically shows prolonged QT intervals.

TREATMENT

Supplement calcium:

- Asymptomatic patients should be given oral calcium (with or without vitamin D).
- Symptomatic patients should be treated with IV calcium (Ca gluconate or Ca chloride).
- When large quantities have to be given, 5% dextrose can be used as carrier fluid for the infusion.
- Caveats:
  - If IV calcium does not relieve symptoms, rule out hypomagnesemia.
  - If hypocalcemia is with metabolic acidosis, correct hypocalcemia before correction of acidosis.
  - Every 4 units of blood will require 10 mL of 10% calcium gluconate.

Potassium

- Potassium is the intracellular cation (98% of total body potassium is intracellular).
- Potassium is excreted primarily in urine (small amount in feces, sweat).
- Renin-angiotensin-aldosterone axis regulates potassium secretion in distal tubules.

A 47-year-old woman presents to the ED stating she has the stomach flu and is feeling tired. Serum chemistry panel reveals she has a potassium of 3.0 mEq/L. How would you treat her electrolyte abnormality?

On average, a reduction of serum potassium by 0.3 mEq/L suggests a total body deficit of 100 mEq/L. (Stated another way, a 1 mEq/L ↓ in serum K equals about 350 mEq/L deficit.) However, note that many factors in addition to the total body potassium stores contribute to the serum potassium concentration. Therefore, this calculation could either overestimate or underestimate the true potassium deficit. For example, a patient with a serum potassium of 2.6 mEq/L has less total body deficit at blood pH of 7.5 than 7.3. The reason for this is that alkaline serum pH (ie, 7.5) can independently lower the serum potassium by intracellular shift. Treatment in this case should begin with IV infusion of 10 mEq/L over 1 hour while patient is on a cardiac monitor. Potassium level can be rechecked in 2 hours to ascertain whether target level is reached.

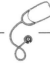

Gluconate = Good

Interpret potassium levels in the context of serum pH: Acidosis causes potassium shift into serum; alkalosis causes potassium shift into cells.

CAUSES AND PATHOPHYSIOLOGY

Three mechanisms for ↓ potassium:

- Intracellular shifts (alkalotic states, administration of insulin and glucose).
- ↓ intake (malnutrition).
- ↑ losses (renal—diuretics, hyperaldosteronism; GI—vomiting, diarrhea, fistulas).

SIGNS AND SYMPTOMS

- Muscle weakness.
- Hyporeflexia.
- Intestinal ileus.
- Respiratory paralysis.
- Nephrogenic diabetes insipidus.
- Dehydration.
- Cardiovascular: Hypokalemia potentiates digitalis and ↑ likelihood of digitalis toxicity (arrhythmias and atrioventricular blocks).

ECG

Cardiac abnormalities on ECG do not correlate well with K+ levels—they include:

- Early changes: Flattened/inverted T waves, U waves (see Figure 2-1), ST segment depression, prolonged QT interval.
- Severe depletion changes: Prolonged PR, low-voltage QRS, widened QRS, premature ventricular contractions (PVCs), and ventricular arrhythmias.

TREATMENT

- K+ levels < 3 mEq/L: Definitive therapy indicated.
- K+ levels 3–3.5 mEq/L: Treat patients at high risk of arrhythmia (eg, CHF patients, patients on digitalis, history of acute myocardial infarction [MI] or ischemic heart disease).

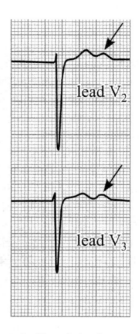

FIGURE 2-1. U waves (arrows) of hypokalemia.

Maximum rate of KCl infusion: 10 mEq/h peripheral IV or 20 mEq/h with central line; 0.5–1 mEq/kg/h in infants.

- K+ levels 3.5–4.5 mEq/L: Oral supplementation. If on diuretics, change to K+-sparing diuretics or ↓ dose.
- Supplement potassium:
  - Mild hypokalemia: Potassium-rich foods (bananas, avocados, passion fruit, orange juice) or oral KCl supplements.
  - Severe hypokalemia: Treat with IV KCl.
- Monitor potassium level closely, especially with IV replacement.

HYPERKALEMIA (> 5.5 MEQ/L)

CAUSES

- When potassium level is high, check ECG and recheck level to rule out false elevation (hemolysis, etc).
- Lab error: Hemolysis, thrombocytosis, leukocytosis, polycythemia ("pseudo-hyperkalemia").
- ↓ excretion: Renal failure, angiotensin-converting enzyme (ACE) inhibitors, K-sparing diuretics, type IV renal tubular acidosis.
- ↑ release: Metabolic acidosis, trauma, burns, rhabdomyolysis, tumor lysis, succinylcholine.
- ↑ intake: Iatrogenic, dietary, salt substitutes.

SIGNS AND SYMPTOMS

- GI: Nausea, vomiting, diarrhea.
- Neurologic: Muscle cramps, weakness, paresthesias, paralysis, areflexia, tetany, focal neurologic deficits, confusion.
- Respiratory insufficiency.
- Cardiac arrest.

- At K = 5.0–6.0 mEq/L, rapid repolarization causes peaked T waves (most prominent in precordial leads) (see Figure 2-2).
- At K = 6.0–6.5 mEq/L, ↓ in conduction causes prolonged PR and QT intervals.
- At K = 6.5–7.0 mEq/L, P waves are diminished and ST segment may be depressed.
- At K = 7.0–8.0 mEq/L, P waves disappear, QRS widens, and irregular idioventricular rhythm appears.
- At K = 8.0–10.0 mEq/L, QRS merges with T wave to produce classic sine wave.
- At K = 10.0–12.0 mEq/L, ventricular fibrillation and diastolic arrest occur.

TREATMENT

- Calcium gluconate: Stabilizes cardiac membrane, onset of action 1–3 minutes.
- Sodium bicarbonate: Alkalosis shifts potassium into cells, onset 5–10 minutes.
- Insulin and glucose: Insulin drives potassium and glucose into cells, onset 30 minutes.
- Nebulized albuterol: Drives potassium and glucose into cells, onset 30 minutes.
- Lasix: Promotes renal excretion of potassium, onset with diuresis.
- Kayexalate: Cation exchange resin (potassium for sodium in GI tract), onset 1–2 hours.
- Dialysis: Peritoneal or hemodialysis removes potassium at time of dialysis.
- Dialysis is indicated for patients in renal failure with hyperkalemia that does not respond to above.

Caution with patients on digitalis; calcium in the setting of digitalis toxicity may induce tetany and "stone heart."

Sodium

- Ninety-eight percent of total body sodium is in extracellular fluid.
- Sodium is the major contributor to serum osmolarity.

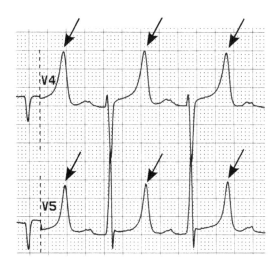

FIGURE 2-2 Peaked T waves (arrows) of hyperkalemia.

- Serum osmolarity = 2(Na) + (glucose/18) + (BUN/2.8).
- Balance between sodium, water, and osmolarity is regulated by kidney (excretion and reabsorption of sodium and water), posterior pituitary (secretion of antidiuretic hormone), and the hypothalamus (thirst center).
- Understanding the relationship between osmolarity (tonicity) and volume is essential:
- Volume status is a clinical diagnosis.
- Tonicity is a laboratory diagnosis.
- Understanding where you are in terms of volume and tonicity allows you to guide therapy appropriately (see Table 2-1).

HYPONATREMIA

A 52-year-old diabetic woman presents because her blood sugar monitor at home read "high." Indeed, her serum glucose is 900 mg/dL. Her serum sodium is 124 mg/dL. In addition to correcting her hyperglycemia, should you also correct her hyponatremia?

No. Her hyponatremia is a pseudohyponatremia, caused by the elevated blood sugar. The sodium "falls" by approximately 1.6 mEq/L for every 100 mg/dL over 200. So in this case, the true sodium is actually 124 + (7 × 1.6) = 135 mEqL, which is normal.

A 6-month-old child is brought in by EMS with seizures. She has had vomiting and diarrhea for 2 days, and her mother has been giving her water to keep her from getting dehydrated. She appears well hydrated, but has a sodium of 118 mEqL. What is the cause of her hyponatremia, and what is the best treatment for her seizures?

This is a case of hyponatremia secondary to inappropriate rehydration with hypotonic free water. The seizure is from the hyponatremia, so the treatment is to correct the sodium with a normal saline bolus (20 mL/kg). Hypertonic (3%) saline can also be considered in this case. Always counsel parents of young infants not to give free water (use breast milk, formula, or electrolyte solutions instead).

TABLE 2-1. Sodium Balance: Volume vs. Tonicity

| | TONICITY | | |
VOLUME	HYPERTONIC	ISOTONIC	HYPOTONIC
Hypervolemic	Iatrogenic	Early CHF, cirrhosis, nephrotic syndrome (no ADH stimulus)	Late CHF, cirrhosis, nephrotic syndrome (with ADH stimulus)
Euvolemic	Early stages of "dehydration"	Normal	Psychogenic polydipsia, SIADH "reset osmostat"
Hypovolemic	Late stages of "dehydration" (H_2O loss > salt loss)	Acute volume loss (ie, burns, bleeding) (no ADH stimulus)	Chronic volume loss (with ADH stimulus) diuretics, Addison's

CAUSES

- *Pseudohyponatremia* is caused by:
    - Hyperglycemia
    - Hyperlipidemia
    - Hyperproteinemia

The serum osmolarity will be normal or high in these cases.

- Causes of hyponatremia may be subdivided based on the fluid status of the patient:
    1. Hypervolemia:
        - ↑ total body free water: CHF, nephrotic syndrome, cirrhosis.
        - ↓ excretion of sodium: Renal failure.
    2. Euvolemic:
        - Hypotonic fluid infusions.
        - Psychogenic polydipsia.
        - Syndrome of inappropriate antidiuretic hormone (SIADH).
    3. Hypovolemic:
        - Renal failure with ↓ excretion of free water.
        - Diuretics.
        - Salt-wasting nephropathies.
        - Extrarenal losses (vomiting, diarrhea, extensive burns, third spacing, pancreatitis, peritonitis).

PATHOPHYSIOLOGY

Severity is dependent on both the magnitude and rapidity of the fall in serum sodium:

- Initial response to low serum sodium is to shift water across blood-brain barrier into the central nervous system (CNS).
- CNS responds by shifting sodium and other osmotic agents from brain into cerebrospinal fluid (CSF) to systemic circulation.
- If hyponatremia is corrected too quickly, CNS loses its ability to retain water (loss of osmotic agents).
- Brain rapidly becomes dehydrated, → osmotic demyelination syndrome, also known as central pontine myelinolysis (seen days after therapy; presents with bulbar dysfunction, quadriparesis, delirium, death).

SIGNS AND SYMPTOMS

- Early: Nonspecific headache, vomiting.
- Late: Confusion, seizures, coma, bradycardia, or respiratory arrest.

TREATMENT

Calculation of sodium deficit:

(Wt in kg)* (0.6)* (140 – measured [Na⁺]) = sodium deficit in mEq

- Normal saline is generally the first line treatment.
- Patients with acute hyponatremia (< 2 days) should be corrected no faster than 1.0 mEq/L/h.
- Patients with chronic hyponatremia (> 2 days) should be corrected no faster than 0.5 mEq/L/h.
- For euvolemic and hypervolemic patients, water restriction may be appropriate.
- In cases of severe (< 120 mEq/L) hyponatremia, consider hypertonic (3%) saline at 25–100 mL/h.

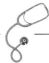

Correcting the sodium too quickly can result in central pontine myelinolysis, seizures, and cerebral edema.

HYPERNATREMIA

CAUSES

- GI losses: Vomiting, diarrhea, ↓ thirst.
- Renal losses: Diabetes insipidus, osmotic diuretics, adrenal/renal disease.
- Insensible losses: Respiratory, skin, hyperthermia.
- Inability to respond to thirst (due to lack of access).

SIGNS AND SYMPTOMS

- Early signs (Na > 158 mEq/L) include irritability, lethargy, anorexia, and vomiting.
- As serum osmolarity rises (350–400 mOsm/L), begin to see ataxia, tremulousness, hypertonicity, and spasms.
- At serum osmolarity > 430 mOsm/L, death usually ensues.

TREATMENT

- First step is to address fluid status: Hydrate with normal saline (NS) until volume is restored.
- Remember, NS will actually be "hypotonic" with hypernatremia.
- Once perfusion is established, may hydrate with hypotonic (0.45%) saline (rarely indicated in the ED).
- Monitor urine output (0.5 mL/kg/h) and check electrolytes every few hours. If adequate urine output cannot be achieved, switch to ½ NS for every liter of water and administer diuretic. This serves to unload excess sodium. For every liter of water lost, the sodium rises by 3–5 mEq/L.
- Target should be to correct sodium over 48–72 hours (max rate of 0.5 mEq/L/h).

Water deficit (liters)
= 0.6 × (weight in kg) ×
{(Na/140) − 1}

The most common cause of hypernatremia is ↓ in total body water (ie, dehydration).

SYNDROME OF INAPPROPRIATE ANTIDIURETIC HORMONE HYPERSECRETION (SIADH)

PATHOPHYSIOLOGY

- Thirst mechanism and ADH work together to control intake/excretion of water.
- Both mechanisms are usually impaired before SIADH becomes clinically apparent (excess ADH → water retention, thirst → ↑ fluid intake).
- ↑ ADH with SIADH; ↓ ADH with diabetes insipidus.

CAUSES

- CNS: Head trauma, tumors, abscesses, meningitis, subarachnoid hemorrhage.
- Tumors: Lung, pancreas, ovaries, lymphoma, thymoma.
- Pulmonary: Pneumonia, chronic obstructive pulmonary disease (COPD), tuberculosis, cystic fibrosis, abscess.
- Drugs: Opiates, nonsteroidal anti-inflammatory drugs, monoamine oxidase inhibitors, tricyclic antidepressants.
- Other: Hypothyroidism, adrenal insufficiency, porphyria, idiopathic.

Diabetes Insipidus
Central: Hypothalamus does not make ADH.
Nephrogenic: Kidneys do not *respond* to ADH.

DIAGNOSIS

SIADH is a diagnosis of exclusion (must rule out other causes of hyponatremia):

- Serum Na < 135 and serum osmolarity < 280.
- Urine is not maximally diluted (urine osmolarity > 100).
- No evidence of dehydration, edema, hypotension.
- No evidence of renal, cardiac, thyroid, or adrenal dysfunction.

TREATMENT

- Treatment generally consists of fluid restriction. (Remember, clinical manifestations of SIADH usually become apparent only when the thirst mechanism → ↑ fluid intake!)
- Hypertonic (3%) saline is appropriate only for patients with neurologic symptoms of hyponatremia.

> Neither respiratory (12 hours) nor metabolic compensation (24–48 hours) will return pH completely to normal.

ACID-BASE DISORDERS

- Assess the acid-base disorder step by step (Figure 2-3):
  - Is the primary disorder an acidosis (pH < 7.40) or alkalosis (pH > 7.40)?
  - Is the disorder respiratory (pH and P_{CO_2} move in opposite directions)?
  - Is the disorder metabolic (pH and P_{CO_2} move in same direction)?
  - Is the disorder a simple or mixed disorder?

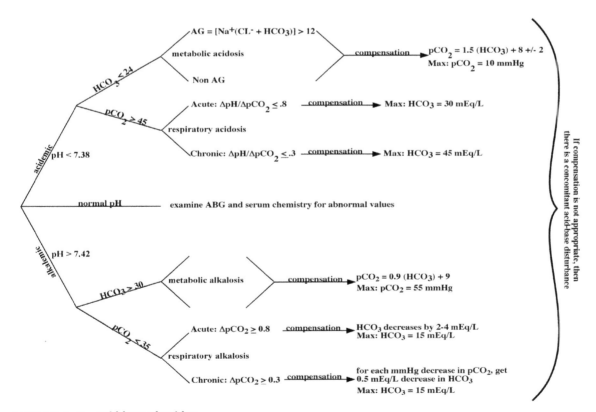

FIGURE 2-3. Acid-base algorithm.

Reproduced, with permission, from Stead L. *BRS Emergency Medicine*. Philadelphia, PA: Lippincott Williams & Wilkins, 2000.

Causes of elevated anion gap metabolic acidosis—

CAT MUDPILES

Cyanide, carbon monoxide
Alcoholic ketoacidosis
Toluene
Methanol, metabolism (inborn errors)
Uremia
Diabetic ketoacidosis
Paraldehyde
Iron, isoniazid
Lactic acidosis
Ethylene glycol
Salicylates, strychnine

Causes of normal anion gap metabolic acidosis—

HARD UP

Hyperparathyroidism
Adrenal insufficiency, **A**nhydrase (carbonic anhydrase) inhibitors
Renal tubular acidosis
Diarrhea
Ureteroenteric fistula
Pancreatic fistulas

Cause of respiratory alkalosis—

MIS[HAP]₃S

Mechanical overventilation
Increased ICP
Sepsis
Hypoxemia, **H**yperpyrexia, **H**eart failure
Anxiety, **A**sthma, **A**scites
Pregnancy, **P**ain, **P**neumonia
Salicylates

- Use the following general rules of thumb for acute disorders:
  - Metabolic acidosis: P_{CO_2} drop ~1.5 (drop in HCO_3)
  - Metabolic alkalosis: P_{CO_2} rise ~1.0 (rise in HCO_3)
  - Respiratory acidosis: HCO_3 rise ~0.1 (rise in P_{CO_2})
  - Respiratory alkalosis: HCO_3 drop ~0.3 (drop in P_{CO_2})

Compensation beyond above parameters suggests mixed disorder.

Metabolic Acidosis

- Two varieties: Anion gap and nonanion gap.
- Calculating the anion gap:

$$AG = Na - [Cl + HCO_3]$$

- Normal $AG \leq 12$ to 14

Metabolic Alkalosis

Two mechanisms:

- Loss of H⁺:
  - Renal: Mineralocorticoid excess, diuretics, potassium-losing nephropathy.
  - GI: Vomiting, gastric drainage, villous adenoma of colon.
- Gain HCO_3: Milk-alkali syndrome, exogenous $NaHCO_3$.

Respiratory Acidosis

Hypercapnia secondary to one of two mechanisms:

- Hypoventilation (brain stem injury, neuromuscular disease, ventilator malfunction).
- Ventilation-perfusion (V/Q) mismatch (COPD, pneumonia, pulmonary embolism, foreign body, pulmonary edema).

Respiratory Alkalosis

- Hyperventilation secondary to anxiety, ↑ intracranial pressure (ICP), salicylates, fever, hypoxemia, systemic disease (sepsis), pain, pregnancy, CHF, pneumonia, asthma, liver disease.
- Alkalosis causes ↓ in serum K and ionized Ca, resulting in paresthesias, carpopedal spasm, and tetany.

ELECTROCARDIOGRAMS (ECGs)

See Cardiovascular Emergencies chapter for a more complete discussion.

- ECGs provide a tremendous amount of information in both the acutely ill patient and for a long-term view of cardiac function.
- To become proficient, one must have a system so as not to miss anything, and one must practice, practice, practice.

* Do not trust the machine's reading; read the ECG yourself first, then look at the reading.

Rate

* Normal
* Bradycardic (< 60 bpm)
* Tachycardic (> 100 bpm)

ECG paper runs at
  25 mm/s.
One small box = 0.040 s
One large box = 200 ms

Rhythm

* Sinus: P waves before every QRS, P upright in I and aVF, all P waves are of same shape (see Figure 2-4 for ECG lead placement).
* Atrial fibrillation: No P waves, irregularly irregular rhythm.
* Atrial flutter: No P waves, sawtooth-shaped waves.
* Ventricular tachycardia: No P wave, no discernible QRS, regular undulating smooth waves.
* Ventricular fibrillation: Grossly irregular waves of varying amplitude, no discernible P or QRS.

Axis

* Normal: 0 to +90
* Rightward: +90 to +270
* Leftward: 0 to –90
* See Figure 2-5 for ECG axes.

Rightward axis frequently seen in asthma and COPD patients.

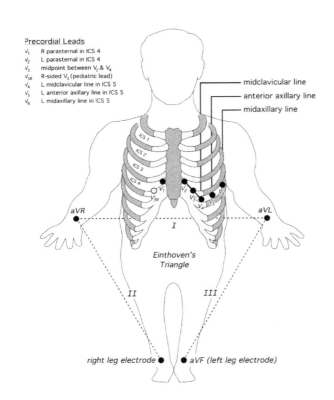

FIGURE 2-4. ECG lead placement.

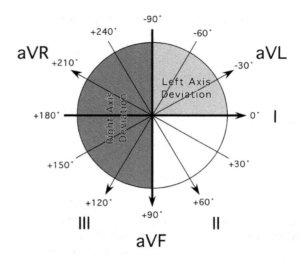

FIGURE 2-5. ECG axes.

Diagnostics

Intervals

Intervals are important to determine if there is an atrioventricular (AV) nodal block, intraventricular conduction delay, or prolonged Q:

- PR interval—normal = 200 ms:
  - Consistently > 200 ms is first-degree AV block (not clinically important).
  - Progressively longer and eventually dropping a beat with a repeated pattern is second-degree Mobitz type I AV block (Wenckebach).
  - Consistent PR with dropped beats in a repeating pattern is second-degree Mobitz type II AV block.
  - No association between P wave and QRS is third-degree AV block.
- QRS duration—normal = < 120 ms; > 120 ms indicates an intraventricular conduction delay or a left or right bundle branch block.
- QT interval—normal varies with rate but corrected QT (QT/√RR) < 450 ms:
  - Must take patient's age and sex into consideration.
  - Prolonged by hypokalemia, hypomagnesemia, hypocalcemia, and certain medications.
  - Risk of torsades de pointes with prolonged QT.

Place transcutaneous pacing pads on all patients with third-degree and Mobitz type II second-degree AV blocks.

Morphology

Morphology of the waves is important as well:

- P wave morphology may indicate right or left atrial enlargement (tall P waves) or ectopic atrial focus (different-looking P waves).
- QRS complex morphology may indicate right ventricular or left ventricular hypertrophy (tall QRS), right bundle or left bundle branch block (M-shaped QRS complex).
- T waves are helpful to determine ischemic changes or hyperkalemia:
  - In general, T waves should have the same deflection as the QRS. If they're flat or inverted, this may be a sign of ischemia or hypertrophic repolarization changes.
  - Peaked T waves are an early ECG change in hyperkalemia.

A new left bundle branch block is considered an acute MI unless proven otherwise.

ST Segments

ST segments are helpful in determining injury or ischemia. In general:

- Elevation means injury.
- Depression means ischemia.

Q Waves

Q waves are pathologic except in aVR, leads III and VI:

- Most commonly used criteria for significant Q waves is > 40 ms wide and at least one-fourth of R wave in same lead.
- Can develop within hours.
- May not be seen in subendocardial infarctions (non–Q wave MI).

Diffuse (across all leads) ST elevations and PR depression are seen in pericarditis.

U Waves

- U waves are sometimes seen after T waves.
- May indicate hypocalcemia or hypokalemia.

Criteria for Cardiac Catheterization or Thrombolysis

Criteria for cardiac catheterization or thrombolysis in acute MI barring contraindications:

- Elevated ST segments > 1 mm in two consecutive leads.
- Chest pain or anginal equivalent consistent with MI.
- New left bundle branch block (LBBB).
- Cardiac catheterization preferred over thrombolysis, when available.
- Contraindications to thrombolysis include recent surgery, active bleeding, recent stroke, suspected dissection, uncontrolled hypertension, or prolonged cardiopulmonary resuscitation.

Remember, have a system and practice, practice, practice. Even senior cardiologists don't agree with each other on some ECGs, so don't be discouraged.

Miscellaneous

- Look for pacemaker spike—may be very subtle.
- S in I, Q in III, inverted T in III—think pulmonary embolus (but not sensitive or specific).
- If injury is evolving, repeat ECGs are very helpful.
- Compare to old ECGs whenever available.

- X-rays are a routine part of the evaluation of emergency patients.
- They are used to detect fractures, foreign bodies, pneumonias, CHF, pneumothoraces, and bowel obstruction.
- X-rays are relatively inexpensive, readily available, and relatively low in radiation exposure, making them an excellent adjunct when used properly.
- The emergency physician must be comfortable reading his or her own radiographs.
- Always ensure the film belongs to the right patient before proceeding

In radiology, "one view is no view." Try to get a lateral when possible.

Loss of costophrenic angle indicates approximately 250 cc of fluid accumulation.

HIGH-YIELD FACTS

Diagnostics

Chest X-Ray

- Use the ABCs for a systematic approach:
  - A—airway: Evaluate the trachea for deviation.
  - B—bones: Evaluate the ribs and other visible bones for evidence of fractures or bony pathology.
  - C—cardiac: Look at the cardiac silhouette. It is considered enlarged when greater than one-half the thoracic diameter.
  - D—diaphragms: Look for free air beneath, flattening, or rising of one side as well as loss of the costophrenic angles.
  - E—everything else: Now look at the lung fields for pathology.
- Know the technique used. You may be fooled thinking of cardiomegaly, which shouldn't be read on a portable anteroposterior (AP) chest x-ray. (See Figure 2-6).
- Small pneumothoraces may be very subtle.

Abdominal Series

- Consist of upright chest, as well as supine and lateral decubitus abdominal x-rays.
- Primarily used to evaluate for bowel obstruction or perforation.
- Look for free air, bowel gas patterns, air-fluid levels, and stool in the intestine.
- Constipation is a clinical diagnosis and does not need an x-ray.

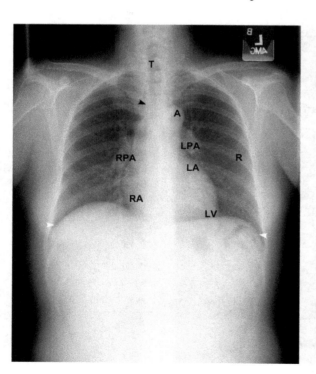
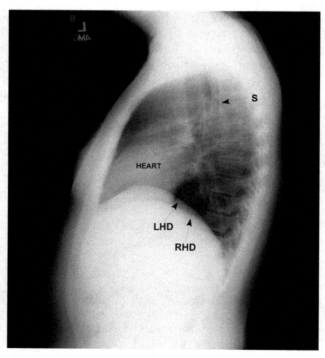

FIGURE 2-6. Normal and PA lateral chest radiograph.

T: trachea; A: aortic knob; RPA: right pulmonary artery; LPA, left pulmonary artery; R, rib; LA, left atrium; RA, right atrium; LV, left ventricle; LHD, left hemidiaphragm; RHD, right hemidiaphragm; S, scapula. On PA view, note superior vena cava (black arrow) and costophrenic angles (white arrows). (Reproduced, with permission, from *First Aid for Radiology*. McGraw Hill, 2008.)

Facial Films

- Useful for trauma and sinus evaluation.
- Complicated fractures are usually followed up with computed tomography (CT) scan.
- Look for opacification of sinuses, air-fluid levels, and mucosal thickening, which are indicative of sinusitis.

Neck Films

Cervical spine series consists of lateral, AP, and open-mouth views:

- Must see from C1 to top of T1 for complete lateral film.
- May try shoulder pull or Swimmer's view for larger patients to expose bottom cervical vertebrae.
- Open-mouth used to evaluate dens and lateral masses.
- Soft tissue of neck useful if suspecting epiglottitis or foreign body.

Extremity Films

- Ordered when suspecting fracture or foreign body.
- Multiple views are better.
- Postreduction views to check for proper positioning are necessary when extremity has been manipulated.
- Can also be used to evaluate for effusions and soft-tissue swelling.

CT SCANS

Computed tomography (CT) scans have become widely available in the United States, with more than 68 million obtained each year. CTs have proven to be invaluable in the diagnosis and treatment of many emergency conditions. However, CT scans are also expensive and expose patients to a significant amount of radiation.

Head CTs

- Useful in atraumatic and traumatic patients.
- Noncontrast CTs can help to see new-onset strokes, bleeds, masses, hydrocephalus, and edema.
- Can also be used to diagnose skull fractures, facial bone fractures, and sinus disease.
- Usually done prior to lumbar puncture to rule out ↑ intracerebral pressure.
- Most head CTs are without contrast; but, if HIV positive and infection is suspected, it is best to do without and with contrast to look for toxoplasmosis, cryptococcosis, and lymphoma.
- C-spine/neck CTs are useful for penetrating trauma to the neck and to further delineate fractures and subluxations seen on plain C-spine films.

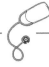
When suspecting epiglottitis, don't send patients to radiology by themselves!

Use **BLT RATS** when describing fractures:
Bone
Location
Type of fracture
Rotation
Angulation
Transposition
Shortening

One abdomen/pelvis CT exposes the patient to as much radiation as 250 chest x-rays!

Acute ischemic strokes may initially present with a negative CT scan.

HIGH-YIELD FACTS

Diagnostics

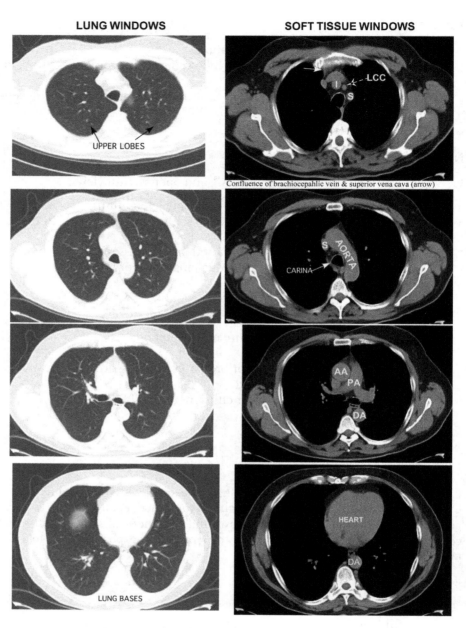

LUNG WINDOWS

SOFT TISSUE WINDOWS

UPPER LOBES

LCC

I

S

Confluence of brachiocepahlic vein & superior vena cava (arrow)

S AORTA

CARINA

AA
PA

DA

HEART

DA

LUNG BASES

FIGURE 2-7. Normal chest CT.

AA, ascending aorta; DA, descending aorta; PA, pulmonary artery; LCC, left common carotid; S. superior vena cava. Reproduced with permission from *First Aid for Radiology*, McGraw Hill, 2008.

Chest CTs

- Newer-generation, high-resolution spiral CTs with IV contrast are useful for diagnosing pulmonary emboli.
- Have high sensitivity for small pleural effusions and small pneumothoraces not picked up by plain films.
- Useful in evaluating aorta and aortic root in suspected dissection or rupture. (See Figure 2-7.)
- Triple rule-out (PE, aortic dissection, acute coronary syndrome). CTs are controversial—high amounts of radiation and low specificity.

Abdominal/Pelvic CTs

- Useful to detect free fluid in the abdomen.
- With IV contrast administered appropriately, excellent test for infectious processes in the abdomen such as appendicitis, diverticulitis, and abscesses.
- Also useful in evaluating intestinal pathology, although not as good for penetrating intestinal trauma.
- Sensitivity not great for pelvic organs. Ultrasound is more useful for gynecologic pathology.

PO AND IV CONTRAST

- IV contrast is helpful to look at vessels and highly vascular areas (inflammation, abscess, etc).
- PO contrast is more controversial: Some radiologists prefer it to look at the bowel while others do not use it routinely.
- PO contrast, if given, needs 1–3 hours to reach the end of the GI tract.
- Risk of allergy and contrast-induced nephropathy with IV contrast. Must weigh risks against benefits.
- May not be able to use IV contrast if creatinine is elevated (> 1.7 mg/dL).
- Contrast is not needed for most head CTs, when looking at bones, and some abdomen/pelvis CTs (eg, kidney stone protocols).

ULTRASOUND

Ultrasound (US) studies have an ever-increasing role in emergency medicine.

- Portable machines have found their way to the bedside, and increased training of residents and attendings in US has helped patients throughout the country.
- Approved uses in the ED are listed in Table 2-2.
- The two most common uses in the ED currently are pelvic sonography and focused abdominal sonogram for trauma (FAST) studies.

Many EM physicians now complete postresidency fellowships in ultrasound.

Pelvic Ultrasound

- Useful in evaluating the pregnant female with pain or bleeding, ruling out ectopic pregnancies, or evaluating the nonpregnant female with pelvic complaints.
- Order of appearance of structures in pregnancy:
  - Double ring sign
  - Double gestational sac
  - Intrauterine fetal pole
  - Fetal heart activity
- Should be able to visualize uterus, ovaries, bladder, and pouch of Douglas for free fluid.

Intrauterine pregnancy (IUP) on transvaginal US is seen at beta-hCG 1000–1500 IU/L. IUP on transabdominal US may not be seen until a beta-hCG around 6000 IU/L.

TABLE 2-2. Uses of Ultrasonography in Emergency Medicine

EXAM	FOR DETECTION OF
FAST	Free intraperitoneal fluid in trauma
Pulmonary	Pneumothorax
Cardiac	Pericardial effusion or heart motion in pulseless electrical activity
Pelvic	Early intrauterine pressure and/or free pelvic fluid
Renal	Hydronephrosis
Aortic	Abdominal aortic aneurysm
Biliary	Cholelithiasis
Ophthalmology	Retinal detachment
Obstetric	Live fetus in second/third trimester
Skin	Foreign body, abscess
Procedures	IVs, central lines, abscess drainage, lumbar punctures

Some consider US the stethoscope of the 21st century.

Focused Abdominal Sonogram for Trauma (FAST)

- Used to detect free peritoneal blood following blunt trauma to the abdomen.
- Has generally replaced more invasive diagnostic peritoneal lavage (DPL).
- Four sites of visualization:
  - Hepatorenal interface (Morison's pouch)
  - Splenic-renal interface
  - Pericardial sac
  - Bladder (pouch of Douglas)
- Sensitivity and specificity vary with experience of user and patient factors.
- Disadvantages:
  - Poor in obese patients or those with lots of bowel gas.
  - Poor in evaluating solid-organ or bowel injury.
  - May not pick up small amounts of fluid (false negative).

HIGH-YIELD FACTS

Diagnostics

- Nuclear medicine studies involve the use of hormones or cells that are labeled radioactively to evaluate the function of different organ systems.
- The two most common studies ordered in the ED are hepato-iminodiacetic acid (HIDA) scans and V/Q scans.

HIDA Scan

- IDA is labeled and taken up by hepatocytes and secreted into bile canaliculi.
- Failure to visualize the gallbladder despite seeing the hepatic and common ducts indicates cystic duct obstruction.
- Ninety-eight percent negative predictive value for cholecystitis.
- Sensitivity as high as 97%.

HIDA scan loses sensitivity as bilirubin levels rise above 5 mg.

V/Q Scan

 A 20-year-old female is 12-weeks pregnant and presents with shortness of breath and pleuritic chest pain. You have a moderate to high suspicion for pulmonary embolism (PE). How should you proceed?

Given the risks of anticoagulation, treating empirically with heparin is not a good option; coumadin is contraindicated (pregnancy classification "X"—highly unsafe). First, obtain bilateral lower extremity US. If positive, presume PE and treat. If negative, should you proceed with V/Q or CT scan?

V/Q scan exposes mother to less radiation, but radioisotope collects in bladder (near fetus) so more radiation exposure to fetus. Therefore, CT (with abdominal shielding) is preferred over V/Q in pregnant patients.

- Has been largely replaced by CT.
- Indicated for patients when pulmonary embolism is suspected and other diagnoses can't be proven.
- Perfusion scan done by labeling albumin.
- Eight views must be obtained for complete scan.
- Perfusion scans alone are not sensitive or specific.
- Ventilation scan performed with radioactive aerosols.
- Four results are reported by radiology:
  - Normal scans have specificity of 96% and sensitivity of 98%.
  - Intermediate probability: 41% sensitive, positive predictive value (PPV) only 30%.
  - Low probability: 16% sensitive, 14% PPV.
  - High-probability scans: 41% sensitive, 87% PPV.
- Low-probability and intermediate-probability scans are considered nondiagnostic: Correlate with clinical suspicion.
- If your clinical suspicion is high enough, go further in workup than V/Q scan (lower-extremity Doppler study, spiral chest CT, angiogram, empiric treatment).

Famous PIOPED study: "Low-probability" V/Q studies miss 16% of pulmonary emboli.

HIGH-YIELD FACTS

Diagnostics

HIGH-YIELD FACTS IN

Trauma

"Golden Hour" of Trauma

Period immediately following trauma in which rapid assessment, diagnosis assessment, diagnosis, and stabilization must occur.

Prehospital Phase

Control of airway and external hemorrhage, immobilization, and rapid transport of patient to nearest appropriate facility.

Preparation

- Gown up, glove up, face shields on!
- Standard precautions.
- Set up: Airway equipment, monitor, O_2, urinary catheter (Foley), IV and blood tubes (complete blood count, chemistry, prothrombin time/partial thromboplastin time, type and cross, human chorionic gonadotropin, +/– toxicologies), chest tube tray, etc.

Primary Survey

- Initial assessment and resuscitation of vital functions.
- Prioritization based on ABCs of trauma care.

ABCs and DEF

- Airway (with cervical spine precautions)
- Breathing and ventilation
- Circulation (and Control of hemorrhage)
- Disability (neurologic status)
- Exposure/Environment control
- Foley

Airway and C-Spine

Quick check: If a patient can talk, his airway is patent.

- Assess patency of airway.
  - Listen for stridor/dysphonia.
  - Look for agitation, obtundation, cyanosis—all of which can suggest hypoxia/hypercarbia.
  - Use jaw thrust initially to open airway.
- Clear foreign bodies.
- Insert oral or nasal airway when necessary. Obtunded/unconscious patients should be intubated. Surgical airway—cricothyroidotomy is used when unable to intubate airway.
  - Patient arriving intubated: Always confirm ET placement—direct visualization, auscultation of symmetric breath sounds, symmetric chest rise, end tidal CO_2 monitor, SaO_2.
  - All patients get supplemental O_2 regardless of SaO_2.

Assume C-spine injury in trauma patients until proven otherwise.

Breathing and Ventilation

- Inspect, auscultate, and palpate the chest and neck.
- Ensure adequate and equal ventilation and identify and treat injuries that may immediately impair ventilation:
  - Tension pneumothorax
  - Flail chest and pulmonary contusion
  - Massive hemothorax
  - Open pneumothorax

Control of Hemorrhage

- Place *two* large-bore (14 or 16G) IVs.
- Assess circulatory status (capillary refill, pulse, skin color) (see Shock section below).
- Control of life-threatening hemorrhage using **direct pressure;** do not "blind clamp" bleeding vessels with hemostats; do not probe deep within a wound.
- If a pelvic fracture is suspected, then pelvic binder to be applied at this stage.

Disability

- Rapid neurologic exam.
- Establish pupillary size and reactivity, and level of consciousness using the Glasgow Coma Scale.
- Check movement of all limbs for a quick assessment of spinal cord function.

AVPU scale:
Alert
Verbal
Pain
Unresponsive

Exposure/Environment/Extras

- Completely undress the patient, most often with the help of your trauma shears.
- Hook up monitors (cardiac, pulse oximetry, blood pressure, etc).
- Remember the hidden places: under collars, splints, axillary folds, and groins.
- Logroll the patient to assess the back—since you are moving the patient, this is a good time to quickly do a rectal examination.

Do not forget to keep your patients **warm**.

Foley Catheter

- Placement of a urinary catheter is considered part of the resuscitative phase, which takes place during the primary survey.
- Important for monitoring urinary output, which is a reflection of renal perfusion and volume status.
- Adequate urinary output:
  - Adult: 0.5 cc/kg/h
  - Child (> 1 year of age): 1.0 cc/kg/h
  - Child (< 1 year of age): 2.0 cc/kg/h
- Foley is contraindicated when urethral transection is suspected, such as in the case of a pelvic fracture. If transection is suspected, perform retrograde urethrogram before Foley (a suprapubic catheter can be placed to empty the bladder).

Examine prostate and genitalia before placing a Foley. Blood at the external meatus is a contraindication for Foley catheterization.

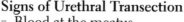

Place OG tube rather than NG tube when fracture of cribriform plate is suspected.

Signs of Urethral Transection
- Blood at the meatus
- A "high-riding" prostate
- Perineal or scrotal hematoma

Gastric Intubation

Placement of nasogastric (NG) or orogastric (OG) tube may reduce risk of aspiration by decompressing stomach, but does not assure full prevention (Figure 3-1).

Trauma History

Whenever possible, take an **AMPLE** history:

- **A**llergies
- **M**edications/**M**echanism of injury
- **P**ast medical history/**P**regnant?
- **L**ast meal
- **E**vents surrounding the mechanism of injury

Trauma resuscitation is a team sport with many different activities overlapping in both time and space.

RESUSCITATION

- Begins during the primary survey.
- Life-threatening injuries are tended to as they are identified.

Intravenous Catheters

The rate of maximal fluid administration is directly related to the internal diameter of the IV catheter (to the fourth power of the radius according to Poiseuille's law) and inversely related to the length of the tubing; for example, a 14-g angiocath in peripheral IV has a higher flow rate then a standard 3-lumen central line. Large-bore "cordis" central line provides the highest flows.

Intravenous Fluid

- Fluid therapy should be initiated with 1–2 L of an isotonic (either lactated Ringer's or normal saline) crystalloid solution (see below).
- Pediatric patients should receive an IV bolus of 20 cc/kg.

Crystalloid versus Colloid

- Crystalloids are sodium-based solutions that provide a transient ↑ in intravascular volume.
- Approximately one-third of an isotonic solution will remain in the intravascular space. The remainder almost immediately distributes to the extravascular and interstitial spaces. This occurs because crystalloid solutions easily diffuse across membranes.
- Colloids have a harder time diffusing across membranes, thus remaining in the intravascular space for longer periods of time, thereby requiring smaller volumes for resuscitation. However, it is costly and carries the risks of transfusion reactions and viral transmission.

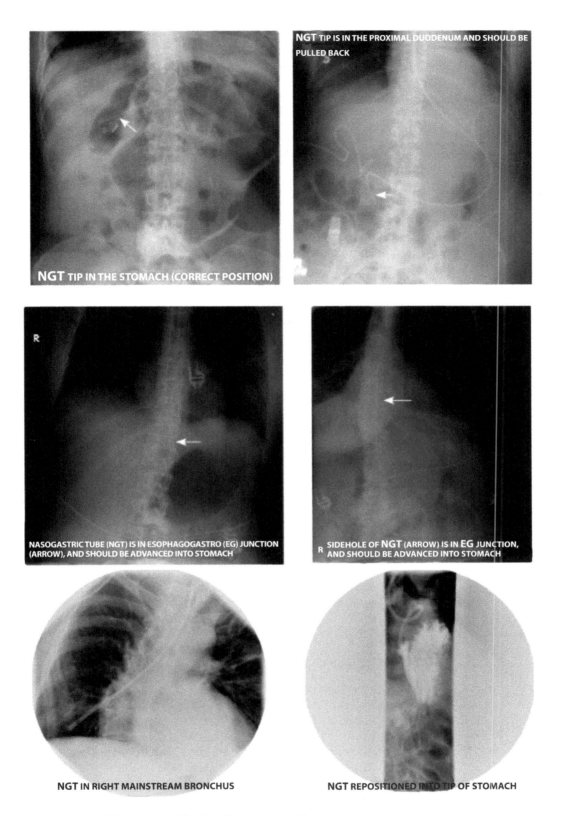

FIGURE 3-1. Correct and incorrect positioning of nasogastric tube.

(Reproduced, with permission, from *First Aid for Radiology*, New York: McGraw-Hill, 2008: Figure 2-41.)

Use **warmed** fluids whenever possible.

Body water:
⅔ Intracellular
⅓ Extracellular
¼ Intravascular
¾ Extravascular

- Crystalloids include saline, Ringer's lactate, and glucose.
- Colloids include blood products such as red blood cells (RBCs) and albumin.

Potential areas of blood loss → shock:
- Chest
- Abdomen
- Pelvis
- Long bones
- External

Hemorrhage is the most common cause of shock in the injured patient. Vasopressors will not help!

- Neither crystalloids nor colloids have been shown to be superior for volume resuscitation. Therefore, volume resuscitation begins with crystalloids (see below).

"3-to-1 Rule"

Used as a rough estimate for the total amount of crystalloid volume needed acutely to replace blood loss.

Shock

- Inadequate delivery of oxygen on the cellular level secondary to tissue hypoperfusion.
- In traumatic situations, shock is the result of hypovolemia until proven otherwise.

HYPOVOLEMIC SHOCK

Caused by the acute loss of blood in most cases. Blood volume estimate based on body weight in kilograms:

- Adults: 7% of weight
- Peds: 8–9% of weight

For example, 70-kg adult ($70 \times 7\% = 4.9$ L of blood).

HEMORRHAGIC SHOCK

CLASSES

Table 3-1 lists the grades of hemorrhagic shock.

TREATMENT

- Response to the initial fluid bolus (eg, change in vital signs, urinary output, and/or level of consciousness) should direct further resuscitative efforts.
- Early blood transfusion and surgical intervention should be considered in patients who fail to respond to initial fluid resuscitation.
- Trauma patients with hemorrhagic shock are typically already "clamped down" and will not benefit from vasopressors. What they need is what they have lost—fluids.

NONHYPOVOLEMIC SHOCK

- **Cardiogenic shock:**
  - After trauma may occur secondary to blunt myocardial injury.
  - Nontraumatic causes include tachy- or bradydysrhythmias, myocardial infarction, and heart failure.
- **Obstructive shock** (some consider this part of cardiogenic shock):
  - After trauma from cardiac tamponade or tension pneumothorax.
  - Pulmonary embolism is another cause of obstructive shock.
- **Distributive shock:**
  - **Neurogenic shock** may occur secondary to sympathetic denervation in patients who have suffered a spinal injury.
  - **Septic shock** is due to infection and is not seen in the acute setting of a trauma. It may be seen when there is a significant delay in patients'

TABLE 3-1. Types of Hemorrhagic Shock

CLASS	BLOOD LOSS (%)	VOL. BLOOD LOSS (CC)	HR	PULSE PRESSURE	sBP	URINE OUTPUT	ALTERED MENTAL STATUS?	TREATMENT
I	Up to 15	Up to 750	< 100	N	N	N	No	Crystalloids (3 to 1 rule); no blood products necessary
II	15–30	750–1,500	↑	↓	↓	↓	No	Crystalloids initially, then monitor response; may or may not need blood products; can wait for type-specific blood.
III	30–40	1,500–2,000	↑↑	↓↓	↓↓	↓↓	Yes	Crystalloids followed by type-specific blood products
IV	> 40	> 2,000	↑↑↑ > 140	↓↓↓	↓↓↓ nil	↓↓↓	Yes Confused lethargic	2-L crystalloid bolus followed by un-crossed (O negative) blood; death is imminent.

N = normal; = increased; ↓ = decreased.

arrival to the emergency department (ED) or during the hospital course of patients with penetrating abdominal injuries, for example.
- Anaphylaxis: A rapid-onset, severe allergic reaction that is not directly associated with trauma, but may result from interventions (eg, medications, IV contrast) during trauma evaluation.
- Distributive shock results in vasodilation and patients respond to fluids and vasopressor medications.

Radiologic and Diagnostic Studies

- X-rays of the chest, pelvis, and lateral cervical spine usually occur concurrently with early resuscitative efforts; however, their procedure should never interrupt the resuscitative process.
- Computed tomography (CT) studies, often of the head, neck, chest, abdomen, and pelvis, have become very commonly used in trauma patients. They are fast and pick up most injuries, but they do expose patients to significant amounts of radiation and pick up some injuries that may not be significant (eg, a small pneumothorax).
- Diagnostic peritoneal lavage (DPL) has generally been replaced by focused abdominal sonogram for trauma (FAST).
- FAST can be done quickly at the bedside for the rapid detection of intra-abdominal bleeding. However, false negative results can occur.

A "trauma series" consists of radiographs of the C-spine, chest, and pelvis.

Secondary Survey

- Begins once the primary survey is complete and resuscitative efforts are well under way.
- Includes a **head-to-toe evaluation** of the trauma patient and **frequent reassessment** of status.
  - HEENT—head, eyes, ear, nose, throat:
    - Always look for skull fractures.
    - Face: Palpate for facial fractures.
    - Do not forget intraoral, intranasal, and intra-aural examinations.
    - Good time to check and document visual acuity.
  - Spine and neck exam.
  - Chest—clavicles ribs, sternum: Look for any bruising, crepitus.
  - Abdomen: Palpate, auscultate.
  - FAST exam: May be part of the primary survey (see Figures 3-16 and 3-17).
  - Back.
  - Extremities, pelvic, and perianal examination.
  - Rectal exam and examination of the external genitalia.
- Neurologic examination, procedures, radiologic examination, and laboratory testing also take place at this time if not already accomplished.

Tetanus Prophylaxis

Immunize as needed.

"Fingers and tubes in every orifice" is often quoted for trauma resuscitation; however, data to support the universal use of the rectal exam in trauma are lacking.

HEAD TRAUMA

Anatomy and Physiology

- Scalp:
  - Consists of five layers.
  - Highly vascular structure.
  - May be the source of major blood loss.
  - The loose attachment between the galea and the pericranium allows for large collections of blood to form a subgaleal hematoma.
  - Disruption of the galea should be corrected and may be done so with single-layer, interrupted 3.0 nonabsorbable sutures through the skin, subcutaneous tissue, and galea.
  - Prophylactic antibiotics are not indicated in simple scalp lacerations (rarely get infected).
- Skull:
  - Rigid and inflexible (fixed volume).
  - Composed of the cranial vault and base.
- Brain:
  - Makes up 80% of intracranial volume.
  - Partially compartmentalized by the reflections of dura (falx cerebri and tentorium cerebelli).
  - *Note:* CN III runs along the edge of the tentorium cerebelli. Most common site of herniation is the inner edge of the tentorium cerebelli—uncal herniation. Cranial nerve III compression from herniation leads to a "blown" pupil.
- Cerebrospinal fluid (CSF):

Layers of the **SCALP:**
Skin
Connective tissue
Aponeurosis (galea)
Loose areolar tissue
Pericranium

- Formed primarily by the choroid plexus at a rate of approximately 500 cc/day with 150 cc of CSF circulating at a given moment.
- Cushions the brain.
- Cerebral blood flow:
  - Brain receives approximately 15% of cardiac output.
  - Brain responsible for ~20% of total body O_2 consumption.
  - Cerebral perfusion pressure (CPP) = mean arterial pressure (MAP) – intracranial pressure (ICP).

> Concept of CPP is important in a hypertensive patient. Lowering the blood pressure too rapidly will also ↓ the CPP, creating a new problem.

Monro-Kellie Hypothesis

- The sum of the volume of the brain, blood, and CSF within the skull must remain constant. Therefore, an ↑ in one of the above must be off-set by a ↓ volume of the others. If not, the ICP will ↑.
- ↑ ICP can thus result in cerebral herniation, or when ICP = systolic blood pressure (BP), cerebral blood flow ceases and brain death occurs.

Assessment

History: Identify mechanism and time of injury, loss of consciousness, seizure activity, concurrent use of drugs or alcohol, medications that may affect pupillary size (eg, glaucoma medications), anticoagulant use, past medical history (especially previous head trauma and stroke with their residual effects, and previous eye surgery, which can affect pupillary size and response), and the presence of a "lucid interval."

Vital Signs

Cushing reflex: Hypertension, bradycardia, and respiratory depression in the setting of ↑ ICP.

> The Cushing reflex is the brain's attempt to maintain the CPP.

Physical Exam

- Search for signs of external trauma such as lacerations, ecchymoses, and avulsions, as these may be clues to underlying injuries such as depressed or open skull fractures. Remember to look for raccoon eyes, Battle sign (mastoid ecchymosis), hemotympanum, blood from the ear, blood or fluid from nose—all these could suggest a basilar skull fracture.
- Anisocoria (inequality of pupils) is found in a small percentage of normal people; however, unequal pupils in the patient with head trauma is pathologic until proven otherwise.

> Hypotension is usually not caused by isolated head injury. Look for other injuries in this setting.

Glasgow Coma Scale (GCS)

GCS (Figure 3-2) may be used as a tool for classifying head injury:

- Severe head injury: GCS ≤ 8
- Moderate head injury: GCS 9–13
- Mild head injury: GCS 14 or 15

Eyes	Open spontaneously	4
	Open to verbal command	3
	Open to pain	2
	No response	1
Best motor response	Obeys verbal command	6
	Localizes pain to painful stimulus	5
	Flexion withdrawal	4
	Decorticate rigidity	3
	Decerebrate rigidity	2
	No response	1
Best verbal response	Oriented and converses	5
	Disoriented and converses	4
	Inappropriate words	3
	Incomprehensible sounds	2
	No response	1
TOTAL		**15**

FIGURE 3-2. Glasgow Coma Scale.

Diagnostic Studies

- Assume C-spine injury in head injury patients and immobilize until cleared.
- Skull films have largely been replaced by CT scan.
- Indications for head/brain CT:
  - Neurologic deficit.
  - Persisting depression or worsening of mental status/focal neurological deficits.
  - Moderate to severe mechanism of injury.
  - Depressed skull fracture or linear fracture overlying a dural venous sinus or meningeal artery groove (as demonstrated with skull x-rays). Risk factors:
    - Loss of consciousness post trauma, vomiting, amnesia for event.
    - History of anticoagulation or coagulopathy.
    - Presence of distracting injuries/intoxication.

Skin staples interfere with CT scanning and should therefore not be used until after CT scanning is complete.

Noxious stimuli for GCS:
- Nail bed pressure
- Sternal pressure/rub

Always quote the individual components of GCS when communicating the score: "The GCS is W with $E_x M_y V_z$." GCS for intubated patients:
- No verbal score given.
- Replace by a T for verbal score.

SKULL FRACTURES

Linear (Nondepressed)

Becomes clinically important if it occurs over the middle meningeal artery groove or major venous dural sinuses (formation of an epidural hematoma), air-filled sinuses, or if associated with underlying brain injury.

Stellate

Suggestive of a more severe mechanism of injury than linear skull fractures.

Depressed

- Carries a much greater risk of underlying brain injury and complications, such as meningitis and posttraumatic seizures.
- Treatment involves surgical elevation for depressions deeper than the thickness of the adjacent skull.

Basilar

- Often a clinical diagnosis and sign of a significant mechanism of injury.
- Symptoms include vertigo. Signs include periorbital ecchymoses (raccoon's eyes), retroauricular ecchymoses (Battle's sign), otorrhea, rhinorrhea, hemotympanum, and cranial nerve palsies (CN VII).
- Recommend initiation of antibiotics.

Open

- A laceration overlying a skull fracture.
- Requires careful debridement and irrigation. Avoid blind digital probing of the wound.
- Obtain neurosurgical consultation.

Ring test for CSF rhinorrhea (in the presence of epistaxis):
- Sample of blood from nose placed on filter paper to test for presence of CSF. If present, a large transparent ring will be seen encircling a clot of blood.
- β_2-transferrin has the highest sensitivity and specificity for diagnosis of a fluid as CSF.

DIFFUSE INTRACRANIAL LESIONS

Cerebral Concussion

> A 20-year-old woman sustains brief loss of consciousness following head injury. She presents to the ED awake but is amnestic for the event and keeps asking the same questions again and again. What will her head CT most likely show?
>
> This patient has had a concussion. Her head CT will most likely be unremarkable with no evidence of intracranial bleeding.

- Transient loss of consciousness that occurs immediately following blunt, nonpenetrating head trauma, caused by impairment of the reticular activating system.
- Amnesia and confusion are typical.
- Recovery is often complete; however, residual effects such as headache may last for some time.
- Cerebral contusion can also occur on the opposite side of the injury (contrecoup injury).

Diffuse Axonal Injury (DAI)

- Caused by microscopic shearing of nerve fibers, scattered microscopic abnormalities.
- Frequently requires intubation, hyperventilation, and admission to a neurosurgical intensive care unit.
- Patients are often comatose for prolonged periods of time.
- Mortality is ~33%.

Cerebral Contusion

- Occurs when the brain impacts the skull; may occur directly under the site of impact (coup) or on the contralateral side (contrecoup).
- Patients usually have focal deficits; mental status ranges from confusion to coma.
- Common locations include frontal poles, subfrontal cortex, and anterior temporal lobes. Contused area is hemorrhagic.

Epidural Hematoma

> A 19-year-old man fell off of a 15-foot ladder and hit his head. He had loss of consciousness followed by a brief lucid interval. He presents to the ED in a coma, with an ipsilateral fixed and dilated pupil and contralateral hemiparesis. What do you expect to see on his brain CT?
>
> This is the classic description of a patient with an epidural hematoma. CT will demonstrate an opacity (blood) between the dura and skull, which will be lenticular in shape. Epidural hematomas comprise ~2% of head injuries, and are less common than subdural hematomas. Prognosis is good with prompt surgical intervention.

- Collection of blood located between the dura and the skull.
- Majority are associated with tearing of the middle meningeal artery from an overlying temporal bone fracture.
- Typically biconvex or lenticular in shape (see Figure 3-3).
- Patients may have the classic "lucid interval," wherein they "talk and die." Requires early neurosurgical involvement.

Subdural Hematoma

Acute subdural hematomas have a high mortality: approximately one-third to two-thirds.

- Collection of blood below the dura and over the brain (see Figure 3-4). Results from tearing of the bridging veins, usually secondary to an acceleration–deceleration mechanism.
- Classified as acute (< 24 hours), subacute (24 hours to 2 weeks), and chronic (> 2 weeks).
- Acute and subacute subdurals require early neurosurgical involvement.
- Alcoholics and the elderly (patients likely to have brain atrophy) have ↑ susceptibility.
- Crescent shaped and may cross suture lines on a CT scan.
- Duration of subdural hematoma is directly proportional to the isodensity of the insult on CT scan because of phagocytosis (greater the duration, the more gray the appearance).

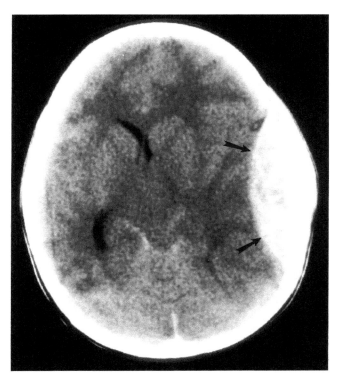

FIGURE 3-3. Epidural hematoma.

Arrows indicate the characteristic lens-shaped lesion. (Reproduced, with permission, from Schwartz SI, Spencer SC, Galloway AC, et al. *Principles of Surgery*, 7th ed. New York: McGraw-Hill, 1999: 1882.)

MANAGEMENT OF MILD TO MODERATE HEAD TRAUMA

- Safe disposition of the patient depends on multiple factors.
- Any patient with a persisting or worsening ↓ in mental status, focal deficits, severe mechanism of injury, penetrating trauma, open or depressed skull fracture, or seizures or who is unreliable or cannot be safely observed at home should be admitted for observation.
- Patients with mild and sometimes moderate head trauma, brief or no loss of consciousness, no focal deficits, an intact mental status, and reliable family members who can adequately observe the patient at home can often be discharged home with proper discharge instructions. Patients with concussions should receive follow-up evaluation and should not return to sports until cleared.
- Discharge instructions should include signs and symptoms for family members to watch for, such as:
  - Persisting or worsening headache
  - Dizziness
  - Vomiting
  - Inequality of pupils (late finding)
  - Confusion
  - If any of the above signs are found, the patient should be brought to the ED immediately.

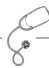

When in doubt, admit the patient with head trauma for observation.

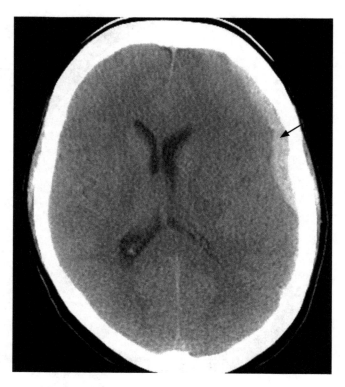

FIGURE 3-4. Head CT showing left subdural hematoma overlying left frontal lobe (arrow) with associated midline shift.

MANAGEMENT OF SEVERE HEAD TRAUMA

Measures to lower ICP—
HIVED
Hyperventilation
Intubation with pretreatment and sedation
Ventriculostomy (burr hole)
Elevate the head of the bed
Diuretics (mannitol, furosemide)

- Patients must be treated aggressively starting with the ABCs.
- Secure the airway via endotracheal intubation using topical anesthesia, intravenous lidocaine, and paralytics when necessary to prevent any further ↑ in the ICP.
- Maintain an adequate BP with isotonic fluids. (Aim for mean arterial pressure [MAP] of 90 mm Hg.)
- Treatment of ↑ ICP:
  - Elevate head of the bed to 30 degrees.
  - Hyperventilation to an arterial P_{CO_2} of 30–35 will ↓ the ICP by approximately 25% acutely. *Note:* This is not recommended prophylactically within the first 24 hours of head injury.
  - Mannitol (1 g/kg in a 20% solution) is an osmotic diuretic and lowers ICP by drawing water out of the brain. Contraindicated in the hypotensive patient.
- Coagulopathy/elevated INR should be reversed with fresh frozen plasma.
- Corticosteroids have not been shown to be useful in the patient with head trauma.
- Consider prophylactic anticonvulsant therapy with phenytoin 18 mg/kg IV at no faster than 50 mg/min (usually at the discretion of the neurosurgeon).
- Acute seizures should be managed with diazepam or lorazepam and phenytoin.
- Emergency decompression via trephination (burr holes) is best left to the neurosurgeon. Ventriculostomy should be done by neurosurgery (usually not in the ED), and drainage is performed in the operating room, because of the ability to convert to open craniotomy if needed.

- Treat the pathology whenever possible (eg, surgical drainage of a hematoma).

General

Described in broad terms as penetrating versus blunt injuries even though considerable overlap exists between the management of the two.

Anatomy

The neck is divided into triangles (anterior and posterior) as well as zones (I, II, and III).

ANTERIOR TRIANGLE

- Bordered by the midline, posterior border of the sternocleidomastoid muscle (SCM) and the mandible.
- Contains vascular and aerodigestive structures

POSTERIOR TRIANGLE

- Bordered by the trapezius, posterior border of the SCM, and the clavicle.
- There is a paucity of vital structures in its upper zone (above the spinal accessory nerve).
- In the lower zone lies the subclavian vessels and brachial plexus. The apices of the lungs are in close proximity.

ROON AND CHRISTENSEN ZONES (FIGURE 3-5)

- Further division of the anterior triangle:
  - Zone I lies between the cricoid cartilage and the clavicle.
  - Zone II lies between cricioid cartilage and the mandible.
  - Zone III lies between the angle of the mandible and base of skull.
- These divisions help to drive the diagnostic and therapeutic management decisions for penetrating neck injuries.

Penetrating Injuries

Any injury to the neck in which the platysma is violated.

Vascular Injuries
- Very common and often life threatening.
- Can → exsanguination, hematoma formation with compromise of the airway, and cerebrovascular accidents (eg, from transection of the carotid artery or air embolus).

Nonvascular Injuries
- Injury to the larynx and trachea including fracture of the thyroid cartilage and dislocation of the tracheal cartilages and arytenoids, for example, → airway compromise and often a difficult intubation.
- Esophageal injury does occur and, as with penetrating neck injury, is not often manifest initially.

Within the anterior triangle lie the majority of the vital structures of the neck.

Fracture of the hyoid bone is suggestive of a significant mechanism of injury.

C-spine injuries are much more common with blunt neck injury.

HIGH-YIELD FACTS

Trauma

Alerting signs of impending airway compromise: dyspnea, dysphonia, stridor, drooling, ↑ in hematoma size, bruit.

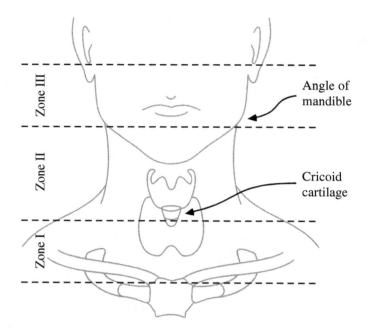

FIGURE 3-5. **Zones of the neck.**

Zone III

Zone II

Zone I

Angle of mandible

Cricoid cartilage

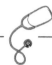

Risks of early intubation must be compared to the possibility of respiratory distress and complicated intubation with a distorted airway later.

Avoid unnecessary manipulation of the neck, as this may dislodge a clot.

Keep cervical in-line stabilization until C-spine fracture has been ruled out.

Resuscitation

Airway
- Special attention should be paid to airway management of the patient with neck trauma.
- Anatomy may be distorted, and an apparently patent airway can rapidly evolve into a compromised, difficult airway.
- Initial attempts at securing the airway should be via endotracheal intubation; however, alternative methods of airway management, such as percutaneous transtracheal ventilation and surgical airway, should be readily available.

Breathing
- Inability to ventilate the patient after an apparently successful intubation should prompt rapid reassessment of that airway.
- Creation and/or intubation of a "false lumen" in the patient with laryngotracheal or tracheal transection may be a fatal error if not identified immediately.
- Look for pneumohemothorax, as the apices of the lungs lie in close proximity to the base of the neck.

Circulation
- Cover open wounds.
- Compress bleeding areas, without occluding the airway.
- If the patient remains unstable after appropriate volume resuscitation, he or she should be taken rapidly to the operating room (OR) for operative control of the bleeding.
- If injury to the subclavian vessels is suspected, IV access should be obtained in the opposite extremity, or more appropriately in the lower extremities.

Secondary Survey

- After stabilization, the wound should be carefully examined.
- Obtain soft-tissue films of the neck for clues to the presence of a soft-tissue hematoma and subcutaneous emphysema, and a chest x-ray (CXR) for possible hemopneumothorax.
- CTA (CT angiogram) is investigative study of choice.
- Surgical exploration is indicated for:
  - Expanding hematoma
  - Subcutaneous emphysema
  - Tracheal deviation
  - Change in voice quality
  - Air bubbling through the wound
- Pulses should be palpated to identify deficits and thrills and auscultated for bruits.
- A neurologic exam should be performed to identify brachial plexus and/or central nervous system deficits as well as Horner syndrome.

Control of hemorrhage in the ED is via direct pressure (no blind clamping).

Management

- Injuries to zones I and III may be taken to the operating room (OR) or managed conservatively using a combination of angiography, bronchoscopy, esophagoscopy, gastrografin or barium studies, and CT scanning.
- Zone II injuries are taken to the OR for exploration.

Never blindly probe a neck wound, as this may → bleeding in a previously tamponaded wound.

SPINAL TRAUMA

GENERAL

- Spinal trauma may involve injury to the spinal column, spinal cord, or both.
- Over 50% of spinal injuries occur in the cervical spine, with the remainder being divided between the thoracic spine, the thoracolumbar junction, and the lumbosacral region.
- As long as the spine is appropriately immobilized, evaluation for spinal injury may be deferred until the patient is stabilized.

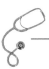

Cardiac arrest unresponsive to fluid resuscitation in penetrating neck trauma may be venous air embolism.
Keep patient in head down, left lateral decubitus position.

ANATOMY

- There are 7 cervical, 12 thoracic, 5 lumbar, 5 sacral, and 4 coccygeal vertebrae.
- The cervical spine is the region that is most vulnerable to injury.
- The thoracic spine is relatively protected due to limited mobility from support of the rib cage (T1–10); however, the spinal canal through which the spinal cord traverses is relatively narrow in this region. Therefore, when injuries to this region do occur, they usually have devastating results.
- The thoracolumbar junction (T11–L1) is a fairly vulnerable region, as it is the area between the relatively inflexible thoracic region and the flexible lumbar region.
- The lumbosacral region (L2 and below) contains the region of the spinal canal below which the spinal cord proper ends and the cauda equina begins.

Patients on a backboard for a prolonged period of time are at risk for the formation of pressure ulcers.

Mechanisms suspicious for spinal injury:
- Diving
- Fall from > 10 feet
- Injury above level of shoulders (C-spine)
- Electrocution
- High-speed motor vehicle crash
- Rugby or football injury (tackling)

Suspicion for Site of Injury

Hypotension tachycardia:
BLEEDING
Hypertension bradycardia:
BRAIN
Hypotension bradycardia:
SPINAL CORD

Deep tendon reflexes and sacral reflexes may be preserved in complete injuries.

- Three spinal columns for stability—anterior, middle, and posterior. Distribution of any two or vertebral body compression of > 50% is suggestive of unstable spine.

PATHOLOGY AND PATHOPHYSIOLOGY

Spinal injuries can generally be classified based on:

- Fracture/dislocation type (mechanism, stable versus unstable).
- Level of neurologic (sensory and motor) and bony involvement.
- Severity (complete versus incomplete spinal cord disability).

Neurogenic Shock

- A state of vasomotor instability resulting from impairment of the descending sympathetic pathways in the spinal cord, or simply a loss of sympathetic tone.
- Signs and symptoms include flaccid paralysis, hypotension, bradycardia, cutaneous vasodilation, and a normal to wide pulse pressure.

Spinal Shock

- State of flaccidity and loss of reflexes occurring immediately after spinal cord injury.
- Loss of visceral and peripheral autonomic control with uninhibited parasympathetic impulses.
- May last from seconds to weeks, and does not signify permanent spinal cord damage.
- Long-term prognosis cannot be postulated until spinal shock has resolved.
- First sign of resolution of spinal shock: Return of bulbocavernous reflex.

Spinal Cord Injuries

Complete versus incomplete:

- Complete spinal cord injuries demonstrate no preservation of neurologic function distal to the level of injury. Therefore, any sensorimotor function below the level of injury constitutes an incomplete injury.
- Sacral sparing refers to perianal sensation, voluntary anal sphincter contraction, or voluntary toe flexion, and is a sign of an incomplete spinal cord injury.

PHYSICAL EXAM

- Classification of spinal cord injuries as complete or incomplete requires a proper neurologic exam.
- The exam should include testing of the three readily assessable long spinal tracts (see Figure 3-6):
  - Corticospinal tract (CST):
    - Located in the posterolateral aspect of the spinal cord.
    - Responsible for ipsilateral motor function.
    - Tested via voluntary muscle contraction.
  - Spinothalamic tract (STT):
    - Located in the anterolateral aspect of the spinal cord.
    - Responsible for contralateral pain and temperature sensation and is tested as such.

- Posterior (dorsal) columns:
  - Located in the posterior aspect of the spinal cord.
  - Responsible for ipsilateral position and vibratory sense and some light touch sensation.
  - Test using a tuning fork and position sense of the fingers and toes.

Spinal Cord Syndromes

Anterior Cord Syndrome
- Pattern seen with injury to the anterior portion of the spinal cord or with compression of the anterior spinal arteries.
- Involves full or partial loss of bilateral pain and temperature sensation (STT) and paraplegia (CST), with preservation of posterior column function.
- Often seen with flexion injuries.
- Carries a poor prognosis.

Brown-Séquard Syndrome
- Pattern seen with hemisection of the spinal cord usually secondary to a penetrating injury, but may also be seen with disk protrusion, hematoma, or tumor.
- Consists of ipsilateral loss of motor function (CST) and posterior column function, with contralateral loss of pain and temperature sensation.

Central Cord Syndrome
- Pattern seen with injury to the central area of the spinal cord often in patients with a preexisting narrowing of the spinal canal.
- Usually seen with hyperextension injuries: Its cause is usually attributed to buckling of the ligamentum flavum into the cord and/or an ischemic etiology in the distribution of branches of the anterior spinal artery.

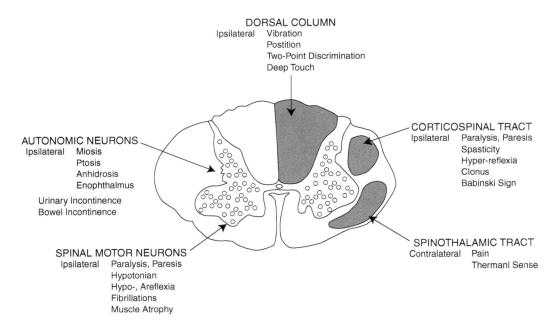

FIGURE 3-6. Effects of lesions in major spinal cord tracts.

(Reproduced, with permission, from Afifi AA, Bergman RA. *Functional Neuroanatomy: Text and Atlas*. New York: McGraw-Hill, 1998: 92.)

A 70-year-old male presents to the ED after a whiplash injury. He is ambulating well but has an extremely weak handshake. *Think: Central cord syndrome.*

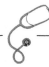

NEXUS Low-Risk Criteria:
C-spine films are indicated for patients with a potential mechanism of C-spine injury and any of the following:
- Posterior midline cervical spine tenderness
- Intoxication
- Altered mental status
- Focal neurologic deficit
- Painful distracting injury

C-spine views:
1. Cross table grid lateral
2. AP view — with 20-degree cephalad angle
3. Swimmer's view — if C7–T1 not visualized
4. Open-mouth odontoid view
5. Oblique views (optional)

- Characterized by weakness greater in the upper extremities than the lower extremities, and distal worse than proximal.
- Has a better prognosis than the other partial cord syndromes with a characteristic pattern of recovery (lower extremity recovery progressing upward to upper extremity recovery, then the hands recover strength).

TREATMENT

- Always start with the ABCs of trauma resuscitation.
- Maintain spinal immobilization throughout the resuscitation.
- Estimate level of neurologic dysfunction during the secondary survey.
- Obtain appropriate diagnostic studies.
- Establish early neurosurgical consultation.
- For penetrating spinal cord injury, administer prophylactic antibiotics and consider high-dose methylprednisolone in consultation with neurosurgeon:
  - Methylprednislone is commonly used for spinal cord injury, but its use is controversial. Loading dose of 30 mg/kg over 15 minutes during hour 1, followed by a continuous infusion of 5.4 mg/kg/h over the next 23 hours.
  - Consider traction devices in consultation with the neurosurgeon.
- Consider early referral to a regional spinal injury center.

C-SPINE FRACTURES AND DISLOCATIONS

GENERAL

As mentioned above, usually classified on the basis of mechanism (flexion, extension, compression, rotation, or a combination of these), location, and/or stability.

IMAGING

- Three views of the cervical spine are obtained (lateral, anteroposterior [AP], and an odontoid view) for best accuracy.
- A lateral view alone will miss 10% of C-spine injuries.
- Adequate AP and lateral films will allow visualization of C1–T1.
- If C1–T1 can still not be adequately visualized, CT scanning is indicated.

READING A C-SPINE FILM

- Most common level of fracture is C5.
- Most common level of subluxation is C5 on C6.
- **Alignment:**
  - Evaluate the alignment of the four lordotic curves (see Figure 3-7):
    - Anterior margin of the vertebral bodies
    - Posterior margin of the vertebral bodies
    - Spinolaminar line
    - Tips of the vertebral bodies: In the adult, up to 3.5 mm of anterior subluxation is considered a normal finding.
- **Bones:** Assess the base of the skull and each vertebral body, pedicle, facet, laminae, and spinous and transverse process for fracture/dislocation.
- **Cartilage:** Assess the intervertebral spaces and posterolateral facet joints for symmetry.

- **Soft tissue:**
  - Assess the prevertebral soft tissue: Wider than 6 mm at C2 or 2 cm at C6 associated with ↑ likelihood of fracture ("6 at 2, 2 at 6").
  - Assess the predental space: Wider than 3 mm in adults and 4 to 5 mm in children is suggestive of a torn transverse ligament and fracture of C1.
  - Assess the spaces between the spinous processes: Any ↑ in distance between the spinous processes is likely associated with a torn interspinous ligament and a spinal fracture.

Atlanto-Occipital Dislocation

- Results from severe traumatic flexion.
- Survival to the hospital setting is rare.
- Traction is not recommended.

Jefferson Fracture (Figure 3-8)

- C1 (atlas) burst fracture.
- Most common C1 fracture.
- Consists of a fracture of both the anterior and posterior rings of C1.
- Results from axial loading such as when the patient falls directly on his or her head or something falls on the patient's head.
- Often associated with C2 fractures.
- Consider all C1 fractures unstable even though most are not associated with spinal cord injury.
- Seen as an ↑ in the predental space on lateral x-ray and displacement of the lateral masses on the odontoid view.

Diagnostic Criteria:
BAI — Basion Axis Interval:
   > 12 mm or ↓ < 4 mm
BDI — Basion Dental
   Interval: > 12 mm

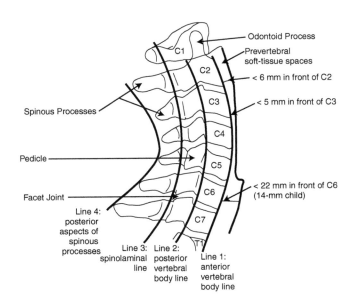

FIGURE 3-7. Lateral view of the cervical spine.

The four "lines" should flow smoothly, without step-up. The prevertebral soft-tissue spaces should be within normal.

C1 Rotary Subluxation

- Seen most often in children or in patients with rheumatoid arthritis.
- Seen as an asymmetry between the lateral masses and the dens on the odontoid view.
- Patients will present with the head in rotation and should not be forced to place the head in the neutral position.

Odontoid Fractures (Figure 3-9)

- Type 1:
  - Involves only the tip of the dens (stable).
  - Incidence ~10%.
- Type 2:
  - Involves only the base of the dens (most common type).
  - Incidence ~60%.
  - Neurologic complications in 20%.
- Type 3:
  - Fracture through the base and body of C2.
  - Neurologic sequelae less common than with type II.
  - Incidence ~30%.
  - Generally unstable.

Hangman's Fracture (Figure 3-10)

- Traumatic spondylolisthesis of C2 over C3.
- Fracture of both pedicles ("posterior elements") of C2 with anterior displacement of C2.
- Usually due to a hyperextension mechanism.
- Unstable fracture; however, often not associated with spinal cord injury because the spinal canal is at its widest through C2.

Burst Fracture of C3–7

- An axial loading mechanism causing compression of a vertebral body with resultant protrusion of the anterior portion of the vertebral body anteriorly and the posterior portion of the vertebral body posteriorly into the spinal canal, often causing a spinal cord injury (usually the anterior cord syndrome).
- Stable fracture when ligamentous structure remains intact.

Simple Wedge Fracture

- A flexion injury causing compression on the anterior portion of the vertebral body.
- Appears as a wedge-shaped concavity, with loss of vertebral height on the anterior portion of the vertebral body.
- Usually stable when not associated with ligamentous damage.

Flexion Teardrop Fracture (Figure 3-11)

- A flexion injury causing a fracture of the anteroinferior portion of the vertebral body.

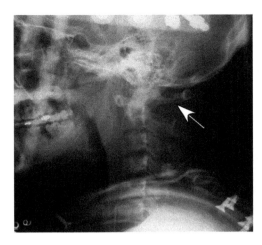

FIGURE 3-8. Jefferson fracture.

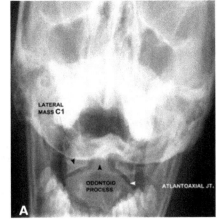
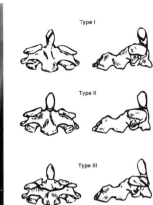

FIGURE 3-9. A. Odontoid view. B. Odontoid fractures.

- Appears as a teardrop-shaped fragment off the anteroinferior corner of the vertebral body.
- Unstable fracture, as it is usually associated with a tearing of the posterior ligament and often neurologic damage.
- Presents clinically with acute anterior cervical cord syndrome.

Extension Teardrop Fracture

- Also appears as a teardrop-shaped fragment on the anteroinferior portion of the vertebral body.
- However, occurs as an extension injury with avulsion of the fragment, rather than a compression mechanism.
- The posterior ligaments are left intact, making this a stable fracture.
- However, differentiation between a flexion versus extension teardrop fracture may be difficult and should be treated initially as if it were unstable.

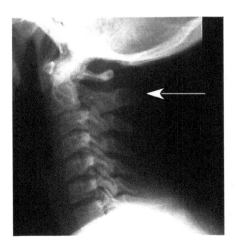

FIGURE 3-10. Hangman fracture.

Clay Shoveler's Fracture (Figure 3-12)

- Usually a flexion injury resulting in an avulsion of the tip of the spinous process (C7 > C6 > T1).
- Mechanism: Abrupt flexion of the head and neck against the tense set of posterior ligaments. May also result from a direct blow.

Unilateral Facet Dislocation

- Occurs as a flexion-rotation injury.
- Usually stable, but is potentially unstable as it often involves injury to the posterior ligamentous structures.
- Often identified on the AP view of the C-spine films when the spinous processes do not line up.
- Radiographic findings:
  - Displacement of dislocated vertebra < 50% AP diameter.
  - Above level of dislocation, vertebra oblique; below, vertebra in true lateral view.
  - Naked facet.

Bilateral Facet Dislocation

- Occurs as a flexion injury and is extremely unstable.
- Associated with a high incidence of spinal cord injury.
- Appears on lateral C-spine films as a subluxation of the dislocated vertebra of greater than one-half the AP diameter of the vertebral body below it.

Subluxation

- Occurs with disruption of the ligamentous structures without bony involvement.
- Potentially unstable.
- Findings on C-spine films may be subtle, and flexion-extension views may be needed.

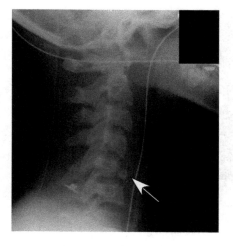

FIGURE 3-11. **Flexion teardrop fracture.**

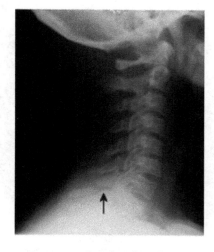

FIGURE 3-12. **Clay shoveler's fracture.**

- As mentioned above, the majority of injuries take place at the junction between the relatively fixed upper thoracic spine and the mobile thoracolumbar region (T10–L5).
- When thoracic fractures do take place, they can be devastating because the spinal canal through this region is relatively narrow and the blood supply to this region of spinal cord is in a watershed area (the greater radicular artery of Adamkiewicz enters the spinal canal at L1 but provides blood flow as high as T4).
- Most thoracic spine fractures are caused by hyperflexion → a wedge or compression fracture of the vertebral body.
- The majority of fractures/dislocations in this area are considered stable because of the surrounding normal bony thorax.
- However, as mentioned, neurologic impairment resulting from injuries in this area is often complete.

THORACOLUMBAR JUNCTION AND LUMBAR SPINE FRACTURES AND DISLOCATIONS

Compression (Wedge) Fracture

- Results from axial loading and flexion.
- Potentially unstable.
- Frequency: L1 > L2 > T1.
- Neurologic injury is uncommon.
- Treatment is symptomatic (patients usually experience pain and are at ↑ risk for the formation of an ileus).

Burst Fracture

- Fracture of the vertebral end plates with forceful extrusion of the nucleus pulposus into the vertebral body causing comminution of the vertebral body.
- Results from axial loading.
- See loss of vertebral height on lateral spine film.

Distraction or Seat Belt Injury

- Frequently referred to as a "chance fracture."
- Horizontal fracture through the vertebral body, spinous processes, laminae, and pedicles and tearing of the posterior spinous ligament.
- Caused by an acceleration-deceleration injury of a mobile person moving forward into a fixed seat belt.

Abdominal injuries frequently coexist with fracture-dislocations.

Fracture-Dislocations

- Result from flexion with rotation.
- Unstable and often associated with spinal cord damage.

- Fractures in this area are relatively uncommon.
- Sacral injuries must often be diagnosed via CT scan.
- Neurologic impairment is rare; however, damage to the sacral nerve roots results in bowel/bladder and sexual dysfunction as well as loss of sensory and motor function to the posterior lower extremities.
- Fractures of the coccyx are usually caused by direct trauma.
- Diagnosis is made upon palpation of a "step-off" on rectal examination, and rectal bleeding must also be ruled out (severe fractures may → a rectal tear).
- Treatment of uncomplicated coccygeal fracture is symptomatic and includes pain management and a doughnut pillow.

THORACIC TRAUMA

Cardiac Tamponade

Beck's tamponade triad:
1. Hypotension
2. JVD
3. Muffled heart sounds

- Life-threatening emergency usually seen with penetrating thoracic trauma, but may be seen with blunt thoracic trauma as well.
- Signs include tachycardia, muffled heart sounds, jugular venous distention (JVD), hypotension, and electrical alternans on electrocardiogram (ECG) (see Figure 3-13).
- Diagnosis may be confirmed with cardiac sonogram if immediately available.
- Requires immediate decompression via **needle pericardiocentesis** (see Procedures chapter, Figure 16-2), pericardial window, or thoracotomy with manual decompression.

Pneumothorax

DEFINITION

Air in the pleural space.

A 19-year-old man who was stabbed in the chest with a knife presents complaining of dyspnea. Breath sounds on the left are absent. *Think: Pneumothorax.*

SIGNS AND SYMPTOMS

- Chest pain
- Dyspnea
- Hyperresonance of affected side
- ↓ breath sounds of affected side

DIAGNOSIS

- Upright chest x-ray is ~83% sensitive, demonstrates an absence of lung markings where the lung has collapsed (see Figure 3-14). Often a deep sulcus can be seen at the costophrenic angle.
- Ultrasound has been suggested to have higher sensitivity for diagnosis of pneumothorax:
  - Lung sliding: 91% sensitive
  - Comet tailing: 77% sensitive
  - Lung point presence: 100% sensitive
- If a hemopneumothorax is suspected and central venous access is necessary, a femoral line is the first option, followed by placement of the access on the side ipsilateral to the "dropped lung" (because the patient doesn't like it when both lungs are down!).

Tracheostomy is the procedure of choice in the patient with laryngotracheal separation.

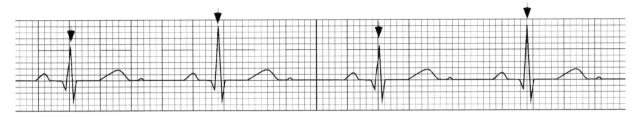

FIGURE 3-13. ECG demonstrating electrical alternans. Note alternating heights of the R (arrow) in the QRS complexes.

TUBE THORACOSTOMY

See Procedures chapter.

Tension Pneumothorax

- Life-threatening emergency caused by air entering the pleural space (most often via a hole in the lung tissue) but being unable to escape.
- Causes total ipsilateral lung collapse, mediastinal shift (**away from injured lung**) impairing venous return and thus ↓ cardiac output, eventually resulting in shock.
- Signs and symptoms include dyspnea, hypotension, tracheal deviation, absent breath sounds, and hyperresonance to percussion.
- Requires immediate needle decompression followed by tube thoracostomy.

A diagnosis of tension pneumothorax via x-ray is a missed diagnosis. Do not delay treatment of a suspected tension pneumothorax in order to confirm your suspicion (ie, tension pneumothorax is a **clinical** diagnosis).

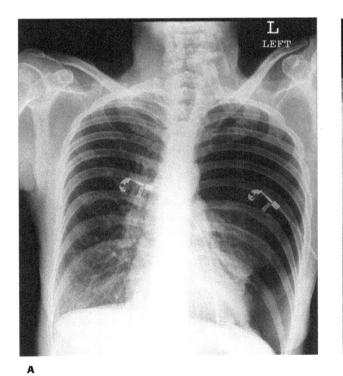

A

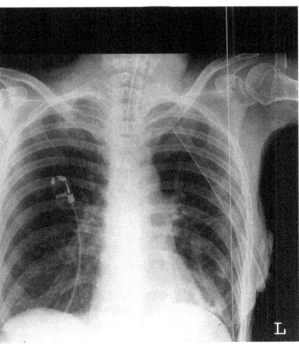

B

FIGURE 3-14. A. CXR demonstrating left-sided pneumothorax. Note lack of lung markings. Notice the deep sulcus sign. B. Same patient, after tube thoracostomy and endotracheal intubation.

Hemothorax

- Defined as the presence of blood in the lungs.
  - > 200 mL of blood must be present before blunting of costophrenic angle will be seen on upright CXR.
  - >1500 mL of blood—massive hemothorax
- Such high volumes can cause:
  - ↓ in blood volume
  - Lung collapse
  - Vena caval compression, causing ↓ in preload
- Treatment involves chest tube placement and drainage.

Indications for Thoracotomy

- 1500 mL initial drainage from the chest tube.
- 200 mL/h continued drainage for 2–4 hours.
- Patients who decompensate after initial stabilization.
- > 50% hemothorax.

Traumatic Aortic Rupture

- Most often seen with sudden deceleration injuries (high-speed motor vehicle crash, falls from > 25 feet).
- Most frequent site of rupture is isthmus of aorta b/w left subclavian and ligamentum arteriosum.
- High-mortality injury: Almost 90% die at the scene, and another 50% of those that survive the scene die within 24 hours.

SIGNS AND SYMPTOMS

- Retrosternal chest pain.
- Dyspnea.
- New systolic murmur.
- Pseudocoarctation syndrome: ↑ BP in upper extremities with absent or ↓ femoral pulses.
- Pulse deficits between upper and lower extremities.
- Findings on CXR (see Figure 3-15):
  - Widened mediastinum
  - Tracheal or NG tube deviation to the right
  - Depression of left main stem bronchus
  - Widening of paratracheal stripe to the right
  - Indistinct aortic knob
  - ↑ right paraspinal interface displacement
  - Indistinct space between pulmonary artery and aorta
  - Presence of left apical cap
  - Multiple rib fractures

DIAGNOSIS

Via transesophageal echocardiography, CT angiogram.

MANAGEMENT

Fluid resuscitation and stat surgical consultation for OR.

Needle decompression involves placing a needle or catheter over a needle into the second intercostal space, midclavicular line, over the rib on the side of the tension pneumothorax, followed by a tube thoracostomy (chest tube).

One-fourth of cases of hemothorax have an associated pneumothorax.

Three-fourths of cases of hemothorax are associated with extrathoracic injuries.

A 16-year-old baseball player presents to the ED after trauma during a game. The patient was playing baseball when he ran into another player injuring his left chest and left upper abdomen. Subsequently, he lost consciousness and upon regaining consciousness, he was diaphoretic, confused, and complained of left chest and upper abdominal pain. He was flown from the scene on a backboard with C-collar immobilization in place. In the ED, patient complained of back and abdominal pain. On exam, he was alert and oriented with stable vitals. There was marked tenderness to palpation in left lower back and over the lumbar spine. FAST scan revealed clear Morison's pouch. Splenorenal window was obscured. CXR was negative. What is the next step in your management?

The fact that the splenorenal window on FAST exam was obscured, and the patient complains of left upper abdominal pain along with being diaphoretic, suggests he has an intra-abdominal injury. The next step would be a CT scan, which is depicted below (Figure 3-16). Abdominal CT scan reveals a large left renal laceration extending into the renal hilum with associated hematoma measuring approximately 12 cm (solid arrow), tracking down the left retroperitoneum into the pelvis with evidence of extravasation. Also noted is a large splenic laceration with moderate-size subcapsular hematoma (open arrow). Lower left three ribs are fractured.

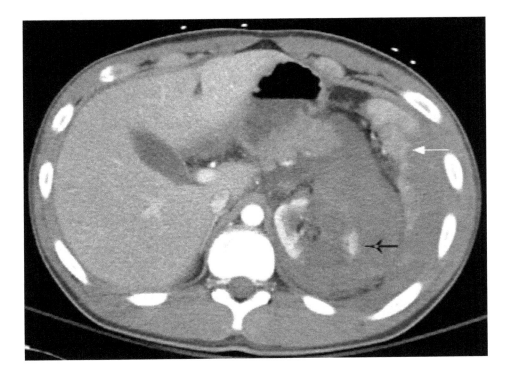

FIGURE 3-16. Abdominal CT scan.

The most frequently injured solid organ associated with penetrating trauma is the liver, followed by the small bowel.

The most frequently injured solid organ associated with blunt trauma is the spleen, followed by the liver.

Stable patient: Consider CT to look for injury regardless of whether FAST is positive or negative.

GENERAL

- Penetrating abdominal injuries (PAIs) resulting from a gunshot create damage via three mechanisms:
  1. Direct injury by the bullet itself
  2. Injury from fragmentation of the bullet
  3. Indirect injury from the resultant "shock wave"
- PAIs resulting from a stabbing mechanism are limited to the direct damage of the object of impalement.
- Blunt abdominal injury also has three general mechanisms of injury:
  1. Injury caused by the direct blow
  2. Crush injury
  3. Deceleration injury that occurs

ANATOMY

- Anterior abdominal wall: Bordered laterally by the midaxillary lines, superiorly by a horizontal line drawn through the nipples and inferiorly by the symphysis pubis and inguinal ligaments.
- The "thoracoabdominal region" is that region below the nipples and above the costal margins and is the area within which the diaphragm travels. Penetrating injuries to this region are more likely to involve injury to the diaphragm.
- Flank: Area between the anterior and posterior axillary lines.
- Back: Area posterior to the posterior axillary lines, bordered superiorly by a line drawn through the tips of the scapulae and inferiorly by the iliac crests.
- Peritoneal viscera: Liver, spleen, stomach, small bowel, sigmoid and transverse colon.
- Retroperitoneal viscera: Majority of the duodenum (fourth part is intraperitoneal), pancreas, kidneys and ureters, ascending and descending colon, and major vessels such as the abdominal aorta, inferior vena cava, renal and splenic vessels.
- Pelvic viscera: Bladder, urethra, ovaries and uterus in women, prostate in men, rectum, and iliac vessels.

PHYSICAL EXAMINATION

- **Seat belt sign:** Ecchymotic area found in the distribution of the lower anterior abdominal wall and can be associated with perforation of the bladder or bowel as well as a lumbar distraction fracture (chance fracture).
- **Cullen's sign** (periumbilical ecchymosis) is indicative of intraperitoneal hemorrhage.
- **Grey Turner's sign** (flank ecchymoses) is indicative of retroperitoneal hemorrhage.
- Inspect the abdomen for evisceration, entry/exit wounds, impaled objects, and a gravid uterus.
- Local wound exploration: Abdominal wounds may be probed or explored if it is unclear if they enter the abdominal cavity. Chest wounds should never be probed.

DIAGNOSIS

- Perforation: Pelvic x-ray for fractures. CXR with both domes of diaphragm included/abdominal x-ray to look for free air.
- Diaphragmatic injury: CXR to look for blurring of the diaphragm, hemothorax, or bowel gas patterns above the diaphragm (at times with a gastric tube seen in the left chest).

FOCUSED ASSESSMENT WITH SONOGRAPHY FOR TRAUMA (FAST)
(FIGURES 3-17 AND 3-18)

- Used as a rapid bedside screening study.
- Noninvasive and not time consuming.
- Positive if free intrathoracic, free intraperitoneal and/or pericardial fluid is seen.

Four views are utilized to search for free intraperitoneal fluid (presumed to be blood in the trauma victim), which collects in dependent areas and appears as hypoechoic areas on ultrasound:

- Morison's pouch in the right upper quadrant: Free fluid can be visualized between the interface of the liver and kidney.
- Splenorenal recess in the left upper quadrant: Free fluid can be visualized between the interface of the spleen and kidney.
- Pouch of Douglas, which lies above the rectum (probe is placed in the suprapubic region).
- Subxiphoid and parasternal views to look for hemopericardium.

Four views of FAST:

- Subxyphoid, four-chamber view: Obtained by placing the probe in the subxyphoid area with the indicator toward the patient's right; assesses the heart for pericardial fluid. If unable to obtain image, you may resort to parasternal long axis view up on the chest, which is obtained by placing the probe upon the chest at the nipple line (approx. 4–5 interspace) on left of sternum with indicator pointing toward the right shoulder.

Role of FAST
Unstable patient:
- Positive FAST: To OR.
- Negative FAST: Look for other sites of bleeding.

Serial abdominal examinations can and should be performed.

HIGH-YIELD FACTS

Trauma

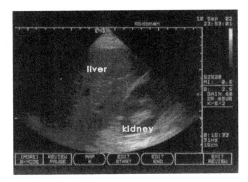
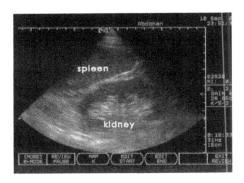
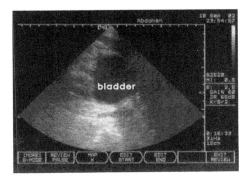
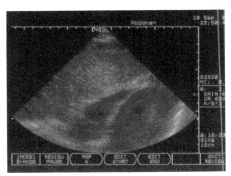

FIGURE 3-17. Normal FAST exam.

(Courtesy of Latha Ganti Stead, MD.)

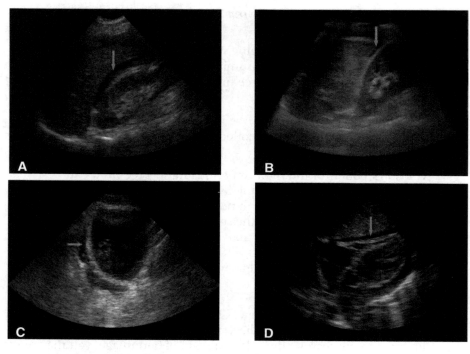

FIGURE 3-18. Abnormal FAST exam.

Panels A, B, C, and D correspond to the RUQ, LUQ, bladder and subxiphioid view as in Figure 3-16. The arrows denote free fluid, seen as a black stripe. (Courtesy of F. Eike Flach, MD.)

EFAST or extended FAST is FAST exam with pneumothorax.

Important point in FAST: Always scan through completely to not miss free fluid.

- RUQ view: Obtained by placing the probe in the midaxillary line, with the indicator toward the patient's head, obtaining a coronal cut through the patient. This assesses right intrathoracic space, Morison's pouch, the interface between the liver and kidney, and the paracolic gutter. These spaces are all along that coronal cut with the chest cavity seen just above the diaphragm, closer to the patient's head (superiorly). Morison's pouch is along that line more inferiorly and paracolic gutter tracking even more inferiorly to tip of kidney. All of these views might be seen in one view, or it may take three separate views to assess them. This is patient dependent.
- LUQ view: Same as RUQ, but on left. Place probe in midaxillary line, indicator toward the patient's head, coronal cut, assessing the left chest cavity, splenorenal interface, and paracolic gutter area.
- Pelvic view: Place probe in suprapubic area in transverse and sagittal positions. With firm pressure, rock back behind the pubic bone, viewing the bladder.
- For PTX, a linear probe is used in M-mode and it is placed sagittal on the anterior chest in a trauma patient just below the clavicular line. Slide probe up and down (superior and inferior) to bring ribs into view, which are hyperechoic horizontal lines with dense shadow beneath. The first hyperechoic line inferior to the ribs running between them is the pleural line. Look for sliding along this line that is very subtle. The stratosphere sign (Figure 3-19) demonstrates the pattern of absent lung sliding against normal lung sliding, consistent with pneumothorax. The seashore sign (Figure 3-20) is a smooth linear pattern indicative of normal lung sliding.

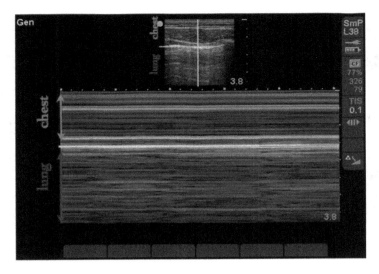

FIGURE 3-19. Stratosphere sign, positive for pneumothorax.

(Courtesy of L. Connor Nickels, MD.)

- Normal RUQ/LUQ: Mirroring, loss of spinal landmark (Figure 3-21A).
- Abnormal RUQ/LUQ: Loss of mirroring, continuation of spine and anechoic fluid collection in intrathoracic space (Figure 3-21B).
- Advantages of FAST: Cheap, repeatable, quantifiable, performed at bedside, fast, safe, noninvasive.
- Disadvantages of FAST: Operator dependent, can miss injuries, cannot evaluate the retroperitoneum, inability to determine etiology of blood, difficulty in interpreting in following scenarios at times due to body habitus, subcutaneous air, excessive bowel gas, intraperitoneal hemorrhage versus ascites.

In the past, diagnostic peritoneal lavage was performed in the trauma setting to evaluate for free fluid. Since the advent of FAST, it is rarely used today, so DPL is not discussed further in this book.

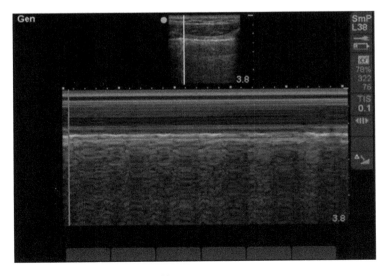

FIGURE 3-20. Seashore sign, normal lung.

(Courtesy of L. Connor Nickels, MD.)

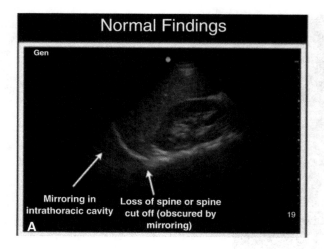

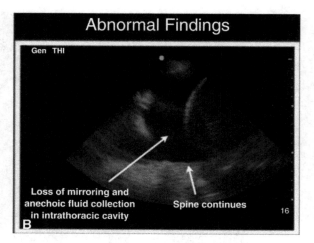

FIGURE 3-21. **A. Loss of spinal landmark, seen in normal RUQ/LUQ view. B. Continuation of spinal landmark, seen in abnormal RUQ/LUQ view.**

(Courtesy of L. Connor Nickels, MD.)

CT SCANNING

- Useful for the hemodynamically stable patient.
- Has a greater specificity than DPL and ultrasonography (US).
- Noninvasive.
- Relatively time consuming when compared with DPL and US.
- Diagnostic for specific organ injury; however, may miss diaphragmatic, colonic, and pancreatic injury.

SERIAL HEMATOCRITS

Serial hematocrits should be obtained during the observation period of the hemodynamically stable patient.

LAPAROTOMY

Indications for exploratory laparotomy:

- Abdominal trauma and hemodynamic instability.
- Bleeding from stomach (not to be confused with nasopharyngeal bleeding).
- Evisceration.
- Peritoneal irritation.
- Suspected/known diaphragmatic injury.
- Free intraperitoneal or retroperitoneal air.
- Intraperitoneal bladder rupture (diagnosed by cystography).
- Surgically correctable injury diagnosed on CT scan.
- Removal of impaled instrument.
- Rectal perforation (diagnosed by sigmoidoscopy).
- Transabdominal missile (bullet) path (eg, a gunshot wound to the buttock with the bullet being found in the abdomen or thorax).

GENERAL

- Often overlooked in the initial evaluation of the multiply injured trauma victim.
- Diagnostic evaluation of the GU tract is performed in a "retrograde" fashion (ie, work your way back from the urethra to the kidneys and renal vasculature).
- Remember to look for blood at the external meatus.

ANATOMY

The GU tract injury is divided into upper (kidney and ureters) and lower tract (bladder, urethra, and genitalia) injury.

SIGNS AND SYMPTOMS

- Flank or groin pain
- Blood at the urethral meatus
- Ecchymoses on perineum and/or genitalia
- Evidence of pelvic fracture
- Rectal bleeding
- A "high-riding" or superiorly displaced prostate

PLACEMENT OF URETHRAL CATHETER

- A Foley or coudé catheter should be placed in any trauma patient with a significant mechanism of injury in the **absence** of any sign of urethral injury.
- Partial urethral tears warrant one careful attempt of a urinary catheter. If any resistance is met or a complete urethral tear is diagnosed, suprapubic catheter placement will be needed to establish urinary drainage.

URINALYSIS

- The presence of gross hematuria indicates GU injury and often concomitant pelvic fracture.
- Urinalysis can be done to document presence or absence of microscopic hematuria, but may result in false-positive results.

RETROGRADE URETHROGRAM

- Should be performed in any patient with suspected urethral disruption (before Foley placement).
- A preinjection KUB (kidneys, ureter, and bladder) film should be taken.
- A 60-cc Toomey syringe (versus a Luer-lok syringe) should be filled with the appropriate contrast solution and placed in the urethral meatus.
- With the patient in the supine position, inject 20–60 cc contrast over 30–60 seconds.
- A repeat KUB is taken during the last 10 cc of contrast injection.
- Retrograde flow of contrast from the meatus to the bladder without extravasation connotes urethral integrity, and Foley may then be placed.
- May be performed in the OR in patients requiring emergency surgery for other injuries.

CT is the most sensitive test for retroperitoneal injury.

Suspect GU trauma with:
- Straddle injury
- Penetrating injury to lower abdomen
- Falls from height

Do not probe perineal lacerations, as they are often a sign of an underlying pelvic fracture, and disruption of a hematoma may occur.

Blood at the urethral meatus is virtually diagnostic for urethral injury and demands early retrograde urethrogram before Foley placement.

HIGH-YIELD FACTS

Trauma

History of enlarged prostate, prostate cancer, urethral stricture, self-catheterization, or previous urologic surgery may make Foley placement difficult or can be confused with urethral disruption.

Bladder Rupture

- **Intraperitoneal:**
  - Usually occurs due to blunt trauma to a full bladder.
  - Treatment is surgical repair.
- **Extraperitoneal:**
  - Usually occurs due to pelvic fracture.
  - Treatment is nonsurgical management by Foley drainage.

RETROGRADE CYSTOGRAM

- Should be performed on patients with gross hematuria or a pelvic fracture.
- Obtain preinjection KUB.
- Fill the bladder with 400 cc of the appropriate contrast material using gravity at a height of 2 feet.
- Obtain another KUB.
- Empty the bladder (unclamp the Foley), then irrigate with saline and take another KUB ("washout" film).
- Extravasation of contrast into the pouch of Douglas, paracolic gutters, or between loops of intestine is diagnostic for intraperitoneal rupture and requires operative repair of the bladder.
- Extravasation of contrast into the paravesicular tissue or behind the bladder as seen on the "washout" film is indicative of extraperitoneal bladder rupture.

Ureteral Injury

- Least common GU injury.
- Must be surgically repaired.
- Diagnosed at the time of intravenous pyelogram (IVP) or CT scan during the search for renal injury.

Renal Contusion

- Most common renal injury.
- Renal capsule remains intact.
- IVP is usually normal and CT scan may show evidence of edema or microextravasation of contrast into the renal parenchyma.
- Often associated with a subcapsular hematoma.
- Management is conservative and requires admission to the hospital.
- Recovery is usually complete unless there is underlying renal pathology.

Renal Laceration

- Classified as either minor (involving only the renal cortex) or major (extending into the renal medulla and/or collecting system).
- Diagnosed by CT scan or IVP.
- Minor renal lacerations are managed expectantly.
- Management of major renal lacerations varies and depends on the surgeon, hemodynamic stability of the patient, and the extent of injury and its coincident complications (ongoing bleeding and urinary extravasation).

Renal Fracture ("Shattered Kidney")

- Involves complete separation of the renal parenchyma from the collecting system.
- Usually → uncontrolled hemorrhage and requires surgical intervention.

SIGNS AND SYMPTOMS

- Tenderness to palpation
- ↓ range of motion
- Deformity or shortening of extremity
- Swelling
- Crepitus
- Laceration or open wound over extremity (open fracture)
- Temperature or pulse difference in one extremity compared to the other
- Loss of sensation in extremity
- Abnormal capillary refill

TREATMENT

- Reduction of fracture or dislocation under sedation.
- Splint extremity.
- Irrigation, antibiotics, and tetanus prophylaxis for open fractures.

COMPLICATIONS

- Compartment syndrome
- Neurovascular compromise
- Fat embolism
- Osteomyelitis
- Rhabdomyolysis (with prolonged crush injuries)
- Avascular necrosis
- Malunion
- Nonunion

Airway

- Smaller airway.
- Relatively large tongue.
- Anterior larynx.
- Narrowest portion is below the vocal cord at the level of the cricoid:

$$\text{ET tube size} = \frac{\text{age} + 16}{4}$$

$$\text{Depth} = \frac{\text{age (years)} + 12}{2}$$

$$\text{Depth} = \text{Internal diameter} \times 3$$

Rhabdomyolysis causes myoglobin release, which can cause renal failure. Maintaining a high urine output together with alkalinization of the urine can help prevent the renal failure by reducing precipitation of myoglobin in the kidney.

Signs of compartment syndrome — The 6 Ps
Pain
Pallor
Paresthesias
Pulse deficit
Poikilothermia
Paralysis

Endotracheal (ET) tube size based on size of cricoid ring rather than glottic opening because narrowest part of the child's airway is beyond the glottic opening.

HIGH-YIELD FACTS

Trauma

	INFANT	CHILD	
Eye opening	Spontaneously	Spontaneously	4
	To speech	To speech	3
	To pain	To pain	2
	No response	No response	1
Best motor response	Spontaneous	Obeys commands	6
	Withdraws from touch	Localizes pain	5
	Withdraws from pain	Same	4
	Decorticate	Same	3
	Decerebrate	Same	2
	No response	Same	1
Best verbal response	Coos, babbles, smiles	Oriented	5
	Crying, irritable	Confused	4
	Cries, screams to pain	Inappropriate words	3
	Moans, grunts	Incomprehensible	2
	No response	No response	1
TOTAL			**15**

FIGURE 3-22. Pediatric Glasgow Coma Scale.

Breathing

- Infants: 40 breaths/min
- Children: 20 breaths/min
- Tidal volume: 7–10 mL/kg

Systolic BP = 80 mm Hg +
2 (age in years)

Circulation

- Child blood volume 80 mL/kg:
  - One-fourth of blood volume must be lost before hypotension occurs.
  - Hypovolemia causes tachycardia long before it causes hypotension.
- Intraosseous cannulation < 6 years.
- Adequate urine output must be maintained:
  - Infant: 2 mL/kg/h
  - Child: 1.5 mL/kg/h
  - Adolescent: 1 mL/kg/h

Neurologic

- Separate Glasgow Coma Scale for infants and children (see Figure 3-22).
- ↑ intracranial pressures may be masked in infants because cranium can expand via open fontanelles.

Neurologic Emergencies

Mental Status

- Orientation: Person (×1), place (×2), time (×3).
- Level of consciousness: Awake, lethargic, comatose.
- Affect: Appropriate, alert, confused.
- Speech: Presence of dysphasia or dysarthria, appropriateness of speech and language content.

Definitions of Expression

- *Dysarthria:* Difficulty in speech secondary to muscle weakness or paralysis.
- *Aphasia:* Disorder in the comprehension or expression of language.
- *Expressive aphasia:* Difficulty in finding words or expression of language without a defect in comprehension.
- *Receptive aphasia:* Problems in understanding words or written language.
- *Fluent aphasia:* Normal rate, meter, quantity of speech, usually abnormal content, poor understanding.
- *Nonfluent aphasia:* Diminished quantity of speech, better understanding, more word-finding difficulties.

- **CN I—olfactory:** Distinguishing two odors (eg, coffee and garlic powder).
- **CN II—optic:** Test visual fields of each eye, visual acuity, fundoscopy, pupillary reactions.
- **CN III—oculomotor:** Check pupillary reactions, ptosis, and extraocular movements.
- **CN IV—trochlear:** Controls Superior Oblique (SO4); predominant movement is down and in. Eye will be elevated and extorted if nerve palsy present.
- **CN V—trigeminal:**
  - Sensation to face (V1, V2, and V3).
  - Check motor function of muscles of mastication (masseter, pterygoids, temporalis).
- **CN VI—abducens:** Controls Lateral Rectus (LR6), abducts the eye.
- **CN VII—facial:**
  - Check motor function of face—ask patients to puff out cheeks (buccinator muscle), smile, close eyes, and raise eyebrows.
  - Check for facial symmetry.
  - **Peripheral versus central CN VII palsy:** In patients with a seventh nerve palsy, ask patient to raise eyebrows and examine forehead for symmetry:
    - Peripheral. lesion: Asymmetrical or absent wrinkles on the side of the lesion.
    - Central lesion: Symmetrical wrinkles due to crossed fibers (innervation from both sides of the cerebral hemispheres).
- **CN VIII—vestibulocochlear:**
  - Check auditory acuity.
  - Look for nystagmus (onset, direction, fatigability).

Fracture of cribriform plate can disrupt odor sensation.

Corneal reflex: Touch side of cornea with cotton wisp. A blink is a normal response indicating normal reflex arc. This reflex requires V1 division of trigeminal nerve (V) for sensory input and motor response from intact facial nerve (VII).

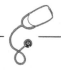

- **CN IX—glossopharyngeal:**
  - Check gag reflex (shared with CN X).
  - Check taste on posterior one-third of tongue.
- **CN X—vagus:** Check for uvula deviation.
- **CN XI—accessory:** Check trapezius and sternocleidomastoid muscles. Ask patient to shrug shoulders, turn head against resistance.
- **CN XII—hypoglossal:** Check for tongue deviation. Deviation indicates ipsilateral lesion.

> If vertical nystagmus is found in a patient, a central lesion within the brain stem or cerebellum must be ruled out.

MOTOR SYSTEM

Posturing

- **Flexor posture:** Abnormal flexion of the arm and wrist, with extension of the leg (lesion above red nucleus).
- **Extensor posture:** Abnormal extension of both the arms and legs (lesion below red nucleus).

Strength

5 = Normal strength
4 = Able to move against resistance
3 = Movement against gravity
2 = Movement with gravity eliminated
1 = Flickers of motion
0 = No movement

Pronator Drift

- Have patient hold arms outstretched, palms upward, with eyes closed.
- Pronation of the hand with downward drift of the arms is considered an abnormal sign, typically an upper motor neuron lesion.
- Normal strength and proprioception is required to prevent arms from drifting.

SENSORY SYSTEM

Symmetry

- Right versus left
- Upper versus lower

Sensation

- Touch—large and small fiber
- Pain—small fiber
- Temperature—small fiber
- Position—large fiber
- Vibratory sensation—large fiber

Level of Reactivity

- Hyperactive reflexes are associated with upper motor neuron lesions.
- Hypoactive reflexes are associated with lower motor neuron lesions or acute spinal injury.

Symmetry

Visualize spinal roots starting from feet up to arms.

Spinal Roots	Reflex
S1–2	Ankle
L3–4	Knee
C5–6	Biceps
C7–8	Triceps

Cerebellar Tests

- Finger to nose.
- Heel to shin.
- Check rapid repetitive motions (dysdiadokinesis).
- Gait.

MENTAL STATUS CHANGES

DEFINITION

Change in mental status is a term used to describe a spectrum of altered mentation including dementia, delirium, psychosis, and coma.

CAUSES

- Infection:
  - Meningitis
  - Neurosyphilis
  - Encephalitis
  - Urosepsis
  - Central nervous system (CNS)
  - Lyme disease
  - Pneumonia
- Metabolic:
  - Uremia
  - B_{12} deficiency
  - Hepatic encephalopathy
  - Electrolyte imbalance
  - Hyper/hypoglycemia
  - Thyroid disease
  - Adrenal disease
- Neurological:
  - Stroke
  - CNS space-occupying lesions (neoplasm)
  - Seizures/postictal state

- CNS trauma
- Hydrocephalus
  - Vascular:
    - Hypertensive encephalopathy
    - Vasculitis
    - Cardiopulmonary:
    - Hypoxic encephalopathy
    - Congestive heart failure (CHF)
    - Chronic obstructive pulmonary disease
    - Pulmonary embolism
  - Toxic:
    - Drug overdose
    - Alcohol withdrawal
    - Respiratory:
    - CO_2 retention
    - Inflammatory/autoimmune:
    - Paraneoplastic syndrome, neurosarcoidosis, lupus, Hashimoto's encephalopathy
  - Environmental:
    - Carbon monoxide exposure
    - Hypo/hyperthermia

Delirium

DEFINITION

- Impairment of brain function secondary to another disease state.
- Delirium is usually transient in nature, reversing with removal or treatment of underlying cause.
- Patients with structural brain damage as cause of delirium may progress to chronic dementia.

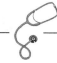

Treatment of delirium —
CAST
Cocktail
Admission
Sedation
Tomography (CT)

CLINICAL PRESENTATION

- Patients usually have difficulty in focusing or sustaining attention.
- Clinical course is usually fluctuating, waxing and waning.
- Onset is usually rapid, from days to weeks.
- Symptoms usually worsen at night.
- Some patients may experience hallucinations, usually visual in nature.
- Patients usually have clinical signs and symptoms suggestive of underlying cause.

DIAGNOSIS

Head computed tomography (CT) and labs to identify underlying cause. Toxic metabolic work up which may include CBC, chemistries, LFTs, CXR, EKG, UA, tox screen, head CT and possibly even lumbar puncture.

TREATMENT

- Coma cocktail: Thiamine, glucose, naloxone, oxygen.
- Sedation as needed for patient comfort. Sedation with haldol or ativan to control agitation, but may worsen delirium.
- Treat underlying cause.

Dementia

DEFINITION

- A chronic, progressive decline in mental capacity that interferes with a patient's normal psychosocial activity.
- The identification of *reversible dementia* is key because progression can be halted.

NONREVERSIBLE CAUSES

- Degenerative:
  - Alzheimer's disease
  - Parkinson's disease
- Vascular:
  - Multiple infarcts
  - Subarachnoid hemorrhage (SAH)
  - Anoxic brain damage

CLINICAL PRESENTATION

- Impairment is gradual and progressive.
- Attention is usually normal, without waxing or waning of consciousness.
- Distant memory is usually preserved.

DIAGNOSIS

Identify *reversible* causes of dementia.

TREATMENT

- Address *reversible* causes of dementia.
- Supportive environmental, psychosocial interventions.

Reversible causes of dementia—
DEMENTIA
Drugs
Electrolyte disturbances, Eye and ear problems
Metabolic abnormalities (uremia, thyroid)
Emotional problems (psych)
Neoplasm, nutritional (vitamin deficiency)
Trauma
Infection, inflammation (lupus)
Alcohol

Differentiating Delirium, Dementia, and Psychosis

See Table 4-1.

Coma

DEFINITION

Diffuse brain failure → impaired consciousness.

MANAGEMENT

- **ABCs:**
  - Airway—intubate if necessary to protect airway.
  - Breathing—oxygen, oral airway.
  - Circulation—intravenous (IV) access, blood pressure.
- **C-spine:** Cervical collar unless absolutely sure no history of trauma.
- **Vitals:** Temperature, oxygen saturation (fifth vital sign), frequent reassessment.
- **Electrocardiogram (ECG)/cardiac monitor:** Arrhythmias, myocardial infarction (MI).

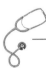

Causes of coma:
AEIOU TIPS
Alcohol
Encephalopathy, endocrine (thyroid disease, etc), electrolyte abnormality
Insulin-dependent diabetes
Opiates, oxygen deprivation
Uremia
Trauma, temperature
Infection
Psychosis, porphyria
Space-occupying lesion, stroke, SAH, shock

TABLE 4-1. Differentiating Delirium, Dementia, and Psychosis

MANIFESTATIONS	DELIRIUM	DEMENTIA	PSYCHOSIS
Onset	Sudden	Insidious	Sudden
Duration	Days to weeks	Permanent	Years (history)
Arousal level	Fluctuating	Normal	Normal
Orientation	Altered	Altered	Normal
Attention	Poorly maintained	Maintained	Varies
Memory	Usually not intact	Distant memory intact	Varies
Hallucinations	Usually visual	Usually absent	Usually auditory
Delusions	Transient	Absent	Sustained
Thought process	Poorly organized	Varies with degree	Varies
Vital signs	Fluctuating	Normal	Variable

HISTORY

- From patient, family member, bystander, or old chart
- Past medical history
- Past psychiatric history
- Medications
- Social history (drug or alcohol use)

PHYSICAL EXAM

- General exam:
  - Check for signs of trauma.
  - Glasgow Coma Scale.
- Respiratory pattern: Cheyne-Stokes: Periodic fluctuations of respiratory rate and depth suggest CNS pathology.
- Ocular exam:
  - Pupillary function: If pupils are **reactive** to light bilaterally, midbrain is probably intact:
    - **Pinpoint pupils** suggest opioid toxicity or pontine dysfunction.
    - **Fixed and dilated pupils** suggest ↑ intracranial pressure (ICP) with possible herniation.
    - **Doll's eyes reflex:** Turn patient's head quickly to one side and observe eye movement. In a normal response, the eyes move in the opposite direction. Absence of motion suggests dysfunction in hemisphere or brain stem function. (Note that this reflex is also absent in a conscious patient.)

- Oculo-vestibular testing: Information about the integrity of brain stem and brain itself. Patient in supine position. Raise head to about 30 degrees, and inject 20 cc cold saline in eternal auditory canal. Interpretation:
  - Both eyes deviate with nystagmus: Slow on side of cold saline, fast on opposite; patient is not comatose.
  - Both eyes deviate toward cold saline: Coma with intact brain stem.
  - No movement in either eye or lack of movement in contralateral eye: Brain stem damaged.
- Neurological exam: Refer to section on neurological examination.

Do not perform doll's eye maneuver in the presence of head or neck trauma.

DIAGNOSIS

- Glucose
- Arterial blood gas: Acid-base disorders can help point to etiology (remember MUDPILES).
- Routine labs: Look for infection or electrolyte abnormalities.
- Urinalysis: Infection, hyperglycemia, ketosis, dehydration, toxicology.
- Toxicology screen: Look for drugs and alcohol.
- Electrocardiogram (ECG).
- X-rays: C-spine in suspected cases of trauma.
- Head CT: Look for intracranial pathology.
- Lumbar puncture (LP): Look for SAH or infection. Remember, CT before LP for mass lesion/cerebral edema/hydrocephalus.

TREATMENT

- Coma cocktail.
- Supportive care.
- Monitoring (cardiac, oxygen saturation).
- Identify specific cause and apply appropriate treatment.
- Appropriate specialty consult as deemed necessary.

Coma cocktail—
DON'T
Dextrose (1 amp)
Oxygen
Naloxone
(To remind you to give thiamine before dextrose)
Thiamine

STROKE

DEFINITIONS

- **Stroke:** Any vascular injury that reduces cerebral blood flow (CBF) to a specific region of the brain, causing neurologic impairment.
- **Ischemic stroke:** Occlusion of cerebral vessels → infarction secondary to lack of perfusion.
- **Hemorrhagic stroke:** Neurologic impairment due to rupture of a blood vessel into the parenchyma of the brain (intracerebral hemorrhage [ICH]) or into the subarachnoid space (subarachnoid hemorrhage [SAH]).
- **Transient ischemic attack (TIA):** A transient episode of neurological dysfunction caused by focal brain, spinal cord, or retinal ischemia, without acute infarction.

ANATOMY

- Anterior circulation:
  - Originates from the carotid system, then → to anterior and middle cerebral artery.

- Supplies blood to the eye, the frontal and parietal lobes, and majority of the temporal area.
  - Posterior circulation:
    - Originates from the vertebral arteries, then forms the basilar artery, cerebellar arteries, then the posterior cerebral artery (PCA).
    - Supplies the brain stem, ears, cerebellum, occipital cortex, and parts of the temporal lobe.

GENERAL CLASSIFICATION

Ischemic Stroke (Figures 4-1 and 4-2)
- 80% of all strokes:
  - Thrombotic stroke
  - Embolic stroke
  - Lacunar stroke
- Systemic hypoperfusion (results in "watershed" infarcts, boundary zones between middle anterior and posterior cerebral arteries; usually bilateral and symmetric)
- 5–10% in-hospital mortality

Hemorrhagic Stroke (Figure 4-3)
- 20% of all strokes
- Intracerebral hemorrhage
- SAH (see section on headaches)
- 45–50% in-hospital mortality

RISK FACTORS

Thrombotic Stroke
- Atherosclerosis (most common cause)
- Hypertension (HTN)
- Hyperlipidemia
- Vasculitis

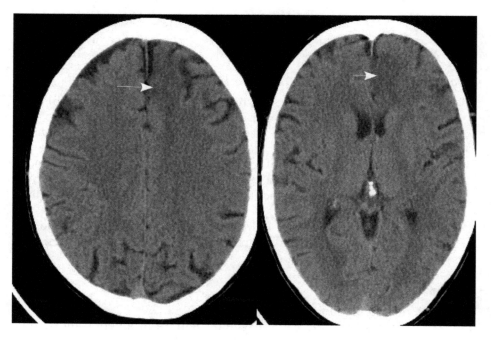

FIGURE 4-1. CT of ischemic stroke in the anterior cerebral artery (ACA) distribution (arrows).

(Photo courtesy of Latha Ganti Stead, MD.)

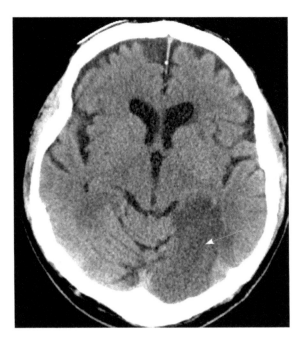

FIGURE 4-2. CT of ischemic stroke in the posterior cerebral artery (PCA) distribution (arrows).

(Photo courtesy of Latha Ganti Stead, MD.)

- Often preceded by TIA
- Pathophysiology: Vessel narrowing and occlusion secondary to plaque formation

Embolic Stroke
- Atrial fibrillation.
- Dilated cardiomyopathy.

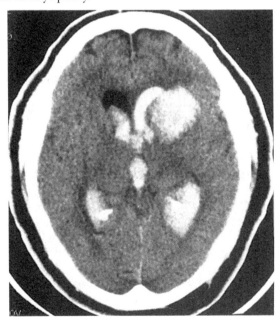

FIGURE 4-3. Hemorrhagic stroke due to hypertension.

Note that the lesion is hyperdense. Note bleeding into the ventricles. Effacement of sulci suggests edema. Mild mass effect is also present. (Reproduced, wth permission, from Lee SH, Zimmerman RA, Rao KC. *Cranial MRI and CT*, 4th ed. New York: McGraw-Hill, 1999.)

- Recent MI.
- Endocarditis.
- IV drug abuse.
- Smoking.
- Hyperlipidemia.
- Pathophysiology: Occlusion from intravascular material (clot, air bubble, fat, etc) from distal sites.
- Sources of emboli:
  - Most common sources of emboli are from heart or ruptured plaque from major vessels.
  - Dislodged vegetation from cardiac valves (fibrin clots, septic vegetations, etc).
  - Dislodged mural thrombi from atrial fibrillation, dilated cardiomyopathy, or recent MI.

Lacunar Stroke
- Chronic HTN
- Diabetes

ICH
- Age
- History of prior stroke
- Smoking
- HTN
- Anticoagulation (eg, warfarin therapy)
- Cerebral amyloidosis
- Cocaine use
- Pathophysiology: Vessel rupture with bleeding into brain parenchyma, causing ↑ ICP

SAH
- Ruptured berry aneurysms
- Arteriovenous malformations
- Pathophysiology:
  - Vessel rupture with blood leaking into subarachnoid space
  - Usually occurs at bifurcation of vessels

*Vertebrobasilar strokes present with **3 D's:** **D**izziness (vertigo) **D**iplopia **D**ysphasia*

PHYSICAL EXAM

- Vitals: Cushing reflex—HTN, bradycardia, and abnormal breathing could represent an ↑ in ICP.
- Eyes:
  - Do funduscopic exam.
  - Papilledema is a sign of ↑ ICP.
  - Subhyaloid hemorrhage is pathognomonic for SAH.
  - Note pupillary function and extraocular movements.
- Neurological exam:
  - Will help with localizing lesion and determining whether current presentation is consistent with imaging findings.
  - The National Institutes of Health Stroke Scale (NIHSS) is a standardized physical exam commonly used for stroke assessment that helps practitioners track changes over time. The scale (Figure 4-4) ranges from 0 (no deficit) to 42 (maximum score). Most stroke interventions are applied to patients with NIHSS scores between 4 and 20.

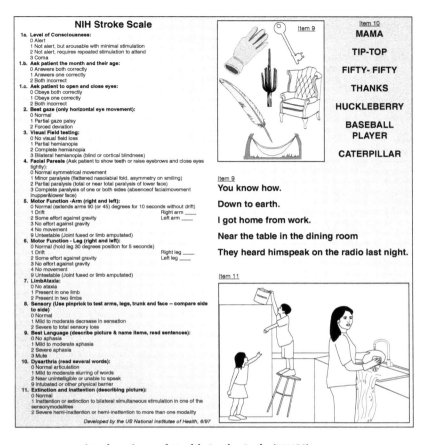

NIH Stroke Scale

1a. Level of Consciousness:
0 Alert
1 Not alert, but arousable with minimal stimulation
2 Not alert, requires repeated stimulation to attend
3 Coma

1.b. Ask patient the month and their age:
0 Answers both correctly
1 Answers one correctly
2 Both incorrect

1.c. Ask patient to open and close eyes:
0 Obeys both correctly
1 Obeys one correctly
2 Both incorrect

2. Best gaze (only horizontal eye movement):
0 Normal
1 Partial gaze palsy
2 Forced deviation

3. Visual Field testing:
0 No visual field loss
1 Partial hemianopia
2 Complete hemianopia
3 Bilateral hemianopia (blind or cortical blindness)

4. Facial Paresis (Ask patient to show teeth or raise eyebrows and close eyes tightly):
0 Normal symmetrical movement
1 Minor paralysis (flattened nasolabial fold, asymmetry on smiling)
2 Partial paralysis (total or near total paralysis of lower face)
3 Complete paralysis of one or both sides (absence of facial movement in upper & lower face)

5. Motor Function - Arm (right and left):
0 Normal (extends arms 90 (or 45) degrees for 10 seconds without drift)
1 Drift   Right arm ____
2 Some effort against gravity   Left arm ____
3 No effort against gravity
4 No movement
9 Untestable (Joint fused or limb amputated)

6. Motor Function - Leg (right and left):
0 Normal (hold leg 30 degrees position for 5 seconds)
1 Drift   Right leg ____
2 Some effort against gravity   Left leg ____
3 No effort against gravity
4 No movement
9 Untestable (Joint fused or limb amputated)

7. LimbAtaxia:
0 No ataxia
1 Present in one limb
2 Present in two limbs

8. Sensory (Use pinprick to test arms, legs, trunk and face -- compare side to side)
0 Normal
1 Mild to moderate decrease in sensation
2 Severe to total sensory loss

9. Best Language (describe picture & name items, read sentences):
0 No aphasia
1 Mild to moderate aphasia
2 Severe aphasia
3 Mute

10. Dysarthria (read several words):
0 Normal articulation
1 Mild to moderate slurring of words
2 Near unintelligible or unable to speak
9 Intubated or other physical barrier

11. Extinction and inattention (describing picture):
0 Normal
1 Inattention or extinction to bilateral simultaneous stimulation in one of the sensory modalities
2 Severe hemi-inattention or hemi-inattention to more than one modality

Developed by the US National Institutes of Health, 6/97

Item 9

Item 10
MAMA
TIP-TOP
FIFTY- FIFTY
THANKS
HUCKLEBERRY
BASEBALL PLAYER
CATERPILLAR

Item 9
You know how.
Down to earth.
I got home from work.
Near the table in the dining room
They heard him speak on the radio last night.

Item 11

FIGURE 4-4. National Institute of Health Stroke Scale (NIHSS).

LOCALIZATION

- Middle cerebral artery:
  - Most common
  - Contralateral weakness and numbness of arms greater than legs
  - Aphasia
  - Homonymous hemianopsia: Loss of vision on right or left side of both eyes
- Anterior cerebral artery:
  - Contralateral weakness of legs greater than arms.
  - Anarthria with paraplegia is a sign of bilateral parasaggital infarction.
- Posterior cerebral artery:
  - Vision changes (diplopia).
  - Sensory changes—fine touch and pin prick.
  - Usually have subtle presentations, often billed as "dizziness."
  - Small penetrating arteries: Lacunar strokes present as "DAMS."
- Vertebrobasilar artery:
  - Syncope
  - Weakness
  - Cranial nerve changes
  - **Crossed findings** (ipsilateral cranial nerve changes with contralateral motor weakness)
  - Ataxia

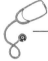

Signs of lacunar stroke:
DAMS
Dysarthria — clumsy hand: Slurred speech with weak, clumsy hands
Ataxic hemiparesis: Ataxia with leg weakness
Pure **M**otor hemiplegia: Motor hemiplegia without sensory changes
Pure **S**ensory stroke: Sensory deficits of face, arms, legs without motor deficits

Cincinnati Pre-Hospital Stroke Scale — for quick identification of stroke:
1. Facial droop
2. Slurred speech
3. Arm drift/Pronator drift

Any one of these positive is indicative of stroke

HIGH-YIELD FACTS

Neurologic Emergencies

Identification of strokes involving the cerebellum is important due to risk of edema and ↑ pressure to brain stem.

- Cerebellar arteries:
  - Central vertigo
  - Headache
  - Nausea and vomiting
  - Loss of posture (inability to sit or stand without support)

DIAGNOSIS

- Stroke labs: Complete blood count (CBC), electrolytes, cardiac biomarkers.
- Coags, UA, CXR.
- ECG for atrial fibrillation.
- CT of the head:
  - Helps differentiate ischemic from hemorrhagic cerebrovascular accident (CVA).
  - CT can be negative in ischemic strokes for 12 hours and may remain equivocal for small strokes.
  - Posterior fossa (brain stem and cerebellum) not as well visualized on CT.
  - Detects ≥ 1-cm ICH (acute bleed looks white on CT scan).
  - Detects SAH 95% of time.
- CT angiography: This modality is gaining some traction in acute stroke imaging. It has the advantage of being fast, not taking the patient out of the department, and the ability to provide information on the carotid vessels. Most importantly, it can differentiate core from penumbra, which is imperative for endovascular intervention. The disadvantage is that is does require intravenous contrast.
- Magnetic resonance imaging (MRI):
  - Can detect subtle ischemic infarcts, particularly diffusion-weighted sequences.
  - Good study for brain stem or cerebellar lesions.
  - Availability of MRI, patient claustrophobia, and taking the patient out of the ED are all limiting factors in the acute setting.

EMERGENCY DEPARTMENT MANAGEMENT OF ISCHEMIC STROKE

1. Determine time of onset of symptoms.
2. STAT brain imaging.
3. ABCs: Give supplemental O_2.
4. Serum glucose control:
   - Hyperglycemia provides more substrate for anaerobic metabolism, worsening acidosis.
   - It is recommended to keep serum glucose < 150 mg/dL.
   - Use sliding scale regular insulin for glucose > 300 mg/dL.
5. Temperature control:
   - Hyperthermia ↑ oxygen demand when the ischemic brain is already hypoxic.
   - Administer acetaminophen for fever.
6. Order stroke labs, CXR, ECG.
7. Call stroke team/neurology consult as appropriate and available.
8. Do stroke physical exam (eg, NIHSS).
9. Blood pressure (BP) control:
   - Since autoregulation is lost in ischemic brain, perfusion is directly dependent on the cerebral perfusion pressure (CPP), which in turn is dependent on the mean arterial pressure (MAP).
     - CPP = MAP – ICP.
     - MAP = ⅓ SBP + ⅔ DBP.
     - Ideally want MAP ≥ 90.

- Use pressors for MAP < 60 or SBP < 90.
- Do not treat MAP < 130.
- Do not treat acutely elevated blood pressure, unless concurrent MI, aortic dissection, ICH, CHF, acute renal failure, hypertensive encephalopathy, or patient receiving tissue plasminogen activator (tPA).

10. Thrombolytic therapy (recombinant tissue plasminogen activator [rtPA]):
    - Only approved specific therapy (Class I within 3 hours of symptom onset). In May 2009, the American Heart Association/American Stroke Association (AHA/ASA) guidelines for the administration of rtPA following acute stroke were revised to expand the window of treatment from 3 to 4.5 hours.
    - Very specific inclusion criteria: Need a clinical diagnosis of stroke with NIHSS score < 22. Stroke needs to be moderate; massive strokes and very mild strokes are not eligible.
    - Contraindications include SBP > 180, history of hemorrhagic stroke, any stroke within past year, suspected aortic dissection, active bleeding.
    - Recently, the European Cooperative Acute Stroke Study 3 (ECASS 3J) study has extended the time window for rtPA administration between 3 and 4.5 hours after acute stroke with the following extra exclusions:
        - Age > 80 years
        - Patients on anticoagulants, irrespective of International Normalized Ratio (INR)
        - NIHSS > 25
        - Patients with a history of stroke and diabetes.
    - Intra-arterial tPA administration: Can be given up to 6 hours post-stroke onset (Class II recommendation)
    - Many new intra-arterial clot extraction, maceration, or lytic drug delivery devices are under investigation.
11. Most patients with acute stroke are hospitalized for further workup.
12. Patients with larger or more severe strokes may be candidates for endovascular neurosurgical intervention, including mechanical embolectomy.

EMERGENCY DEPARTMENT MANAGEMENT OF TIA

Same as for ischemic stroke as detailed above, *plus:*
1. Imaging of the carotids (ultrasonography, CTA, or MRA).
2. Education regarding subsequent risk of stroke, stroke risk factors.
3. Evaluation for further workup within 48 hours including MRI, echocardiogram, and special blood (eg, lupus anticoagulant, factor V Leiden deficiency) tests as appropriate.
4. Sometimes a historical score such as the ABCD2 (**A**ge, **B**lood pressure, **C**linical features, symptom **D**uration, **D**iabetes) can help to risk-stratify patients when acute evaluation or transfer is not available. It has little utility when the patient can be adequately evaluated in the ED.
5. Patients who have a negative CT, clean carotids, normal ECG, normal labs, and are completely back to baseline can be discharged home with an aspirin and follow up within 48–72 hours.

EMERGENCY DEPARTMENT MANAGEMENT OF HEMORRHAGIC STROKE

1. ABCs: Consider early intubation.
2. BP control:
    - Treat systolic BP (sBP) > 160 mm Hg and diastolic BP (dBP) > 105 mm Hg.
    - Agents of choice: Nitroprusside, labetalol, nicardipine.

Optimization for ischemic stroke:
- Supplemental O_2
- BP: MAP ≥ 60, SBP ≥ 90
- Serum glucose: < 150
- Normal temperature
- Screen for thrombolytics
- For HTN, do not treat until MAP > 130.

The possibility of carotid or vertebral dissection should be considered in young patients with stroke and in patients with headaches and neck pain with acute stroke.

3. Control seizures with lorazepam acutely, followed by fosphenytoin. Consider seizure prophylaxis, especially in patients with lobar hemorrhage; use fosphenytoin 18 mg/kg.
4. Reversal of anticoagulation with protamine sulfate (to reverse heparin) and vitamin K with clotting factor replacement (to reverse warfarin).
5. Control elevated ICP with graded measures: Starting at elevation of head, analgesia, sedation, going to more aggressive measures like osmotic diuresis with mannitol, extraventricular cerebrospinal fluid (CSF) drainage, neuromuscular blockade, and hyperventilation. Goal is to maintain a CPP > 70 mm Hg.
6. Nimodipine (Ca^{2+} channel blocker) to ↓ vasospasm in SAH.
7. Serum glucose to be lowered at least below 300 mg/dL if elevated.
8. Prompt neurosurgical evaluation.

PREVENTION

- Antiplatelet therapy for ischemic strokes
- Anticoagulation with warfarin for embolic strokes
- Smoking cessation
- Strict HTN control
- Control of hyperlipidemia
- Control of diabetes

HEADACHE

Primary Headache Syndromes

- Migraine
- Tension headache
- Cluster headache

Secondary Causes

- CNS infection:
  - Meningitis
  - Encephalitis
  - Cerebral abscess/tumor
- Non-CNS infection:
  - Sinusitis (overrated)
  - Fever
  - Herpes zoster
  - Ear infections
  - Dental infections
- Vascular:
  - SAH
  - Subdural hematoma
  - Epidural hematoma
  - Intracerebral hemorrhage
  - Temporal arteritis
  - Carotid or vertebral artery dissection
  - Ophthalmologic:
  - Glaucoma
  - Iritis
  - Optic neuritis

- Toxic/metabolic:
  - Carbon monoxide (CO) poisoning
  - Nitrates and nitrides
  - Hypoglycemia
  - Hypoxia
  - Hypercapnia
  - Caffeine withdrawal
  - Withdrawal from chronic analgesics (rebound headache)
  - Malignant HTN
  - Preeclampsia
  - Pseudotumor cerebri
  - Post-LP/CSF leak
  - HTN

DIAGNOSTIC APPROACH

- Differentiate between primary headache syndromes and secondary causes of headache.
- Recognize critical life-threatening causes of headache.
- Treat primary causes of headache.

HISTORY

- Pattern:
  - First episode or chronic in nature.
  - In chronic headache, assess duration, severity, or associated symptoms.
  - Onset: Gradual versus sudden or severe.
- Location:
  - Migraines typically unilateral.
  - Tension headache usually bilateral.
  - SAH headache usually occipital.
- Associated symptoms:
  - Syncope
  - Changes in mental status
  - Fever
  - Vision changes
  - Seizures
  - Neck pain and stiffness
  - History of head trauma
- Past medical history:
  - HTN
  - CVA
  - Migraines
  - Human immunodeficiency virus (HIV)
- Medications:
  - Nitrates
  - Analgesics
  - Anticonvulsants
- Family history:
  - Migraines
  - SAH
- Age: Look for secondary causes in elderly.

Consider CO poisoning if similar symptoms of headache, nausea, vomiting in other members of household (more common in winter/cold climates due to space heaters).

Remember, LP is required in patients suspected of SAH with negative CT of head.

PHYSICAL EXAM

- Vitals: Fever, BP, Cushing reflex (systemic response to ↑ ICP, HTN, tachycardia, bradypnea).
- Eyes: Funduscopic exam may reveal absence of venous pulsations or papilledema, suggesting ↑ ICP.
- Neurological exam: Refer to section on neurological exam.

LABS/RADIOLOGY

- Routine labs:
  - Check glucose.
  - Erythrocyte sedimentation rate (ESR): Positive if > 50 mm/h.
- CT scan of the brain helps to identify:
  - Mass lesions
  - Midline shift of intracranial contents
  - CNS bleeds
  - ↑ ICP (↑ size of ventricles, cerebral edema)
- Contrast is useful for:
  - Cerebral toxoplasmosis
  - Small brain mass
  - Intracranial abscess
- LP indications (do not perform LP until CT is negative for mass lesion or obstructive hydrocephalus):
  - Meningitis
  - Encephalitis
  - SAH

Migraine Headache

EPIDEMIOLOGY

- Onset in adolescence.
- ↑ frequency in females.
- Migraine headaches are more common in women and are influenced by hormonal factors.
- Preeclampsia can present as migraine headache in pregnant women.

PATHOPHYSIOLOGY

Not completely understood; involves:

- Trigeminal innervation of meningeal vasculature.
- Sterile inflammatory changes in meningeal vessel walls.
- In aura, posterior to anterior spreading depression of brain metabolism.

SIGNS AND SYMPTOMS

- Frequently associated with aura (should not last > 1 hour). Aura can be any neurologic symptom; paresthesias are common.
- May have visual auras (scintillating scotoma, or flashing lights).
- Slow onset.
- Last 4–72 hours.
- Worsen with exertion.
- Unilateral and pulsating.
- Nausea, vomiting, photophobia, phonophobia, osmophobia.
- Neurological deficits (history of similar deficits in prior episodes). Focal deficits contraindicate treatment with triptans or dihydroergotamine (DHE).

- Tricyclics (amitriptyline, nortriptyline)
- Gabapentin
- Valproic acid
- Topiramate
- Beta blockers (propranolol)
- Calcium channel blockers

TREATMENT

- Whatever worked in the past
- Metoclopramide
- Compazine
- DHE (not with focal deficit)
- Nonsteroidal anti-inflammatory drugs (NSAIDs) such as ketorolac
- Opioid analgesia (beware of creating iatrogenic narcotic dependence)
- Triptans (not with focal deficit)

Cluster Headache

EPIDEMIOLOGY

- More common in men
- Onset usually > 20 years old

PATHOPHYSIOLOGY

Mechanism unknown.

SIGNS AND SYMPTOMS

- Short lived.
- Severe, unilateral, lasting up to 3 hours.
- Appear in clusters, multiple attacks in same time of day or month.
- Patients appear restless.
- Associated with ipsilateral conjunctival injection, lacrimation, nasal congestion, rhinorrhea, miosis, and ptosis.
- Precipitated/exacerbated by EtOH.

PROPHYLAXIS

- Verapamil
- Lithium
- Topiramate
- Valproic acid
- Gabapentin

TREATMENT

- 100% oxygen
- NSAIDs
- Steroids
- EtOH cessation

Hunt and Hess classification for SAH

Grade I: Asymptomatic, mild headache, mild nuchal rigidity.

Grade II: Moderate to severe headache, nuchal rigidity, cranial nerve palsy may be present.

Grade III: Drowsiness, confusion, or mild focal neurologic deficit.

Grade IV: Stupor, hemiparesis, early decerebration or vegetative state

Grade V: Coma, decerebrate, moribund.

Tension Headache

PATHOPHYSIOLOGY

Muscle tension has been theorized as the causative factor.

SIGNS AND SYMPTOMS

- Bilateral
- Nonpulsating
- Not worsened with exertion
- Usually no nausea or vomiting
- Associated neck or back pain

PROPHYLAXIS

- Tricyclics
- Gabapentin
- Good posture, exercise

TREATMENT

- Exercise, massage
- NSAIDs
- Muscle relaxant

Subarachnoid Hemorrhage (SAH)

EPIDEMIOLOGY

- 1–2/10,000 incidence
- Slight male preponderance

CAUSES

- Trauma is the most common etiology.
- Spontaneous SAHs are usually secondary to ruptured aneurysms (80%) or arteriovenous malformations (AVMs—5%).
- AVM.
- Idiopathic.

SIGNS AND SYMPTOMS

- Severe headache with a "thunderclap" onset.
- Classically: "This is the worst headache of my life!" but there is significant variability in the description.
- Nausea, vomiting, meningismus, photophobia, possible syncope.
- Focal and diffuse neurologic deficits common (CN III palsy, ↓ level of consciousness, coma).

DIAGNOSIS

Head CT without contrast: > 95% sensitivity for acute hemorrhage (see Figure 4-5).

- Blood in perimesencephalic cisterns ("star" or "crab"), along the falx, or in the Sylvian fissure.
- If head CT is equivocal but there is clinical suspicion of SAH, perform an LP to look for RBCs in tubes 1 and 4 and xanthochromia. Xanthochromia requires at least 6 hours to develop; may be negative before that time.
- ECG may demonstrate deep inverted T waves (Figure 4-6).

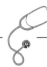

> Sudden, severe headache described as "worst headache of my life" should be considered SAH until proven otherwise (do CT + LP).

TREATMENT

- To prevent vasospasm: Nimodipine 60 mg PO q 4 hours × 21 days, start within 96 hours of SAH.
- For cerebral edema: Dexamethasone 10 mg IV × 1.
- Prevent hypo- or hypertension.
- To prevent seizures: Phenytoin 15–18 mg/kg loading dose. Recommended prophylactically.
- Elevate head of the bed to 30 degrees if C-spine is not a concern.
- Admit patients to ICU for observation.
- Unless traumatic, evaluate for AVM or aneurysm with angiogram.

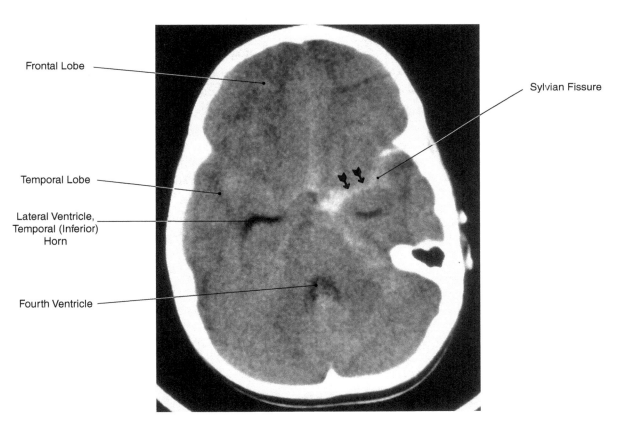

Frontal Lobe

Sylvian Fissure

Temporal Lobe

Lateral Ventricle, Temporal (Inferior) Horn

Fourth Ventricle

FIGURE 4-5. SAH.

Arrows indicate fresh blood in the Sylvian fissure. (Reproduced, with permission, from Afifi AK, Bergman RA. *Functional Neuroanatomy: Text and Atlas.* New York: McGraw-Hill, 1998: 554.)

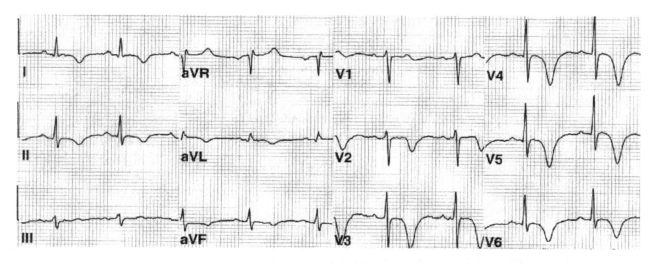

FIGURE 4-6. ECG demonstrating inverted T waves in intracerebral hemorrhage.

Temporal Arteritis

> A 57-year-old woman presents with severe headache of 3 days duration. Headache encompasses the entire back of the head including the temples. She also reports fatigue, malaise, a "tired tongue," subjective low grade fever, and anorexia. Review of systems is negative for arthralgia, vision loss, rash, motor or sensory deficits, neck stiffness, nausea, vomiting, diarrhea, chest pain, abdominal pain, and head or neck trauma. The patient's daily medications include atenolol, aspirin, an HMG-CoA inhibitor, and ibuprofen. She does not smoke, drink, or take illicit drugs. Physical demonstrates tender temporal arteries with nodules that are nonpulsatile. What diagnosis are you worried about?
>
> Temporal arteritis. This patient should be treated with prednisone until diagnosis can be confirmed with temporal artery biopsy. Delaying or not treating can lead to vision loss.

EPIDEMIOLOGY

- More common in women and persons over age > 60 years.
- About 50% of patients with temporal arteritis also have polymyalgia rheumatica.

PATHOPHYSIOLOGY

Systemic panarteritis affecting temporal artery.

SIGNS AND SYMPTOMS

- Headache (4–100%)
- Scalp or TA tenderness (28–91%)
- Weight loss (16–76%)
- Jaw or tongue claudication (4–67%)
- Anorexia (14–69%)
- Proximal muscle weakness (28–86%)

- Fever (not all HA + fever = meningitis!)
- Fatigue, malaise (12–97%)
- Leg claudication (2–43%)

DIAGNOSIS

- ESR > 50 mm/h.
- Temporal artery biopsy showing giant cells is definitive—do not await biopsy results before initiating treatment.

TREATMENT

Prednisone. If left untreated, can → vision loss.

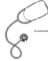

- New headache
- Temporal artery abnormality
- Jaw claudication
→ 94.8% specificity and 100% sensitivity for temporal arteritis

Subdural Hematoma

- History of head trauma (see Trauma chapter).
- Disruption of bridging vessels intracranially.
- High-risk patients include alcoholics, elderly, and patients on anticoagulants.
- Can present like TIA.

Cerebral Ischemia/Infarct

Rarely produces headaches.

Intracerebral Hemorrhage

- Commonly produces headache.
- Neurologic exam usually abnormal.
- Refer to section on stroke for more detail.

Brain Tumor

- Commonly presents with insidious headache.
- Headache positional and worse in morning.
- Neurologic abnormalities usually present on physical exam.

Pseudotumor Cerebri (Idiopathic Intracranial Hypertension)

EPIDEMIOLOGY

- Occurs in young, obese females.
- History of headaches in past.

ETIOLOGY

Unknown; should exclude venous sinus thrombosis, antibiotics, vitamin A intoxication, endocrine dysfunction, chronic meningitis.

SIGNS AND SYMPTOMS

- Papilledema
- Absent venous pulsations on funduscopic exam
- Headache, nausea, vomiting
- Visual loss

DIAGNOSIS

- Usually normal CT of head.
- LP reveals elevated CSF opening pressures.
- Response of headache and visual symptoms to large-volume LP.
- Visual field testing.

TREATMENT

- Acetazolamide +/– other diuretic
- LP to remove CSF
- Optic nerve fenestration
- CSF shunt in refractory cases

Cervical Artery Dissection

A 37-year-old woman tax attorney presents with a 3-day history of severe left-sided occipital headache and neck stiffness. She has been putting in 18-hour days at work, with no time to go to the gym in the past few weeks. She has tried some desk exercises, and reports she "threw out" her neck. Now she complains of dizziness and numbness of her left face and side. She has no PMH, and the only medication she takes is an oral contraceptive. She does not drink, smoke, or take illicit drugs. Physical examination demonstrates a well-appearing female in no acute distress, but who sounds hoarse. The head is atraumatic, and there are no signs of meningismus. Pupils are equal and reactive to light and accommodation. There is horizontal nystagmus present. She also has ↓ sensation to pinprick of left face, arms, and legs. Are you worried about her headache?

Yes! This patient has signs and symptoms consistent with internal carotid artery dissection. She should have brain and neck imaging to rule this out.

EPIDEMIOLOGY

Two main sites: Internal carotid artery dissection (ICAD) and vertebral artery dissections (VAD). See Table 4-2.

- Together, account for one-fifth of strokes in persons < 45 years.
- Less frequent (~2.5%) in elderly population.
- Risk of recurrence is 1%, usually in a different vessel.
- ICAD 3.5 times more common than VAD.
- ICAD 1.5 times more common in men; VAD 3 times more common in women.
- Incidence estimated at 2.6/100,000.
- History of trauma elicited 40% of the time.
- Headache and pain are part of chief complaint 65% of the time.

ETIOLOGY

- History of antecedent neck trauma (including chiropractic manipulation, sudden head turning, minor neck trauma from MVC and weight lifting) may be elicited ~40% of time.
- Another 15–20% have underlying disease such as fibromuscular dysplasia, cystic medial necrosis, or Marfan syndrome.

- Pain is part of the chief complaint 60–85% of the time.
- Signs of cerebral ischemia can be delayed hours to days after initial headache, which likely signals initial intimal tear.

DIAGNOSIS

CT angiography.

TREATMENT

Neurosurgical consultation for repair.

TABLE 4-2. Features of Internal Cartoid Artery Dissections

	INTERNAL CAROTID ARTERY DISSECTION (ICAD)	VERTEBRAL ARTERY DISSECTION (VAD)
Side	U/L (ipsilateral)	Usually ipsilateral; can be B/L 30–60% of time
Location	Frontal orbital, periorbital, and anterior neck	Occipital area and posterior neck
Typical presentation	▪ Unilateral headache ▪ Ipsilateral oculosympathetic paresis (incomplete *painful* Horner) ▪ Signs of cerebral ischemia localizing to opposite side	▪ Severe unilateral posterior headache ▪ Gradual neck pain ▪ Signs of ischemia to medulla

PE clues	▪ 46% have audible carotid bruit or at least patient reports pulsatile tinnitus
	▪ 2–8% have CN palsies
	▪ 12th CN palsy is the most common CN palsy considered sensitive for ICAD
	▪ Transient monocular visual loss (7%)
	▪ < 5% have massive stroke as initial presentation
		▪ Headache may precede neuro symptoms by up to 2 weeks, mean is 3 days
		▪ Signs of posterior circulation ischemia:
		  ▪ Vertigo
		  ▪ Nystagmus (including vertical)
		  ▪ Limb ataxia
		  ▪ Dysphagia, hoarseness
		  ▪ Contralateral loss of pain and temperature sensation
		  ▪ Ipsilateral arm, trunk, or leg weakness

Epidemiology	Spontaneous cases two times more frequent	More common in women
Prognosis	▪ Overall good ▪ Worse when associated with SAH, stroke as initial presentation, older age, or presence of underlying disease	▪ 10% die in acute phase ▪ For those that survive, most (~80%) make complete recovery

HIGH-YIELD FACTS

Neurologic Emergencies

Cerebral Venous Thrombosis

A 33-year-old woman who is 12 days postpartum presents with a throbbing headache. She does have a history of migraines, but "this one feels different." Delivery was normal. Patient has no other symptoms except some nausea, which she used to get with her migraines as well. She had no migraines during pregnancy. She had a DVT 10 years ago, after being started on OCPs (oral contraceptive pills). Physical examination reveals no papilledema, no photophobia, EOMI, no nystagmus, normal tandem gait, normal cranial nerve exam, negative Rhomberg.

The patient received 10 mg of metaclopramide IV, and her headache resolves completely. The MD theorizes that this is a migraine, which is back now that patient is no longer pregnant. The patient is discharged home from the ED with instructions to follow up with PMD if symptoms worsened.

She returns one week later. Headaches have worsened, and she has developed expressive aphasia. What is your next step in management?

This patient has cerebral venous thrombosis, and requires CT imaging with contrast and/or advanced neuro imaging such as MR venogram or CT venogram.

EPIDEMIOLOGY

- Considered uncommon in the United States (3 per million/year).
- More common in other parts of the world (eg, India).

SIGNS AND SYMPTOMS

- Headache is presenting symptoms in 70–100% of cases.
- Most common sinus affected is saggital sinus.
- Symptoms can vary based on sinus involved, in general due to resultant ↑ ICP, and can include:
  - Seizures
  - Papilledema
  - Altered mental status
  - Psychiatric symptoms
  - Fever
  - Elevated opening pressure on LP
  - Focal neuro deficits (palsies, internuclear ophthalmoplegia (Figure 4-7), visual disturbances)

RISK FACTORS

- Hypercoagulable states:
  - Deficiencies of protein S, C, antithrombin III
  - Factor V Leiden mutation
  - Lupus anticoagulant
- Hematologic diseases:
  - Thrombotic thrombocytopenic purpura
  - Polycythemia
  - Sickle cell anemia
- Miscellaneous disorders:
  - Nephrotic syndrome
  - Cirrhosis
  - Sarcoidosis
  - Dehydration

- Medications:
  - Oral contraceptives
  - Steroids
  - Aminocaproic acid
  - L-asparaginase
- Inflammatory diseases:
  - Crohn disease
  - Ulcerative colitis
  - Behçet disease
- Pregnancy

DIAGNOSIS

- CT with contrast is normal in 30% of cases.
- It can also show pattern of infarct or hemorrhage that does not follow arterial anatomy.
- Sometimes an empty delta sign is seen, which is a filling defect within the lumen of the thrombosed dural sinus, along with enlargement of medullary veins and other collateral venous channels.

TREATMENT

- Anticoagulation
- Supportive care

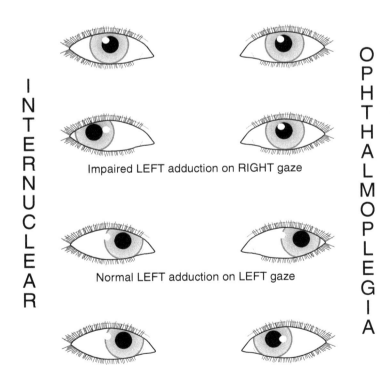

INTERNUCLEAR OPHTHALMOPLEGIA

Impaired LEFT adduction on RIGHT gaze

Normal LEFT adduction on LEFT gaze

FIGURE 4-7. Internuclear ophthalmoplegia.

Post-LP Headache

- Occurs within 24–48 hours post LP.
- Headache secondary to persistent CSF leak.
- Mild cases are treated with caffeine analgesics.
- Severe cases are treated with blood patch (epidural injection of patient's blood to patch leak).

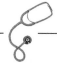

The approach in the emergency department is to first distinguish between true vertigo and syncope, presyncope, or weakness. Once *true* vertigo is differentiated, one must distinguish between *central* and *peripheral* vertigo. Consider all clinical information, including age and comorbidities.

VERTIGO AND DIZZINESS

DEFINITIONS

- **Dizziness** is a nonspecific term that should be clarified. It can be used to describe true vertigo or other conditions such as syncope, presyncope, light-headedness, or weakness.
- **Vertigo** is the perception of movement when there is no movement. The patient typically describes the room as spinning or the sensation of falling.
- **Nystagmus** is the rhythmic movement of eyes with two components (fast and slow). The direction of nystagmus is named by its fast component. Activation of the semicircular canals causes the slow component of the nystagmus to move away from the stimulus. The fast component of nystagmus is the reflex counter movement back to the desired direction of gaze by the cortex.

Distinguishing Peripheral from Central Vertigo

See Table 4-3.

Peripheral Vertigo

Causes:

- Benign paroxysmal positional vertigo
- Ménière's disease
- Vestibular neuronitis
- Labyrinthitis
- Ototoxicity (drugs)
- Eighth (vestibulocochlear) CN lesion
- Posttraumatic vertigo
- Middle ear disease
- Cerebellopontine angle tumors

BENIGN PAROXYSMAL POSITIONAL VERTIGO

EPIDEMIOLOGY

- Common
- Can occur at any age

PATHOPHYSIOLOGY

Transient vertigo precipitated by certain head motions.

TABLE 4-3. Peripheral versus Central Vertigo

	PERIPHERAL VERTIGO	CENTRAL VERTIGO
Pathophysiology	Disorders affecting the vestibular apparatus or the eighth (vestibulocochlear) cranial nerve	Disorder affecting the brain stem or cerebellum
Severity	Intense	Less intense
Onset	Sudden	Slow, insidious
Pattern	Intermittent	Constant
Nausea/vomiting	Usually present	Usually absent
Positional (worsened by motion)	Usually	Usually not
Hearing changes or physical findings on ear exam	May be present	Usually absent
Focal neurologic findings	Absent	Usually present
Fatigability of symptoms	Yes	No
Nystagmus	Horizontal, vertical, rotary	Vertical

SIGNS AND SYMPTOMS

- Sudden onset
- Nausea
- Worse in morning, fatigable
- Normal ear exam, no hearing changes

DIAGNOSIS

Dix-Hallpike maneuver:

- Have patient go from sitting to a supine position with eyes open and head rotated to the side you want to test.
- Positive test entails reproduction of vertigo and nystagmus that resolves within 1 minute.
- Not to be performed on patients with carotid bruits.

TREATMENT

- Antiemetics
- Antihistamines (meclizine)
- Benzodiazepines
- Epley maneuver (canalith repositioning)

MÉNIÈRE DISEASE

EPIDEMIOLOGY

Occurs between the ages of 30 and 60 years.

PATHOPHYSIOLOGY

Etiology unknown; postulated that symptoms are due to extravasation of endolymph into the perilymphatic space. Excess production of endolymph is also known as *endolymphatic hydrops*.

SIGNS AND SYMPTOMS

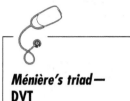

Ménière's triad—
DVT
Deafness
Vertigo
Tinnitus

- Deafness, tinnitus, vertigo.
- Nausea, vomiting, diaphoresis.
- Recurrent attacks.
- Deafness between attacks.
- Attacks occur several times a week to months.

TREATMENT

Symptomatic treatment with antihistamines, antivertigo and antiemetic agents, hydrochlorothiazide.

LABYRINTHITIS

DEFINITION

Infection of labyrinth.

SIGNS AND SYMPTOMS

- Hearing loss
- Peripheral vertigo
- Middle ear findings

DIAGNOSIS

Head CT or clinical.

TREATMENT

Symptomatic treatment with antihistamines, antivertigo and antiemetic agents.

POSTTRAUMATIC VERTIGO

PATHOPHYSIOLOGY

- Injury to labyrinth structures
- History of head trauma

SIGNS AND SYMPTOMS

- Peripheral vertigo
- Nausea, vomiting

DIAGNOSIS

CT of head to check for intracranial bleed or hematoma.

TREATMENT

Symptomatic treatment with antihistamines, antivertigo and antiemetic agents.

VESTIBULAR NEURONITIS

PATHOPHYSIOLOGY

Viral etiology.

SIGNS AND SYMPTOMS

- Sudden onset, lasts several days.
- Upper respiratory tract infection.

TREATMENT

Symptomatic treatment with antihistamines, antivertigo and antiemetic agents.

Other Causes of Central Vertigo

- Cerebellar hemorrhage or infarct
- Lateral medullary infarct (**Wallenberg syndrome**)
- Vertebrobasilar insufficiency
- Multiple sclerosis
- Neoplasm

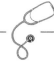

Obtain neurology consult in all cases of central vertigo or cases in which you are unsure.

OTOTOXICITY

Many drugs such as aminoglycosides, furosemide, and PCP cause ototoxicity.

HERPES ZOSTER OTICUS (RAMSAY HUNT SYNDROME)

Presents as deafness, facial nerve palsy, and vertigo with vesicles present in auditory canal.

CEREBELLOPONTINE ANGLE TUMORS

Present with multiple findings (cerebellar signs, ataxia, vertigo, and loss of corneal reflex).

CEREBELLAR HEMORRHAGE OR INFARCTION

- Acute vertigo
- Profound ataxia or inability to stand or sit without support
- Cerebellar findings
- Headache

WALLENBERG SYNDROME

- Occlusion of posterior inferior cerebellar artery
- Acute onset
- Nausea, vomiting
- Nystagmus
- Ipsilateral facial pain or numbness, Horner syndrome
- Contralateral pain and temperature loss

VERTEBROBASILAR VASCULAR DISEASE

- Vertebrobasilar vascular insufficiency can produce symptoms of vertigo.
- Other findings include diplopia, dysphagia, dysarthria, ataxia, **crossed findings** (refer to section on CVA—localizing the lesion).

MULTIPLE SCLEROSIS (FIGURE 4-8)

- Demyelinating disease that can also affect the brain stem, causing vertigo.
- May present with optic neuritis, ataxia, weakness, incontinence, facial pain, or paresthesias.
- Best clue is inability to explain multiple neurologic symptoms and deficits by a single lesion.
- CSF may reveal oligoclonal banding.

CNS INFECTIONS

Meningitis

DEFINITION

Inflammation of the membrane surrounding the brain and spinal cord.

CAUSES

- The majority of meningitides are caused by an infectious etiology, which varies according to age group (see Table 4-4).
- Noninfectious causes of meningitis include neoplasms and sarcoidosis.

SIGNS AND SYMPTOMS

Altered mental status, photophobia, headache, fever, meningeal signs (nuchal rigidity, Kernig and Brudzinski signs).

DIAGNOSIS

Kernig sign: Pain or resistance with passive extension of knee with hip flexed 90 degrees.

- Diagnosis made by LP: Obtain four (three for infants) tubes containing 1–2 mL each of CSF.
- Make sure there is no risk of herniation prior to performing LP. (Head CT scan can support this.)
- CSF findings suggestive of bacterial meningitis include ↑ white blood cells with a high percentage of polymorphonuclear leukocytes, low glucose, and high protein.

TREATMENT

Brudzinski sign: Passive flexion of neck causes flexion of the hips.

- Mainstay of treatment in adults is ceftriaxone, which has good CSF penetration.
- If resistance is an issue for *Streptococcus pneumoniae*, vancomycin or rifampin can be added to the regimen.
- Ampicillin should be added to any age group at risk for *Listeria monocytogenes.*
- Vancomycin and ceftazidime are used in post–head trauma patients, neurosurgical patients, or ventriculoperitoneal shunts.
- Antifungal agents should be considered in HIV-positive and other immunocompromised patients.

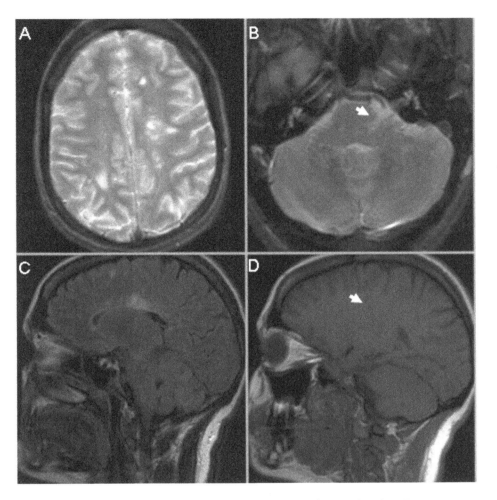

FIGURE 4-8. MRI demonstrating findings associated with multiple sclerosis.

Figure B shows Dawson's fingers. Figure D arrow shows black holes.

CNS Encephalitis

DEFINITION

Inflammation of the brain parenchyma secondary to infection.

CAUSES

Usually viral in origin.

SIGNS AND SYMPTOMS

- Abnormal behaviors and "personality changes"
- Seizures
- Headache
- Photophobia
- Focal neurologic findings
- Signs of peripheral disease:
  - Herpes—skin vesicles, rash
  - Rabies—animal bite
  - Arboviruses—bug bite

Causes of encephalitis:
HEAR
Herpes
Epstein-Barr virus
Arboviruses
Rabies

TABLE 4-4. Bugs in Meningitis by Age

	< 2 Months (Require Follow-up LP in 24–36 Hours)	2 Months to 50 Years	> 50 Years Debilitated or Immunocompromised
Organisms	▪ Group B strep ▪ Listeria ▪ Escherichia coli ▪ Klebsiella ▪ Enterobacter ▪ Staphylococcus aureus ▪ Haemophilus influenzae	▪ Streptococcus pneumoniae ▪ Neisseria meningitidis ▪ H influenzae	▪ S pneumoniae ▪ Listeria ▪ Gram-negative bacteria
Treatment (IV)	▪ Ampicillin 50 mg/kg q 8 h AND ▪ Cefotaxime 50 mg/kg q 8 h ▪ Generally considered good to treat early with steroids in any possible bacterial meningitis	▪ Cefotaxime 2 g q 4–6 h OR ▪ Ceftriaxone 2 g q 12 h ▪ Vancomycin 15 mg/kg q 6 h (until sensitivity known)	▪ Ampicillin 2 g q 4 h AND ▪ Cefotaxime 2 g q 4–6 h OR ▪ Ceftriaxone 2 g q 12 h
Penicillin-allergic Rx (IV)	▪ TMP/SMZ 5mg/kg q 12 h AND ▪ Vancomycin 15 mg/kg q 6 h	▪ Vancomycin 15 mg/kg q 6 h AND ▪ Gentamicin 2 mg/kg loading then 1.7 mg/kg q 8 h AND ▪ Rifampin 10–20 mg/kg qd	

DIAGNOSIS

Primarily diagnosed via CSF culture or serology: Blood in the CSF is a nonspecific clue but suggests herpes.

Do not delay antibiotics for LP or head CT when meningitis is suspected.

TREATMENT

▪ Mainly supportive
▪ Acyclovir for herpes

Brain Abscess

DEFINITION

A focal purulent cavity, covered by granulation tissue located in the brain.

CAUSES

Brain abscesses develop secondary to:

▪ Hematogenous spread
▪ Contiguous infections (sinuses, ears)
▪ Direct implantation via penetrating trauma or neurosurgery

SIGNS AND SYMPTOMS

▪ Headache
▪ Fever

- Focal neurologic findings
- Signs of primary infection
- History of trauma

DIAGNOSIS

CT scan of head with contrast (see Figure 4-9).

TREATMENT

Antibiotics tailored to suspected source of primary infection.

Guillain-Barré Syndrome

DEFINITION

- Ascending peripheral neuropathy
- Can affect all ages
- History of viral illness

CAUSES

Idiopathic.

SIGNS AND SYMPTOMS

- Loss of deep tendon reflexes.
- Distal weakness greater than proximal (legs greater than arms).
- Weakness is symmetrical.
- Numbness or tingling of the extremities.
- Risk of respiratory failure.

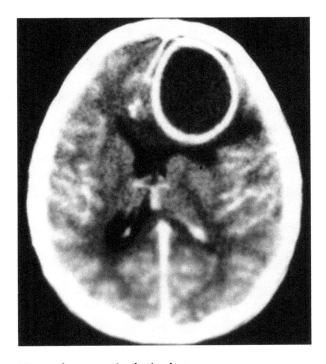

FIGURE 4-9. CT scan demonstrating brain abscess.

(Reproduced, with permission, from Schwartz SI, ed. *Principles of Surgery*, 7th ed. New York: McGraw-Hill, 1999: 1902.)

DIAGNOSIS

LP reveals ↑ CSF protein with a normal glucose and cell count.

TREATMENT

- Plasmapheresis.
- IV immunoglobulin.
- Intubate if there is respiratory compromise.

Myasthenia Gravis

DEFINITION

- Autoimmune disease of the neuromuscular junction.
- Affects old males and young females.

PATHOPHYSIOLOGY

- Acetylcholine receptor antibodies bind acetylcholine receptors, preventing binding of acetylcholine and subsequent muscular stimulation.
- Failure of neuromuscular conduction causes weakness.
- Association with thymoma.

SIGNS AND SYMPTOMS

- Generalized weakness.
- Usually proximal weakness affected more than distal weakness.
- Weakness relieved with rest.
- Ptosis and diplopia usually present.
- Symptoms may fluctuate, but usually worsen as the day progresses.
- Overuse of specific muscle groups can cause specific weakness of those muscle groups.

DIAGNOSIS

- Edrophonium test: Edrophonium is an anticholinesterase that prevents the breakdown of acetylcholine. ↑ level of acetylcholine overcomes the receptor blockage from autoantibodies. There is rapid return of muscle strength. Since the duration is short acting, this is only used as a diagnostic modality.
- Myasthenia gravis can be diagnosed by detection of acetylcholine receptor antibodies in the serum.
- Repetitive stimulation on nerve conduction studies, single-fiber electromyocardiogram (EMG) for ↑ jitter.

TREATMENT

- Anticholinesterase
- Plasma exchange
- Immunoglobulins
- Respiratory support (intubate as needed)
- Thymectomy (with or without thymoma or thymic hyperplasia)

A 37-year-old female presents with severe weakness of respiratory muscles, diplopia, ptosis, and proximal muscle weakness. *Think: Myasthenic crisis.*

DEFINITION

Abnormal electrical discharge of neurons causing a clinical episode of neurologic dysfunction.

EPIDEMIOLOGY

- 1% of adult ED visits
- 2% of pediatric ED visits
- Most common ED etiologies are not epilepsy related:
  - Alcoholism
  - Stroke
  - Trauma
  - CNS infection
  - Metabolic/toxin
  - Tumor
  - Fever in children
- 50,000–100,000 ED cases of status epilepticus annually; 20% mortality

CLASSIFICATION

See Table 4-5.

MANAGEMENT

- **Position:** Patients having a seizure should be rolled to a semiprone position to allow gravity to pull the tongue and secretions out of the airway. The head should be aligned with the body, and nothing should be put in the mouth.
- **ABCs:**
  - **A**irway: Maintain adequate airway with nasal trumpet.
  - **B**reathing: Administer oxygen. If properly positioned, cyanosis and apnea are rare.
  - Circulation: Obtain IV access.

HISTORY

- Important history can be obtained from bystanders or witnesses.
- Include **syncope** as part of your differential diagnosis.
- Seizures can cause loss of bladder control.
- Differentiate between partial and generalized seizure (ask patient if they can recall event).
- First seizure or known seizure history.
- Baseline seizure history (frequency and last seizure episode).
- Recent history of trauma.
- Consider factors that may lower seizure threshold (alcohol/drug withdrawal, illness, sleep deprivation).

SIGNS AND SYMPTOMS

Physical exam:

- Check for injuries caused as a result of seizure activity.
- Look for signs of infection, especially CNS infections.
- Assess and reassess mental status for signs of deterioration.

Factors that lower seizure threshold—
I **AM H⁴IP** Infection
Alcohol withdrawal, drugs
Medication (changes in dosing or compliance)
Head injury, **H**ypoxia
Hypoglycemia
Hypertension
Hyponatremia (and other electrolyte abnormalities [Ca+ Mg])
Intracranial lesions
Pregnancy (eclampsia)

TABLE 4-5. Classification of Seizures

TYPE	DESCRIPTION
Generalized	All generalized seizures involve loss of consciousness.
Tonic-clonic (grand mal)	Loss of consciousness immediately followed by tonic (rigid) contraction of muscles, then clonic (jerking) contraction. Patients may be cyanotic or apneic. Urinary incontinence may occur. Postictal period: Confusion, fatigue, or hypersomnolence following seizure; tongue biting may occur.
Absence (petit mal) (usually < 30 seconds)	Loss of consciousness without loss of postural tone; eye flutter common. Patients do not respond to verbal stimuli, nor do they lose continence. No postictal period.
Myoclonic	Loss of consciousness with brief muscular contractions.
Clonic	Loss of consciousness with repetitive clonic jerks.
Tonic	Loss of consciousness with sustained, prolonged contraction of body.
Atonic	Loss of consciousness with sudden loss of postural tone ("drop attacks").
Partial (focal)	Usually involve focal area of abnormal electrical discharge in cerebral cortex. Partial seizures may progress to generalized seizure ("secondary generalization").
Simple partial	Abnormal focal neurological discharge in which consciousness remains intact.
Complex partial (usually 1–2 minutes)	Frequently of temporal lobe origin. Consciousness is altered. Patient usually has an abrupt termination of ongoing motor activity ("staring spell"). Postictal period.
Aura	Simple partial seizure that becomes more obviously a seizure as it spreads; patients interpret it as a warning rather than a seizure.

Seizures can cause posterior shoulder dislocations, as well as intraoral lacerations.

Todd's paralysis: Focal neurological deficit persisting from seizure, which usually resolves within 48 hours.

DIAGNOSIS

- Routine labs. Work up depends on whether new onset seizure requires a more extensive evaluation, and a breakthrough seizure.
- Magnesium, calcium, toxicology screen, alcohol level, liver function tests.
- Consider LP.
- Consider CT scan of head.

TREATMENT

- Prevention of injury and adequate oxygenation in the actively seizing patient.
- Benzodiazepines are the mainstay of treatment in the seizing patient.
- Correct subtherapeutic levels of anticonvulsants.
- Treat underlying causes (meningitis, hypoglycemia, etc).
- Most often, treatment is mainly supportive.
- IV fosphenytoin, valproic acid, or phenobarbital if benzodiazepines fail.

Primary Seizure Disorder

- Some due to genetic defect in channel proteins.
- 0.5 to 1% of population has disease.
- *Epilepsy:* Diagnosed after two or more unprovoked seizures.

Secondary Seizure Disorder

DEFINITION

Seizures that occur as a result of another disease condition.

CAUSES

- Metabolic:
  - Hyper/hypoglycemia
  - Hyper/hyponatremia
  - Uremia
  - Hypocalcemia
- Infection:
  - Meningitis
  - Encephalitis
  - Intracerebral abscess
- Trauma:
  - Subdural hematoma
  - Epidural hematoma
  - ICH
  - SAH
- Toxic:
  - Theophylline
  - Amphetamines
  - Cocaine
  - Tricyclic antidepressants
  - Alcohol withdrawal
  - CO
  - Cyanide
  - Eclampsia
- Neurologic:
- Cortical infarction
- Intracranial hemorrhage
- Hypoxia
- Hypertensive encephalopathy
- Congenital cerebral malformation or cortical dysplasia

Causes of secondary
seizures —
MITTEN
Metabolic
Infection
Trauma
Toxins
Eclampsia
Neurologic lesions

Status Epilepticus

A 39-year-old male is brought to the ED by EMS because of a seizure at home. The patient had a generalized tonic-clonic seizure prior to going to bed. The seizure lasted for approximately 10 minutes, followed by a period of unresponsiveness during EMS transport. The patient has a long history of post-traumatic seizures that are managed with phenytoin and phenobarbital. There has been neither recent illness nor recent head trauma. In the emergency department, the patient is still unresponsive. What is the patient's status?

This patient is in status epilepticus, and should be treated with an antiepileptic drug as noted below. Also consider EEG monitoring.

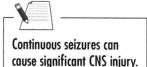

Continuous seizures can cause significant CNS injury.

Patients may still have CNS neuronal discharge despite neuromuscular blockade. Electroencephalogram will be required to detect seizure in this circumstance.

DEFINITION

Seizures occurring continuously for > 10 minutes, or two or more seizures occurring without full recovery of consciousness between attacks.

TREATMENT

- Treat generalized convulsive status epilepticus with IV benzodiazepines (lorazepam or diazepam first line) followed by, fosphenytoin, if necessary.
- Treat non convulsive status epilepticus with valprocic acid and phenobarbital. General anesthetics are last-line agents.

Eclampsia

- Usually occurs in patients > 20 weeks' gestation.
- Present with hypertension, edema, proteinuria, headache, vision changes, confusion, and seizure.
- Treatment includes magnesium sulfate and emergent delivery (unless postpartum).

Delirium Tremens

- Seizures can occur in alcohol withdrawal.
- Associated with autonomic hyperactivity.
- Seizures can occur within 6 hours after last drink.
- Treat with benzodiazepines and supportive care.

Head and Neck Emergencies

Inflammation of the paranasal sinuses of < 3 weeks' duration: There are one sphenoidal, two maxillary, and two frontal sinuses, along with the ethmoid air cells, which compose the paranasal sinuses. Acute sinusitis, also known as rhinosinusitis, can occur when there is drainage obstruction of the sinuses.

PATHOPHYSIOLOGY AND ETIOLOGY

- Edema causes obstruction of the drainage pathways followed by reabsorption of the air in the sinuses.
- The resultant negative pressure causes transudate collection within the sinuses.
- Most acute rhinosinusitis is viral.
- When bacteria is present, a suppurative infection can occur.

RISK FACTORS

- Viral upper respiratory infection (URI)
- Allergic rhinitis

ETIOLOGY

Streptococcus pneumoniae causes 37% of bacterial sinusitis, with *Haemophilus influenzae* causing 38%. Other common URI bacteria are also implicated.

SIGNS AND SYMPTOMS

- Pain over the sinuses.
- ↓ sense of smell.
- Fever.
- Purulent nasal discharge.
- Headache (may be aggravated by coughing, sneezing, and leaning forward).
- Maxillary tooth pain.
- Tenderness to palpation or percussion over the affected area.
- Nasal canal may be inflamed, and purulent exudates may drain from the ostia.

DIAGNOSIS

- Usually clinical based on history and physical:
  - Purulent rhinorrhea
  - Facial tenderness or pressure
  - Nasal congestion
- There is no defined role for sinus plain radiography in diagnosis.
- Role of computed tomography (CT) is unclear, as there are many false negatives and false positives.

TREATMENT

- Most patients should be managed symptomatically.
- Over-the-counter decongestant nasal sprays can provide symptomatic relief (do not use for > 3 consecutive days).
- Antibiotics: Reserve for patients who don't improve with symptomatic management or those who are at high risk.

Approximately 70% of human immunodeficiency virus (HIV) patients will develop sinusitis, which may be caused by opportunistic bacteria, viruses, or fungi.

Most patients with sinusitis can be treated without antibiotics.

- Amoxicillin or amoxicillin with clavulanate is first-line therapy.
- Macrolides and trimethoprim-sulfamethoxasole (TMP/SMX) are alternatives.

COMPLICATIONS

- The infection can extend beyond the sinuses and, in the case of ethmoidal involvement, may enter the CNS.
- Bony destruction can also occur and may result in facial deformity.
- Direct extension from sinuses to the venous or lymphatic system can cause cavernous sinus thrombosis.

ADMISSION CRITERIA

Presence of complications, toxicity, fever with neurologic signs, or orbital or periorbital cellulitis all warrant admission.

EPISTAXIS

DEFINITION

Nosebleed.

EPIDEMIOLOGY

- Anterior epistaxis is more common in younger patients.
- Posterior epistaxis is more common in the elderly population.

ANATOMY

- The nose humidifies and warms air and has a rich blood supply.
- The internal and external carotid arteries supply blood to the nasal mucosa through a number of smaller branches.

Anterior Epistaxis

- Comprise 90% of nose bleeds.
- Most commonly originates from Kiesselbach's plexus (a confluence of arteries on the posterior superior nasal septum).

Kiesselbach's plexus is located in the "picking zone."

ETIOLOGY

- Trauma to the nasal mucosa (usually self-induced)
- Foreign body
- Allergic rhinitis
- Nasal irritants (such as cocaine, decongestants)
- Pregnancy (due to engorgement of blood vessels)
- Infection (sinusitis, rhinitis)
- Osler-Weber-Rendu syndrome (telangiectasias)

DIAGNOSIS

- Labs are not routinely required if there are no comorbidities.
- Facial or nasal films may be considered in the setting of nasal trauma.

In anterior epistaxis, the bleeding is unilateral and the patient generally denies a sensation of blood in the back of the throat.

TREATMENT

- **Direct pressure:** Compress the elastic portions of the nose between the thumb and middle finger. Hold continuously for 10–15 minutes.
- **Vasoconstrictive agents:**
  - Phenylephrine or oxymetazoline can be instilled into the nasal cavity in conjunction with other treatment methods.
  - Cotton-tipped applicators can be used to apply vasoconstrictive agents if the bleed can be visualized.
- **Anterior nasal packing:**
  - Nasal tampons, gauze packing, or balloon catheters.
  - Should be performed on any patient in which vasoconstrictive agents and direct pressure have failed.
  - Coating the tampon with bacitracin may ↓ risk of toxic shock syndrome.
  - The use of prophylactic systemic antibiotics to prevent toxic shock is unproven.
  - Nasal packs should be removed at ear, nose, and throat (ENT) follow-up after 2–3 days.
- **Chemical cautery** with silver nitrate-tipped applicators.
- **Electrocautery** performed by an otolaryngologist.

PROCEDURE FOR ANTERIOR NASAL PACKING

Nasal tampons or balloon catheters can be inserted along the floor of the nasal canal. They expand to several times their original size when instilled with saline (tampons) or when inflated (balloon catheters).

Posterior Epistaxis

DEFINITION

- Comprises approximately 10% of epistaxis in the emergency department (ED).
- More common in older patients and is thought to be secondary to atherosclerosis of the arteries supplying the posterior nasopharynx.

ETIOLOGY

- Hypertension
- Anticoagulation therapy
- Liver disease
- Blood dyscrasias
- Neoplasm
- Atherosclerosis of nasal vessels

CLINICAL FEATURES

- Blood may be seen effluxing from both nares or down the posterior oropharynx.
- Visualization of the bleeding usually requires use of a fiber-optic laryngoscope.
- Bleeding is often more severe than with an anterior bleed.

Twenty-five percent of properly placed nasal packs fail to control bleeding. In this case, an emergent ENT consult is indicated.

Approximately 50% of patients presenting with posterior epistaxis have a systolic blood pressure ≥ 180 mm Hg or a diastolic pressure > 110 mm Hg.

DIAGNOSIS

Routine labs including complete blood count (CBC), prothrombin time, and activated partial thromboplastin time may be drawn to look for possible coagulopathies and to assess for anemia.

TREATMENT

- **Posterior nasal packing:** Commercial nasal packs and specialized hemostatic balloon devices are available and are more efficacious than the traditional methods of posterior nasal packing. The procedure for inserting a commercial nasal hemostatic balloon is described below:
  1. Prepare the nasal cavity with vasoconstrictors and anesthetic agents.
  2. Insufflate 25 cc of saline into the anterior balloon to test for leakage. The posterior balloon is tested with 8 cc of saline.
  3. Lubricate the device with 4% lidocaine jelly and insert it into the nasopharynx. Advance until the distal balloon tip is visible in the posterior oropharynx when the patient opens his mouth.
  4. Fill the posterior balloon tip with 4 to 8 cc of saline and pull the device anteriorly such that it wedges in the posterior nasopharynx.
  5. Fill the anterior balloon with 10 to 25 cc of saline while maintaining traction on the device.
  6. It may be necessary to pack both nares to obtain adequate hemostasis.
  7. Many patients require sedation following the procedure.
- **Embolization and ligation:** These treatments are indicated when the other treatments fail and should be performed by ENT specialists.
- All patients with posterior bleeds should have an emergent ENT consult and require admission to a monitored setting. Posterior packing can → bradycardic episodes.

OTITIS EXTERNA

DEFINITION

Infection of the external ear or external canal: Can be localized (furuncle) or can affect the entire canal.

Otitis externa is also known as "swimmer's ear."

ETIOLOGY

The most common causes are *Pseudomonas aeruginosa* and *Staphylococcus aureus*.

EPIDEMIOLOGY

It is more common in moist environments (summer, swimming pools, and the tropics).

A 16-year-old swim team captain presents with a greenish discharge from his ear and complains that his ear feels "full." He withdraws as you tug on his ear to examine it. *Think: Otitis externa.*

SIGNS AND SYMPTOMS

- Sense of fullness in the ear
- White or green cheesy discharge
- Pain on retraction of pinna
- Itching
- ↓ hearing
- Fever
- A bulging or erythematous tympanic membrane

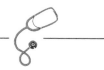

TREATMENT

- Cleanse ear canal thoroughly.
- Polymyxin-neomycin-hydrocortisone ear drop suspension.

COMPLICATIONS

Malignant external otitis media:

- Seen in diabetics and immunocompromised hosts.
- Results in destruction of bone underlying the external ear canal.
- Characterized by excruciating pain, fever, friable granulation tissue in external ear canal, and facial palsies.
- Treated with antipseudomonal antibiotic drops.

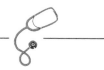

Patients with otitis externa should avoid getting water into their ears for 2–3 weeks after treatment.

ACUTE OTITIS MEDIA (AOM)

A 4-year-old previously healthy boy presents with fever, cough, and runny nose for 1 day. On exam, he is well appearing and nontoxic. His right ear is dull appearing without effusion. He has never had an ear infection. His parents are wondering whether he needs antibiotics for an ear infection. What are the treatment options?

The patient probably has a viral URI. The diagnosis of acute otitis media is equivocal. The patient may be a good candidate for observation without antibiotics. He should be treated with acetaminophen or ibuprofen. A "wait and see" approach could be employed, where the parents are given a prescription for antibiotics but told to fill it only if the symptoms are not improved in 48 hours.

DEFINITION

A bacterial or viral infection of the middle ear, usually secondary to a viral URI. Diagnosis of AOM requires:

1. History of acute onset of symptoms.
2. Presence of a middle ear effusion.
3. Signs and symptoms of middle ear inflammation.

ETIOLOGY

- S pneumoniae, nontypeable H influenzae, and Moraxella catarrhalis are the most common causes.
- Newborns can also get suppurative otitis with Escherichia coli and S aureus.

EPIDEMIOLOGY

- More common in colder months.
- Most common age is ages 6 months to 3 years.

PATHOPHYSIOLOGY

Dysfunction of the eustachian tube → retention of secretions, which → bacterial colonization.

Secondhand smoke is a risk factor for otitis media in children.

138

SIGNS AND SYMPTOMS

- Ear pain and sense of fullness
- Perception of gurgling or rumbling sounds inside the ear
- ↓ hearing
- Dizziness
- Fever
- Poor feeding and irritability in infants

DIAGNOSIS

- Middle ear effusion:
  - Bulging of the typanic membrane (TM)
  - Limited or absent mobility of TM
  - Air-fluid level behind TM
  - Otorrhea
- Middle ear inflammation:
  - Distinct erythema of TM
  - Distinct otalgia

TREATMENT

- Acetaminophen or ibuprofen for analgesia.
- Topical anesthetic drops (eg, benzocaine) can provide additional analgesic relief.
- First-line antibiotic choice is amoxicillin 80–90 mg/kg/day for 5–7 days for mild cases in children over age 2. For those under age 2, standard therapy is 10 days. For severe cases, amoxicillin–clavulanic acid can be used instead.
- Observation option (48–72 hours):
  - For healthy children ages 6 months to 2 years who have nonsevere symptoms at presentation and in whom diagnosis is uncertain.
  - For healthy children over age 2 with any (severe or nonsevere) symptoms *or* an uncertain diagnosis.
  - This option is further limited to those who have ready access to follow-up health care and a caregiver who agrees.
- Failure of observation: Start antibiotics.
- Failure of initial antibiotics: Change antibiotic.

COMPLICATIONS

- Serous otitis media—an effusion of the middle ear resulting from incomplete resolution of otitis media.
- Acute mastoiditis.

ACUTE MASTOIDITIS

DEFINITION

Bacterial infection of the mastoid process resulting in coalescence of the mastoid air cells: It is usually a complication of acute otitis media in which the infection has spread into the mastoid antrum.

SIGNS AND SYMPTOMS

- Swelling, erythema, tenderness, and fluctuance over the mastoid process
- Displacement of pinna laterally and inferiorly
- Fever
- Earache
- Otorrhea
- ↓ hearing

DIAGNOSIS

CT scan of the mastoid air cells reveals cell partitions that are destroyed, resulting in coalescence.

TREATMENT

- Antibiotics should cover the common acute otitis media pathogens and be resistant to beta-lactamase.
- Third-generation cephalosporins are preferred because they offer good penetration into the CNS at the proper doses.
- This therapy is usually effective in preventing neurological sequelae.

COMPLICATIONS

Subperiosteal abscess requires mastoidectomy.

LUDWIG'S ANGINA

DEFINITION

Cellulitis of bilateral submandibular spaces and the lingual space: This is a potentially life-threatening infection.

ETIOLOGY

- Usually a result of spread of a bacterial odontogenic infection into the facial tissue spaces.
- Most common bug is mouth anaerobe *Bacteroides*.

RISK FACTORS

- Oral trauma
- Dental work
- Salivary gland infection

SIGNS AND SYMPTOMS

- Fever
- Drooling
- Trismus
- Odynophagia
- Dysphonia
- Elevated tongue
- Swollen neck
- Labored breathing

Soft-tissue radiographs of the neck can be obtained, but they should not delay treatment or place the patient in an area where emergent airway management is difficult.

TREATMENT

- Secure airway potential for difficult airway. Consider fiberoptic intubation.
- IV antibiotics (penicillin and metronidazole or clindamycin).
- Definitive treatment is incision and drainage, then excision of fascial planes in the operating room (OR).
- ENT or oral and maxillofacial surgery consult.

PHARYNGITIS

DEFINITION

Infection of the pharynx and tonsils that rarely occurs in infants and is uncommon under 2 years of age.

EPIDEMIOLOGY

Peak incidence is between 4 and 7 years old but occurs throughout adult life.

ETIOLOGY

- **Viruses:**
  - Most common cause of all pharyngeal infection.
  - Rhinoviruses and adenoviruses are the most common viral causes.
  - Epstein-Barr virus, herpes simplex virus, influenza, parainfluenza, and coronaviruses also contribute.
- **Bacteria:**
  - *Streptococcus pyogenes* (group A, beta-hemolytic strep) is the most common cause of bacterial pharyngitis.
  - *Mycoplasma, Chlamydia,* and *Corynebacterium* also occur.
- **Fungal and parasitic:** Can also occur in the immunocompromised host.

SIGNS AND SYMPTOMS

- Erythematous tonsils.
- Tonsillar exudates.
- Enlarged and tender anterior cervical lymph nodes.
- Palatal petechiae.
- Incubation period is 2–5 days, after which patients develop sore throat, dysphagia, chills, and fever.
- Headache, nausea, vomiting, and abdominal pain can also occur.

Signs and symptoms are the same for viral and bacterial pharyngitis. One cannot differentiate between the two causes without microbiology testing.

DIAGNOSIS

- Throat culture: Still the most effective means of diagnosis. There is a delay in obtaining results while the culture grows, and a good sample must be obtained.
- Rapid antigen detection tests (RADTs): Detect streptococcus; > 95% specific. A negative RADT should be confirmed with a throat culture.
- See Figure 5-1.

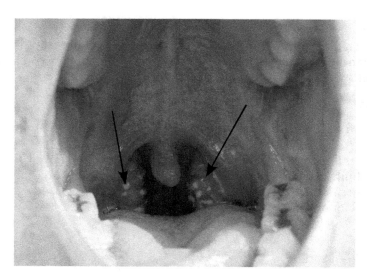

FIGURE 5-1. Streptococcal pharyngitis.

Note white exudates (arrows) on top of erythematous swollen tonsils. (Reproduced, with permission, from Nimishikavi S, Stead LG. Streptococcal pharyngitis. *N Engl J Med* 2005 (Mar 17);352(11): e10. Copyright © 2005 Massachusetts Medical Society. All rights reserved.)

TREATMENT FOR STREPTOCOCCAL PHARYNGITIS

- A one-time intramuscular injection of penicillin (benzathine penicillin 1.2 million units) or a 10-day course of oral penicillin is the treatment of choice.
- Erythromycin is an alternative for penicillin-allergic patients.

COMPLICATIONS

- Post-streptococcal glomerulonephritis (PSGN).
- Rheumatic fever (RF)
- Cervical lymphadenitis
- Peritonsillar abscess
- Retropharyngeal abscess
- Sinusitis
- Otitis media

Treatment algorithm for strep pharyngitis:

- RADT positive: Treat
- RADT negative: Culture and treat until culture results are available.
- If culture is negative, discontinue antibiotics.
- No RADT available: Culture and treat until culture results are known. If negative, discontinue antibiotics.

EPIGLOTTITIS

DEFINITION

A life-threatening inflammatory condition (usually infectious) of the epiglottis and the aryepiglottic folds and periglottic folds.

ETIOLOGY

- *H influenzae* type B (Hib) is the most common cause.
- *Streptococcus* is the next most common cause.
- Can also be caused by other bacteria and rarely viruses and fungi.

EPIDEMIOLOGY

- The incidence in children has ↓ dramatically after the introduction of the Hib vaccine.
- Most cases are now in adults and unimmunized children.

Epiglottitis now occurs more often in adults than children.

SIGNS AND SYMPTOMS

- Prodromal period of 1–2 days.
- High fever.
- Dysphagia.
- Stridor.
- Drooling.
- Secretion pooling.
- Dyspnea.
- Erect or tripod position.
- Pain on movement of the thyroid cartilage is an indicator of supraglottic inflammation.

DIAGNOSIS

- High clinical suspicion is necessary.
- Radiographs of the neck soft tissue can aid in diagnosis (Figure 5-2), as can fiberoptic laryngoscopy.
- Direct laryngoscopy is contraindicated because it may induce fatal laryngospasm.
- Do not examine the oropharynx unless surgical airway capability is available at the bedside.

"Thumbprint sign" (Figure 5-2) is seen on lateral neck radiograph and demonstrates a swollen epiglottis obliterating the vallecula.

TREATMENT

- Intubation as needed to protect airway
- Ceftriaxone
- Intensive care unit admission

COMPLICATIONS

Airway obstruction and resultant respiratory arrest.

CROUP

A 5-year-old girl is brought into the ED by her mother at 2 A.M. with a severe cough and difficulty breathing. She has had fevers, a runny nose, and a cough for 3 days. She became much more short of breath this morning, so her mother brought her in. She is breathing at 30 breaths per minute with a pulse of 135. Her oxygen saturation is 95% on while receiving room air. She is restless in appearance with a barky sounding cough and stridor at rest. The stridor becomes severe with agitation. What should be done to treat her symptoms?

She has moderate to severe croup. She should be given steroids (dexamethasone 0.6 mg/kg) and be started on racemic epinephrine. She will require hospital admission or ED observation for at least 2 hours after the epinephrine to ensure she does not have a return of her symptoms.

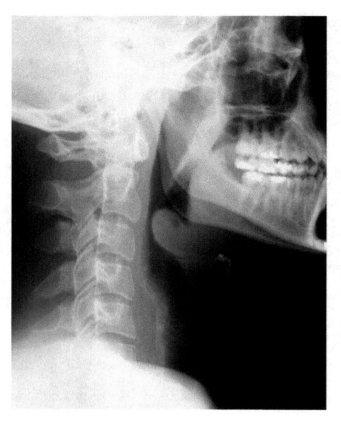

FIGURE 5-2. Epiglottitis.

Arrow indicates classic "thumbprint" sign of enlarged, inflamed epiglottis.

- Viral infection of the upper respiratory tract
- Age: 6 months to 6 years

SIGNS AND SYMPTOMS

- Stridor
- Barking cough
- Hoarse voice
- Fever

DIAGNOSIS

- Clinical suspicion.
- Anteroposterior soft-tissue neck radiograph may show the "steeple sign," which is indicative of subglottic narrowing (Figure 5-3).

TREATMENT

- Cool mist does not appear to be helpful.
- Steroids: Dexamethasone 0.15–0.6 mg/kg IV, IM, or PO.
- Racemic epinephrine if severe.

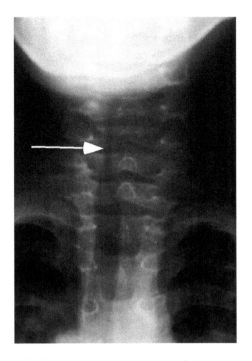

FIGURE 5-3. Radiograph demonstrating steeple sign of croup.

Note narrowing of airway (arrow).

PERITONSILLAR ABSCESS

SIGNS AND SYMPTOMS

- Sore throat
- Muffled voice
- ↓ oral intake
- Tilting of head to affected side
- Trismus
- Deviation of uvula to affected side
- Swollen erythematous tonsils
- Fluctuant soft palate mass
- Cervical lymphadenopathy

DIAGNOSIS

By physical exam.

TREATMENT

- Antibiotics against gram-positive oral flora (including anaerobes).
- Consider steroids to ↓ inflammation.
- Needle aspiration of most perotonsillar abscesses can be accomplished in the ED. Caution to avoid the carotid which lies deep to the peritonsillar space.
- ENT consultation for complicated abscesses.

A 29-year-old man who had been treated for strep throat the previous week presents with progressive difficulty swallowing. Physical exam reveals a fluctuant mass on the right side of the soft palate and deviation of the uvula to the right. *Think: Peritonsillar abscess.*

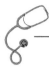

Patients with epiglottitis prefer to sit leaning forward with the neck slightly flexed. Patients with retropharyngeal abscess prefer recumbency and hyperextension of the neck.

DEFINITION

Abscess in the pharyngeal spaces.

SIGNS AND SYMPTOMS

- Difficulty breathing
- Fever, chills
- Severe throat pain
- Toxic appearance
- Hyperextension of neck
- Stridor
- Drooling
- Swollen, erythematous pharynx
- Tender cervical lymph nodes

DIAGNOSIS

- Radiograph of the soft tissues of the neck (see Figure 5-4): Exaggerated swelling in the pharyngeal spaces is indicative of abscess.
- CT with IV contrast can be helpful if the diagnosis is unclear and can differentiate abscess from cellulitis.
- Ultrasound may also be utilized and does not expose the patient to ionizing radiation or IV contrast.

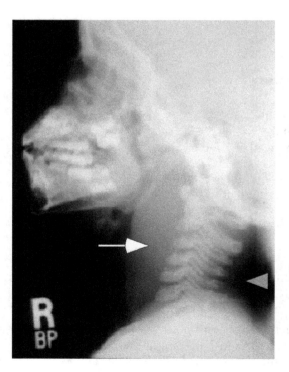

FIGURE 5-4. Retropharyngeal abscess.

Lateral radiograph of the soft tissue of the neck. Note the large amount of prevertebral edema (solid arrow), and the collection of air (dashed arrow). (Photo courtesy of Dr. Gregory J. Schears.)

TREATMENT

Same as for peritonsillar abscess, except that all parapharyngeal and retropharyngeal abscesses are drained in the OR.

BACTERIAL TRACHEITIS

- Caused by *S aureus*, *S pneumoniae*, *H influenzae*, others
- Age: 1–5 years

SIGNS AND SYMPTOMS

- Preceding URI.
- Fever.
- Stridor.
- May initially look like croup, but will not respond to treatment.

DIAGNOSIS

Clinical suspicion.

TREATMENT

- Airway intervention—may require intubation
- IV antibiotics

HIGH-YIELD FACTS

Head and Neck Emergencies

Respiratory Emergencies

> A 27-year-old patient presents with pneumonia, bullous myringitis, and a chest film that looks worse than expected. What is the likely diagnosis?
> *Mycoplasma* pneumonia is the most common cause of pneumonia in healthy adults under the age of 40 years. The causative organism is *Mycoplasma pneumoniae,* which is considered an atypical pathogen. *Mycoplasma* can also cause bullous myringitis. Complications include hepatitis, immune thrombocytopenic purpura, and hemolytic anemia. Treatment is with a macrolide or a respiratory flouroquinolone.

EPIDEMIOLOGY

- Most common cause of death from infectious disease in the United States; sixth most common cause of death in the United States overall.
- Community-acquired pneumonia (CAP) is an acute infection in patients who have not been recently hospitalized or residing in a nursing home.
- Hospital-acquired (or nosocomial) pneumonia (HAP) occurs in those who have recently been hospitalized and are caused by different organism than CAP.
- Ventilator-associated pneumonia (VAP) is a form of HAP that occurs > 48 hours after endotracheal intubation.
- Health care–associated pneumonia (HCAP) occurs in nonhospitalized patients with significant health care exposure, such as residing in a nursing home.

ETIOLOGY

> A patient with human immunodeficiency virus (HIV) has a CD4 count of 52, does not take antiretroviral medications or trimethoprim-sulfamethoxazole, is hypoxic on room air, has an elevated lactic dehydrogenase (LDH), and has diffuse bilateral infiltrates (see Figure 6-1) on chest x-ray (CXR). What is the diagnosis?
> *Pneumocystis* pneumonia (PCP). PCP pneumonia was originally thought to be caused by protozoan called *Pneumocystis carinii;* however, the organism was later identified as fungus *Pneumocystis jirovecii.* In order to avoid confusion, the acronym PCP has been retained, referring to the name *Pneumocystis* pneumonia.

- Bacterial:
  - *Streptococcus pneumoniae:* The most common causative organism
  - *Haemophilus influenzae*
  - *Klebsiella pnuemoniae*
  - *Mycoplasma pneumoniae*
  - *Legionella pneumophila*
  - *Moraxella catarrhalis*
  - *Chlamydia pneumoniae*
  - *Staphylococcus aureus*
  - Gram-negative bacilli *(Pseudomonas)*

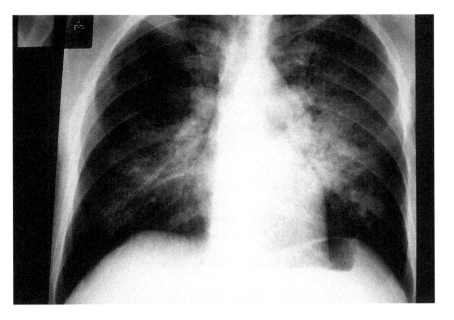

FIGURE 6-1. Chest x-ray of patient with *Pneumocystis jiroveci* pneumonia (PCP).

Photo contributed by Edward C. Oldfield III, MD. (Reproduced, with permission, from Knoop KJ, Stack LB, Storrow AB, Thurman RJ. *The Atlas of Emergency Medicine*, 3rd ed. New York: McGraw-Hill, 2010: 644.)

- Viral:
  - Influenza.
  - Parainfluenza.
  - Adenovirus.
  - *Mycobacterium tuberculosis* and endemic fungi are rare causes of community-acquired pneumonia.

SIGNS AND SYMPTOMS

- Tachypnea
- Tachycardia
- Rales
- Diaphoresis
- Dyspnea
- Chest pain
- Cough
- Hemoptysis
- Physical findings associated with ↑ risk:
  - Respiratory rate > 30/min
  - Heart rate > 140 bpm
  - Blood pressure, systolic < 90 or diastolic < 60 mm Hg
  - Temperature > 101°F
  - Change in mental status
  - Extrapulmonary infection

DIAGNOSIS

- CXR may show a lobar consolidation or patchy infiltrates.
- Elevated WBC often present.
- Hyponatremia (commonly *Legionella*).
- Sputum Gram stain and cultures are low yield and often do not identify an organism.
- Blood cultures should be obtained in admitted patients prior to antibiotics.

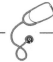

If you see **currant jelly sputum** on physical exam or **bulging fissure** on CXR, think *Klebsiella.*

TREATMENT AND DISPOSITION

- Treatment of viral pneumonia is supportive.
- Antibiotic selection for bacterial pneumonia depends on the organism involved. Empiric therapy and hospital admission are based on the patient's age, comorbidities, severity of symptoms, and particular risk factors.
- Antibiotics for community acquired pneumonia should include coverage for S pneumoniae and M pneumoniae. Common inpatient regimens include ceftriaxone and azithromycin together or a levofloxacin as single agent.
- Antibiotics for nosocomial infections or requiring admission to ICU should include coverage for *Pseudomonas.*
- The Pneumonia Patient Outcomes Research Team (PORT) has proposed a severity index (see Table 6-1) that can be used to guide the decision of outpatient versus inpatient therapy.

Antibiotics should be administered for pneumonia as soon as the diagnosis is made.

ASPIRATION PNEUMONIA

DEFINITION

- Pathogens can enter the lung by inhalation of aerosols, by hematogenous spread, or by aspiration of oropharyngeal contents.
- Up to half of normal adults aspirate oropharyngeal contents during sleep. Individuals with swallowing disorders, intoxication, impaired level of consciousness, or an impaired gag reflex are more likely to aspirate material into the lungs. The chances of developing a pneumonia depend on the volume aspirated and the virulence of the material.
- Different organisms can be present in the aspirate depending on the individual.

Pulmonary pathogens that can be found in the oropharynx:
- S pneumoniae
- M pneumoniae
- H influenzae
- Streptococcus pyogenes
- M catarrhalis

TABLE 6-1. Pneumonia Severity Index ("PORT Score")

CHARACTERISTIC	POINTS ASSIGNED
Demographic factor	
Age (men)	Age (years)
Age (women)	Age (years) − 10
Nursing home resident	+10
Coexisting illnesses	
Neoplastic disease	+30
Liver disease	+20
Congestive heart failure	+10
Cerebrovascular disease	+10
Renal disease	+10
Physical examination findings	
Altered mental status	+20
Respiratory rate ≥ 30 bpm	+20
Systolic blood pressure < 90 mm Hg	+20
Temperature < 35°C (95°F) or 40°C (104°F)	+15
Pulse ≥ 125 beats/min	+10
Laboratory and radiographic findings (if study performed)	
Arterial blood pH < 7.35	+30
Blood urea nitrogen level ≥ 30 mg/dL	+20
Sodium level < 130 mmol/L	+20
Glucose level ≥ 250 mg/dL	+10
Hematocrit < 30%	+10
Partial pressure of arterial O_2 < 60 mm Hg or O_2 sat < 90%	+10
Pleural effusion	+10

CLASS	POINTS	MORTALITY*
I	< 51	0.1%
II	51–70	0.6%
III	71–90	0.9%
IV	91–130	9.5%
V	> 130	26.7%

Patients in classes I–III can usually be managed as outpatients.

(Adapted, with permission, from Fine MJ et al. A prediction rule to identify low-risk patients with community acquired pneumonia. *N Engl J Med* 1997;336(4):247. Copyright © 1997 Massachusetts Medical Society. All rights reserved.)

PATHOPHYSIOLOGY

- Anaerobic pulmonary pathogens colonize dental plaque and gingiva; aspiration can cause pneumonia or lung abscess.
- Common pulmonary pathogens can colonize the nasopharynx of normal individuals.
- Aerobic gram-negative bacilli can colonize the stomach and reach the oropharynx in vomit or by spreading colonization in debilitated individuals.
- Mucociliary dysfunction, common in smokers, and alveolar macrophage dysfunction will reduce the clearing of aspirate and ↑ the chances of infection.
- Presence of foreign bodies in the aspirate will also ↑ the chances of infection.
- Aspiration can → the development of a lung abscess.

Aspiration pneumonia is most commonly seen in the right lower lobe.

A 75-year-old male stroke victim is brought in by his home health aide, who states she has been having to shove food down his throat the past few days because he refuses to eat. Today, she noted he had trouble breathing and was making gurgling sounds. *Think: Aspiration pneumonia.*

APE may be a presentation of acute MI.

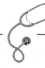

An 81-year-old woman is brought in by EMS gasping for breath. Rales are noted almost all the way up her lungs bilaterally. She has pink frothy sputum and her skin is also wet. *Think: APE.*

Treatment of APE—
NOt **BAD**
Nitroglycerin
Oxygen therapy
BiPAP (or CPAP)
Aspirin
Diuretics

TREATMENT

- Supportive:
  - Oxygen
  - Suctioning
- Bronchoscopy for large foreign body aspirates.
- Antibiotic coverage should be reserved for signs of pneumonia and should include anaerobic coverage with clindamycin or metronidazole in addition to standard coverage.
- No role for prophylactic steroids or antibiotics.

PULMONARY EDEMA

DEFINITION

Pulmonary edema is the accumulation of fluid in the interstitial space of the lung. The most common cause of pulmonary edema is cardiogenic in nature, which results from ↑ pulmonary capillary pressure.

CARDIOGENIC CAUSES

- Left ventricular (LV) failure (myocardial infarction [MI], ischemia, cardiomyopathy).
- ↑ pulmonary venous pressure without failure (valvular disease).
- ↑ pulmonary arterial pressure.

NONCARDIOGENIC CAUSES

- Hypoalbuminemia (↓ oncotic pressure).
- Altered membrane permeability (adult respiratory distress syndrome).
- Lymphatic insufficiency.
- High-altitude pulmonary edema.
- Opiate overdose.
- Neurogenic pulmonary edema.

CONGESTIVE HEART FAILURE (CHF)

Acute pulmonary edema (APE) secondary to LV failure and/or volume overload is commonly known as CHF.

DIAGNOSIS

- Often based on physical exam.
- CXR: Bilateral insterstitial pattern, Kerley B lines, cardiomegaly.
- Elevated B-natriuretic peptide.

TREATMENT

- Nitroglycerin to promote preload reduction and venodilation.
- Oxygen.
- Continuous positive airway pressure (CPAP) or bilevel positive airway pressure (BiPAP).
- Diuretics (furosemide).
- Aspirin: Antiplatelet agent, protective against MI.

- Morphine has traditionally been used to relieve anxiety, but there is no supportive evidence for its use in APE. A low-dose benzodiazapine may be preferred for patients who are very anxious.

PULMONARY EMBOLUS (PE)

A 53-year-old woman presents with dyspnea and tachycardia and appears extremely anxious. She complains of some sharp pain in her right lower chest when she takes a deep breath in. She is currently undergoing chemotherapy for ovarian cancer. She is afebrile and her pulse is 110 bpm, respiratory rate is 24 bpm, and her oxygen saturation is 94% on oxygen 4L by nasal cannula. Her CXR reveals an elevated right hemidiaphragm and her ECG sinus tachycardia. Her troponin is slightly elevated, and her creatinine is normal. What should you do next?

She has at least a moderate risk of PE and would not be a good candidate for a D-dimer. She has normal kidney function and should undergo a PE protocol computed tomography (CT) of the chest. Her elevated troponin is more likely from a PE (typical symptoms) than an acute coronary syndrome (atypical symptoms).

RISK FACTORS

- Genetic predisposition
- Age
- Obesity
- Cigarette smoking
- Hypertension
- Oral contraceptives
- Hormone replacement therapy
- Neoplasm
- Immobilization
- Pregnancy and postpartum period
- Surgery and trauma
- Hypercoagulable state

SIGNS AND SYMPTOMS

- Tachypnea
- Tachycardia
- Hypoxia
- Rales
- Diaphoresis
- Bulging neck veins
- Heart murmur
- Dyspnea (seen up to 90% of the time)
- Chest pain (seen up to 66% of the time)
- Apprehension
- Cough
- Hemoptysis
- Syncope

There are no signs, symptoms, laboratory values, CXR, or electrocardiographic (ECG) findings that are diagnostic of PE or are consistently present. The absence of any of these should not be used to rule out PE. Diagnosis requires a high index of suspicion.

Remember, PE is one of the causes of pulseless electrical activity.

PERC Score

Can be used to obviate the need for further testing in low-risk patients who have none of the following criteria:

- Age ≥ 50 years
- HR ≥ 100 bpm
- O_2 sat on room air < 95%
- Prior history of DVT/PE
- Recent trauma or surgery
- Hemoptysis
- Exogenous estrogen
- Unilateral leg swelling

Source: Kline JA, et al. Clinical criteria to prevent unnecessary diagnostic testing in emergency department patients with suspected pulmonary embolism. *J Thromb Haemost* 2004; 2: 1247–1255.

DIAGNOSIS

- ECG pattern of S1Q3T3 (Figure 6-2) is seen in less than one-fourth of patients. The most common rhythm is sinus tachycardia.
- Arterial blood oxygen levels are not useful in predicting the absence of PE, and a-A gradient is not considered a suitable screening test.
- Lower extremity venography studies are of value when positive but do not exclude PE when negative.
- The gold standard for the diagnosis of PE is pulmonary angiography. However, it is invasive, takes the patient away from the department, and has an up to 5% morbidity and mortality rate.
- Ventilation-perfusion scan can be a useful test in patients who cannot undergo spiral CT (eg, renal insufficiency). However, 15% of patients with low-probability ventilation-perfusion scans have had angiographically proven PE.
- Spiral CT is being used more often as the diagnostic test of choice. One advantage of spiral CT is its ability to identify alternative diagnoses.
- Enzyme-linked immunosorbent assay (ELISA) D-dimer tests are 90% sensitive but nonspecific. False positives occur with malignancy, pregnancy, trauma, infection, recent surgery, many inflammatory states, and advanced age. For this reason, it is most often restricted to use in young patients with low pretest probability of PE.

TREATMENT

- All patients should get oxygen.
- Anticoagulation is the mainstay of therapy and may consist of heparin (or a low-molecular-weight heparin such as enoxaparin) and coumadin.
- Thrombolytics should be considered for hemodynamically unstable patients.

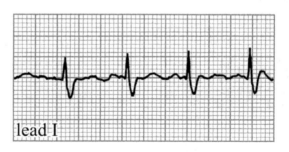

lead I

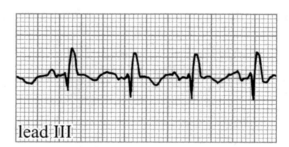

lead III

FIGURE 6-2. Classic $S_1Q_3T_3$ pattern of pulmonary embolism.

- Surgical options include an inferior vena cava filter (good for patients with contraindications to anticoagulation or who develop PE despite anticoagulation) and embolectomy (poor prognosis).

PLEURAL EFFUSION

DEFINITION

- The pleural space lies between the chest wall and the lung and is defined by the parietal and visceral pleuras. A very small amount of fluid is normally present, allowing the two pleural membranes to slide over each other during respiration. An abnormal amount of fluid (> 15 cc) in the pleural space is known as a pleural effusion.
- Pleural effusions are divided into transudates and exudates. Transudative effusions happen when there is either an ↑ in capillary hydrostatic pressure or a ↓ in colloid osmotic pressure. Both of these conditions will cause a net movement of fluid out of capillaries into the pleural space.

Most common causes of pleural effusion:
- CHF
- Bacterial pneumonia
- Malignancy

CAUSES OF TRANSUDATIVE EFFUSIONS

- CHF
- Hypoalbuminemia
- Cirrhosis
- PE
- Myxedema
- Nephrotic syndrome
- Superior vena cava obstruction
- Peritoneal dialysis

CAUSES OF EXUDATIVE EFFUSIONS

- Infection (pneumonia, tuberculosis [TB], fungi, parasites)
- Connective tissue diseases
- Neoplasm
- PE
- Uremia
- Pancreatitis
- Esophageal rupture
- Intra-abdominal abscess
- Post surgery or trauma
- Drug induced

DIAGNOSIS

Pleural fluid analysis:

- Transudate:
  - LDH < 200 U.
  - Fluid-to-blood LDH ratio < 0.6.
  - Fluid-to-blood protein ratio < 0.5.
- Exudate:
  - Glucose < 60 mg/dL in infection, neoplasm, rheumatoid arthritis, pleuritis.
  - Amylase: Elevated in esophageal rupture, pancreatitis, pancreatic pseudocyst, and some neoplasms.
  - Cell count.
  - Gram stain and culture.
  - Cytology.

TREATMENT

- Treat underlying cause.
- A thoracocentesis can be both diagnostic and therapeutic.

ASTHMA

Steroids are given in asthma to ↓ the late inflammatory response.

DEFINITION

Asthma is a disease in which the tracheobronchial tree is hyperreactive to stimuli, resulting in variable, reversible airway obstruction.

EPIDEMIOLOGY

- Incidence greater in men than women.
- Incidence greater in African-Americans.
- Half of cases develop by age 17 and two-thirds by age 40 years.

EXTRINSIC ASTHMA

- Sensitivity to inhaled allergens.
- Immunoglobulin E response.
- Causally related in a third of asthma cases and a contributing factor in another third.
- Frequently seasonal.
- Early asthmatic response is mast cell dependent and results in acute bronchoconstriction.
- Late asthmatic response is an inflammatory reaction that → prolonged airway responsiveness.

Drugs most commonly associated with acute asthma exacerbations are aspirin and beta blockers.

NONIMMUNOLOGIC PRECIPITANTS OF ASTHMA

- Exercise
- Infections
- Pharmacologic stimuli
- Environmental pollution
- Occupational stimuli
- Emotional stress
- Diet

SIGNS AND SYMPTOMS

- Dyspnea.
- Wheezing.
- Cough.
- Chest tightness.
- Severe exacerbation: Use of accessory muscles, tripod position, hypoxia, tachypnea, impending respiratory failure.

Early asthmatic response lasts a few hours. Late asthmatic response hyperresponsiveness can persist for weeks to months.

EMERGENCY TREATMENT

- The mainstay of therapy is oxygen and beta agonist (albuterol) nebulizers.
- Corticosteroids are added for moderate asthma.
- Severe asthma may require epinephrine or terbutaline, magnesium sulfate and heliox.
- Consider BiPAP (or CPAP) to help prevent need for intubation.
- Impending respiratory failure will require intubation.
- Peak flows may be measured to monitor response to therapy.

OUTPATIENT MANAGEMENT OPTIONS

- Leukotriene inhibitors (eg, zafirlukast, montelukast)
- Mast cell stabilizing agents (eg, cromolyn sodium)
- Methylxanthines (eg, theophylline, aminophylline)

CHRONIC OBSTRUCTIVE PULMONARY DISEASE (COPD)

DEFINITIONS

- Three separate disease entities are part of the classification of COPD. These are asthma, bronchitis, and emphysema. Asthma is discussed above.
- Chronic bronchitis is defined as a condition in which excessive mucus is produced. The mucus production is enough to cause productive cough for a minimum of 3 months out of the year in at least 2 consecutive years.
- Emphysema is a disease in which there is distention of the air spaces distal to the terminal bronchioles and destruction of alveolar septa. Alveolar septa are important for providing support of the bronchial walls. Their destruction → airway collapse, especially during expiration

EPIDEMIOLOGY

Third most common cause of hospitalization and fourth most common cause of death (after stroke) in the United States.

RISK FACTORS

- Smoking
- Air pollution
- Occupational exposure
- Infection
- Genetic (eg, α_1-antitrypsin deficiency)

SIGNS AND SYMPTOMS OF CHRONIC BRONCHITIS

- History of cough and sputum production
- History of smoking
- Commonly overweight
- Cyanosis
- Right ventricular (RV) failure
- Normal total lung capacity
- ↑ residual volume
- Normal to slightly ↓ vital capacity

SIGNS AND SYMPTOMS OF EMPHYSEMA

- Exertional dyspnea.
- Thin to cachectic.
- Tachypnea.
- Prolonged expiratory phase often with pursed lips.
- Use of accessory muscles of respiration.
- ↑ total lung capacity and residual volume.
- ↓ vital capacity.

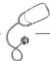

ED treatment of asthma—

BIOMES
Beta agonists
Ipratropium
Oxygen
Magnesium sulfate
Epinephrine
Steroids

Patients with chronic bronchitis are sometimes referred to as "blue bloaters."

Patients with emphysema are sometimes referred to as "pink puffers."

HIGH-YIELD FACTS

Respiratory Emergencies

159

- **Acute:**
  - Oxygen (correct to at least > 90%).
  - Nebulized beta agonist.
  - Intravenous or oral corticosteroids.
  - Antibiotics if underlying pneumonia is suspected.
- **Chronic:**
  - Smoking cessation
  - Optimize nutrition
  - Regular exercise
  - Home O_2 if needed
  - Control of respiratory infections

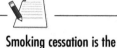

Smoking cessation is the most important treatment for COPD.

TUBERCULOSIS (TB)

TB infection and subsequent scarring of the fallopian tubes used to be a common cause of infertility.

DEFINITION

Mycobacterium tuberculosis is an intracellular, aerobic, acid-fast bacillus that infects humans. It is primarily spread through the respiratory route.

PATHOPHYSIOLOGY

- Bacillus normally enters through the lungs.
- Macrophage phagocytoses bacillus.
- Bacillus multiplies intracellularly in the macrophage until it lyses the macrophage and repeats the process.
- Cell-mediated immunity, through T-helper cells, activates macrophages, destroying infected cells.
- Epithelioid cell granulomas are produced that wall off the primary lesion; remaining bacilli can survive within granulomas for years.
- Months to years later, bacilli can reactivate.

SIGNS AND SYMPTOMS

- Primary TB is usually asymptomatic.
- Reactivation pulmonary TB is the syndrome most commonly seen:
  - Cough
  - Fever
  - Night sweats
  - Weight loss
  - Hemoptysis
  - Fatigue
  - Anorexia
- Extrapulmonary TB occurs in 15% of cases and can be seen in the pericardium, skeletal system, gastrointestinal/genitourinary systems, adenoids, peritoneum, adrenal glands, and skin.

- **Purified protein derivative (PPD) testing:**
  - \> 5-mm induration considered positive in:
    - Persons with HIV or risk factors and unknown HIV status.
    - Close household contacts of person with active TB.
    - Persons with evidence of primary TB on x-ray.
  - \> 10 mm positive in high-risk groups:
    - Intravenous drug users who are HIV negative.
    - Persons from high-prevalence areas.
    - Persons with other medical conditions that render them debilitated or immunocompromised.
  - \> 15 mm is considered positive in all other individuals.
- **CXR:**
  - Most useful test in the emergency department (ED).
  - Active TB usually presents with parenchymal infiltrates. Most common locations for TB in the lung include apices and posterior segments of upper lobes (areas of highest blood flow and oxygen tension).
  - Miliary TB presents as small diffuse nodules (millet seed appearance).
  - Pulmonary lesions can be calcified or cavitated. Cavitation implies higher infectivity.
- Sputum and blood can be cultured for *M tuberculosis* via acid-fast staining (results not available for a few weeks).
- Mantoux/PPD testing result also not available immediately; usually read 48–72 hours after placement. A positive test does not necessarily imply active TB; rather, it detects latent, prior, and active TB, so it is not that useful in the ED. Note that immunocompromised patients may have false-negative Mantoux tests; in this case an "anergy panel" is applied.

Tuberculous adenitis is known as *scrofula*.

A Ghon complex is a calcified lesion of *primary* pulmonary TB.

TREATMENT

- Patient with suspected TB should be masked and placed in respiratory isolation (negative pressure) room.
- Health care workers should wear respiration masks when feasible.
- Initial therapy consists of four drugs, usually isoniazid, rifampin, pyrazinamide, and ethambutol or streptomycin for a 2-month period (see Table 6-2 for adverse effects).
- Patients with active multidrug-resistant TB should be admitted to the hospital.
- Patients with reliable follow-up who are clinically stable with adequate socioeconomic situation may be discharged home. Patients at risk for noncompliance may require directly observed treatment (DOT) wherein a health care worker physically administers the medication to the patient daily.
- Bacille Calmette-Guérin (BCG) vaccine: Given frequently in countries outside the United States. Interferes with the Mantoux test (false positive). In the United States, should be considered only for select persons in consultation with a TB expert.

Miliary TB results from hematogenous spread.

Tuberculosis of the spine is known as Pott disease.

HIGH-YIELD FACTS

Respiratory Emergencies

TABLE 6-2. Potential Adverse Effects of First-Line TB Medications

DRUG	POTENTIAL ADVERSE EFFECTS
Isoniazid	Hepatitis, peripheral neuropathy, drug interaction with phenytoin and carbamazepine
Rifampin	Orange body fluids, hepatitis, gastrointestinal (GI) intolerance, thrombocytopenia, cholestatatic jaundice, significant drug interactions
Pyrazinamide	Hepatitis, hyperuricemia, rash, GI intolerance, thrombocytopenia, cholestatic jaundice, significant drug interactions
Ethambutol	Retrobulbar optic neuritis, color blindness, headache
Streptomycin (IM only)	Ototoxicity, nephrotoxicity

Patients die of massive hemoptysis secondary to *asphyxiation*, rather than *exsanguination*.

Bronchiectasis is persistent and progressive dilation of bronchi or bronchioles as a consequence of chronic infections, tumor, or cystic fibrosis. Coughing, fetid breath, and expectoration of mucopurulent matter are hallmarks.

HEMOPTYSIS

DEFINITION

Coughing up of blood due to bleeding from the lower respiratory tract. Minor hemoptysis is < 5 mL blood in a 24-hour period. Massive hemoptysis is > 600 mL of bleeding in a 24-hour period, or bleeding that results in clinical impairment of respiratory function.

ETIOLOGY

See Table 6-3.

TREATMENT

- Supplemental oxygen.
- Have patient sit up with head of the bed elevated.
- Place patient with radiographically abnormal lung (presumably bleeding side) down when recumbent.
- Codeine to control coughing.
- Massive hemoptysis may require surgical intervention and/or invasive measures such as endobronchial cold saline or epinephrine, bronchial artery embolization, and mainstem bronchus intubation in the good lung (eg, tube in right mainstem bronchus if bleeding is on the left).

VENTILATOR MECHANICS

The O_2 saturation of a patient with a pneumonia who is on a ventilator is dropping slightly. What should be done?

The FIo_2 should be ↑ or PEEP should be added in order to improve oxygenation. Increasing the respiratory rate or the tidal volume will not affect oxygenation but will improve ventilation. The cause of the ↑ oxygen should be explored. Consider issues with obstruction, the ventilator settings, sedation, pneumothorax, or worsening disease. When in doubt, take the patient off the ventilator and bag the patient.

TABLE 6-3. Causes of Hemoptysis

PULMONARY

Airway diseases	▪ Bronchitis
	▪ Bronchiectasis
	▪ Cystic fibrosis
Neoplasms	▪ Bronchogenic carcinoma
	▪ Bronchial carcinoid
Infections	▪ Tuberculosis
	▪ Pneumonia
	▪ Lung abscess
	▪ Aspergilloma
Pulmonary vascular diseases	▪ Pulmonary thromboembolism
	▪ Pulmonary vasculitis
	▪ Arteriovenous malformations
	▪ Bronchovascular fistula
Pulmonary renal syndromes	▪ Wegener granulomatosis
	▪ Goodpasture syndrome
	▪ Systemic lupus erythematosus
Cardiovascular	▪ Mitral stenosis
	▪ Congestive heart failure
Miscellaneous	▪ Use of anticoagulants or fibrinolytics
	▪ Bleeding diathesis
	▪ Factitious hemoptysis (bleeding from nasopharynx or gastrointestinal tract)
	▪ Pulmonary contusion/trauma
	▪ Iatrogenic (pulmonary artery rupture secondary to pulmonary arterial catheterization)
	▪ Idiopathic pulmonary hemosiderosis

TYPES OF VENTILATORS

- Noninvasive ventilation such as BiPAP or CPAP uses a facemask to ventilate the patient.
- Pressure-cycled ventilation delivers volume until a preset peak inspiratory pressure is reached.
- Volume-cycled ventilation delivers a preset tidal volume.
- Time-cycled ventilation delivers volume until a preset time is reached.

Ventilatory rate is initially set at 12–14 bpm.

HIGH-YIELD FACTS

Respiratory Emergencies

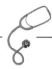

Tidal volume is initially set at 6–10 mL/kg. If concern for developing adult respiratory distress syndrome (ARDS), use lower volumes of 6 mL/kg.

PEEP improves oxygenation by keeping alveoli open during expiration.

CMV is useful in patients with no spontaneous respirations, heavily sedated patients, and paralyzed patients.

VENTILATOR SETTINGS

- Ventilator mode
- Ventilatory rate
- Tidal volume
- Inspired oxygen concentration
- Positive end-expiratory pressure (PEEP)
- Inspiratory-expiratory ratio

VENTILATOR MODES

- Controlled mechanical ventilation (CMV): The patient is ventilated at a preset rate; the patient cannot breathe between the delivered breaths.
- Assist-control ventilation: A minimum rate is set, but if the patient attempts to take additional breaths, the machine will deliver a breath with a preset tidal volume.
- Intermittent mandatory ventilation and synchronized intermittent mandatory ventilation (SIMV): The machine delivers a preset number of breaths at the preset tidal volume; additional breaths initiated by the patient will have a tidal volume dependent on the patient's effort. In SIMV, the machine breaths are synchronized so as not to interfere with spontaneous breaths.
- Pressure support: Patient determines respiratory rate, and tidal volume depends on both the patient's pulmonary compliance and the preset inspiratory pressure.

ADULT RESPIRATORY DISTRESS SYNDROME (ARDS)

- ARDS or acute lung injury occurs in response to an insult to the lung which leads to capillary leakage producing severe hypoxia and reduced lung compliance.
- Conditions that may lead to ARDS include trauma, sepsis, shock, toxic exposures, and aspirations.
- Treatment is targeted at the underlying cause and mainly supportive.

FOREIGN BODY

SIGNS AND SYMPTOMS

- Cough
- Wheezing
- May be asymptomatic

DIAGNOSIS

Inspiratory/expiratory CXR.

TREATMENT

Removal by direct laryngoscopy or bronchoscopy.

- Most commonly caused by respiratory syncytial virus (RSV).
- Primarily children < 1 year of age.
- Most severe in premature children < 6 months.

SIGNS AND SYMPTOMS

- Respiratory distress
- Cough
- Wheezing
- Tachypnea
- Apnea

DIAGNOSIS

- Clinical suspicion
- Interstitial infiltrates on CXR
- Nasal swabs for RSV

TREATMENT

- Supportive:
  - Oxygen
  - Beta-agonist bronchodilators (not proven to be helpful)
  - Suctioning
- Ribavirin:
  - Theoretical risk to health care workers
  - Reserved for severe disease

HIGH-YIELD FACTS

Respiratory Emergencies

Cardiovascular Emergencies

■ Chest pain (CP) is one of the most common emergency department (ED) complaints. The differential is broad (see Figure 7-1), but the eight most emergent causes include:
1. Acute coronary syndrome (ACS)
2. Aortic dissection
3. Pericarditis/myocarditis
4. Tension pneumothorax (see Trauma chapter)
5. Pulmonary embolus (see Respiratory Emergencies chapter)
6. Esophageal rupture (see Gastrointestinal Emergencies chapter)
7. Perforated peptic ulcer (see Gastrointestinal Emergencies chapter)
8. Pneumonia (see Respiratory Emergencies chapter)

■ ED evaluation of CP consists of rapid determination as to whether the CP represents a potentially life-threatening cause. The history and physical can provide helpful clues.

■ Features of history that ↑ likelihood that CP is due to ACS (in order of decreasing probability):
  ▪ Substernal location of CP.
  ▪ Pain lasts from 30 minutes to 3 hours, of gradual onset.
  ▪ Pain is described as crushing, squeezing, tightness or pressure ("like an elephant sitting on my chest"), rather than knifelike, sharp, stabbing, or pins and needles.
  ▪ Pain is accompanied by diaphoresis or "impending sense of doom."
  ▪ Pain is similar to previous anginal pain.
  ▪ Family history of first-degree male relative with ACS at age 50 years or younger.
  ▪ Pain radiating to left, right, or both arms.

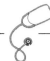

Levine sign: A patient puts a clenched fist to his chest to describe the pain of myocardial ischemia.

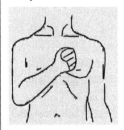

HIGH-YIELD FACTS

Cardiovascular Emergencies

Cardiac	**Pulmonary**
Myocardial ischemia/acute coronary syndrome	Pulmonary embolism
Coronary vasospasm	Pleuritis
Dissecting aortic aneurysm	Mediastinitis
Pericarditis	Spontaneous pneumothorax
Myocarditis	Pneumonia
Aortic stenosis	Neoplasm
Hypertropic cardiomyopathy	Bronchitis
Mitral valve prolapse	
	Musculoskeletal
	Herpes zoster
GI	Costochondritis
Esophageal rupture (Boerhaave's)	Rib fracture
Esophageal tear (Mallory–Weiss)	Myalgia
Esophageal spasm	Chest wall pain
Reflux esophagitis	
Cholecystitis/biliary colic	
Pancreatitis	

FIGURE 7-1. Differential diagnosis of chest pain.

Contraindications to NTG:

- Patients who have taken phosphodiesterase inhibitors such as sildenafil (Viagra), vardenafil (Levitra), or tadalafil (Cialis) in the preceding 24 hours.
- Patients with inferior wall MI.
- Severe hypotension can result in these cases.

Contraindications to beta blockers:

- Heart rate (HR) < 60 bpm
- Systolic BP < 100 mm Hg
- Second- or third-degree heart block
- Moderate to severe left ventricular (LV) dysfunction
- Severe chronic obstructive pulmonary disease (COPD) or asthma
- Signs of peripheral hypoperfusion
- PR interval > 0.24 msec
- Acute MI due to cocaine

- Features of physical exam that ↑ likelihood that CP is due to ACS (in order of decreasing probability):
  - Diaphoresis
  - Nausea/vomiting
  - New S3 sound
  - Hypotension (systolic blood pressure < 80 mm Hg)
  - Lung crackles
- **Women,** the **elderly,** and **diabetics** tend to present with *atypical* symptoms, including:
  - Dyspnea alone
  - Nausea/vomiting
  - Palpitations
  - Syncope
  - Weakness
  - Fatigue
  - Cardiac arrest
- Chest pain may or may not be present in these populations.

EVALUATION OF ACUTE CORONARY SYNDROME (ACS)

An 85-year-old woman presents to the emergency department with 8 hours of epigastric burning and nausea. She also feels weak and tired. She is afebrile, with a pulse of 85 bpm and BP 174/92 mm Hg. Her physical exam reveals clear lungs and benign abdomen. Her electrocardiogram (ECG) reveals ST elevation in leads II, III, and F with reciprocal depressions in V_1–V_3. What is the next step in the management of this patient?

The patient is presenting with an acute STEMI. Women and the elderly often present with atypical symptoms, as in this case. Diabetics also can infarct without experiencing chest pain. The ECG represents ST elevations in the inferior leads represents an inferior MI. Inferior ischemia can often present with abdominal/GI symptoms. The treatment of choice is emergent percutaneous transluminal coronary angioplasty in < 90 minutes from time of presentation. Thrombolytic therapy is an alternative to angioplasty, but comes with high risk in an older patient.

Acute coronary syndromes can be classified as ST segment elevation myocardial infarction (STEMI), non–ST segment elevation myocardial infarction (NSTEMI), or unstable angina (UA). NSTEMI and UA are thought to represent the ends of the same disease process spectrum.

Angina is considered "unstable" if:

1. It lasts longer than 20 minutes or frequency is ↑ from baseline.
2. It is new onset and markedly limits physical activity.
3. Onset occurs at rest.

Unstable angina with elevated serum cardiac biomarkers is NSTEMI.

MANAGEMENT OF ACS

1. Airway, breathing, circulation (ABCs) assessed.
2. Intravenous (IV) O_2 monitor.
3. 12-lead electrocardiogram (ECG) obtained. If evidence of STEMI, see section on reperfusion therapy below.
4. Laboratory analyses obtained: cardiac biomarkers (see Table 7-1), complete blood count (CBC), electrolytes, coagulation studies, and drug levels (eg, digoxin) if relevant.
5. Chewable aspirin 162–325 mg unless patient is allergic or had it prior to arrival.
6. Sublingual (SL) nitroglycerin (NTG) provides analgesia and coronary dilatation; 0.4 mg should be given SL q 5 minutes up to total of three doses. If patient transiently responds to NTG but pain returns, IV NTG can be started.
7. IV morphine 4 mg should be administered for analgesia with titrated increments of 2–10 mg repeated in 5- to 15-minute intervals. Reduces excess catecholamine release.
8. Unfractionated heparin or low molecular weight heparin may be used in high risk patients.
9. **Other antiplatelet agents like glycoprotein** *2b3a inhibitors and* clopidogrel maybe used for patients undergoing percutaneous intervention.

DISPOSITION

Patients suspected of having ACS will require further diagnostic testing, which includes serial biomarkers and possible stress testing or coronary CT angiography.

DIAGNOSIS OF STEMI

- Elevation of > 1 mm in ST segments of two or more contiguous segments (Figure 7-2).
- New left bundle branch block (LBBB).

REPERFUSION THERAPY FOR STEMI

- Reperfusion therapy is given for STEMI within 12 hours of onset. There are two options: pharmacologic thrombolytics (eg, alteplase, reteplase, tenecteplase, streptokinase, urokinase) and percutaneous coronary intervention (PCI or "cardiac catheterization").

Sgarbossa Criteria for Impending MI in LBBB:
1. ST elevation > 1 mm in leads with dominant R waves (concordant with QRS complex)
2. ST elevation > 5 mm in leads with dominant S waves (discordant with QRS complex)
3. ST depression > 1 mm in V_1, V_2, or V_3

Absolute contraindications to thrombolytic therapy:
- History of intracranial hemorrhage
- History of ischemic stroke > 3 hours but < 3 month
- Cerebral vascular malformation
- Intracranial malignancy
- Symptoms or signs suggestive of an aortic dissection
- Bleeding diathesis
- Active bleeding
- Significant closed-head or facial trauma < 3 months

TABLE 7-1. Cardiac Biomarkers

ENZYME/CARDIAC BIOMARKER	RISE (HOURS POST AFTER CP)	PEAK (HOURS)	RETURN TO BASELINE
Myoglobin	1–2 h	4–6 h	24 h
Troponin	3–6 h	12–24 h	7–10 days
Creatine kinase, total and MB fraction	4–6 h	12–36 h	3–4 days
Lactate dehydrogenase	6–12 h	24–48 h	6–8 days

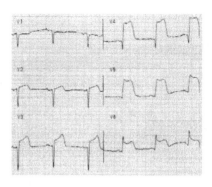

FIGURE 7-2. Anterolateral STEMI.

Relative contraindications to thrombolytic therapy
- History of chronic, severe, poorly controlled hypertension (HTN)
- Severe uncontrolled hypertension on presentation >180/110 mm Hg
- Recent (within 2–4 week) internal bleeding
- Traumatic or prolonged (>10 min) CPR
- Major surgery within the preceding 3 weeks
- Current use of anticoagulant (eg, warfarin) with INR 1.7
- Pregnancy

- The American College of Cardiology (ACC)/American Heart Association (AHA) class I recommendation for reperfusion therapy is as follows: primary PCI is preferred to thrombolytics when it can be performed within 90 minutes of presentation and if the patient is in severe congestive heart failure (CHF) or cardiogenic shock. If primary PCI is > 90 minutes away, thrombolytics should be administered unless any contraindications exist (see box).

RISK STRATIFICATION IN ACS

The TIMI Risk Score is a stratification tool developed by the Thrombolysis in Myocardial Infarction (TIMI) group that can be helpful to categorize patients into high- and low-risk groups. This score has been prospectively validated in several studies. Separate scores have been developed for UA/NSTEMI and STEMI. For UA/NSTEMI, the TIMI Risk Score may be helpful for disposition decisions (hospital admission vs. observation unit vs. discharge home). A score of 5 or more is considered high risk, 3–4 intermediate risk, and 0–2 low risk (see Figure 7-3 and 7-4).

Age > 65 years
Presence of three or more cardiac risk factors:
    Male gender
    MI in male relatives < 50 years of age
    Cigarette smoking
    Hypertension
    Diabetes mellitus
    Hypercholesterolemia
Aspirin use within last 7 days
Two or more anginal events within last 24 hours
ST segment elevation on initial ECG
Elevated cardiac biomarkers
Prior coronary artery stenosis > 50%

FIGURE 7-3. TIMI Risk Score for UA/NSTEMI (1 point for each).

(Data from Antman EM, Cohen M, Bernink PJ, et al. The TIMI Risk Score for unstable angina/non-ST elevation MI: A method for prognostication and therapeutic decision making. *JAMA* 2000;284:835–842.)

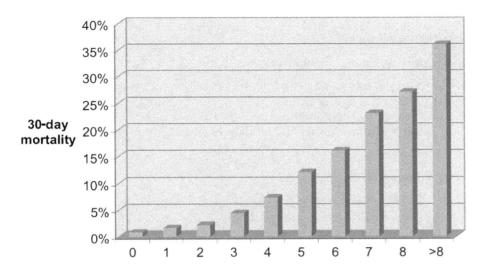

FIGURE 7-4. Risk of death at 30 days for STEMI based on ED TIMI score.

PACEMAKERS

DEFINITION

- Most pacers use a three-letter code; advanced functions are described by a fourth/fifth letter:
  1. Pacing chamber: V (ventricular), A (atrial), or D (dual)
  2. Sensing chamber: V, A, or D
  3. I (inhibited), T (triggered), D (dual)
  4. P (programmable rate), C (communications stored), R (rate responsive)
  5. P (pacing), S (shock), D (dual), 0 (neither)

- Transcutaneous pacing: Indicated in refractory bradycardia with hypotension when a transvenous pacemaker cannot be placed quickly.
- Transvenous pacing: Pacemaker wire is passed through central venous access line into heart for pacing.

EMERGENT PACEMAKER PLACEMENT INDICATIONS

Symptoms of cardiovascular compromise associated with:

- New bi-/trifascicular block with acute ischemia:
  - Mobitz type II AV block
  - Third-degree or complete AV block
- Significant bradycardia (< 40 bpm)

MOST COMMON PROBLEMS

- Failure to capture
- Failure to sense
- Undersensing
- Oversensing

First-Degree AV Block

First degree (prolonged PR interval—see Figure 7-5):

- Prolonged conduction of atrial impulses without loss of any impulses
- PR interval > 0.20 second
- Benign and asymptomatic
- Doesn't warrant further ED workup or treatment

Second-Degree AV Block, Type I

Second-degree, Mobitz type I (Wenckebach—see Figure 7-6): Progressive prolongation of PR interval with each successive beat until there is a loss of AV conduction and hence a dropped beat or failure of ventricles to depolarize (P wave but no QRS). RR interval appears irregular.

Second-Degree AV Block, Type II

Second degree, Mobitz type II (see Figure 7-7):

- Random loss of conduction and beat below the AV node without change in PR interval (His-Purkinje system) (P, no QRS). RR interval regular except for drop beats.
- Potentially serious pathology present.
- Can be seen with anterior wall MI.
- Often progresses to complete AV block (third degree).

Third-Degree AV Block

Third degree (complete AV dissociation [see Figure 7-8]):

- No conduction of atrial signal and P wave through to the ventricle, and hence independent atrial and ventricular rhythms.
- Either congenital (with associated anatomic anomalies) or acquired (many causes—idiopathic fibrosis most common).
- Patients present with tachypnea, dyspnea on exertion, cyanosis, or syncope.
- ECG shows no correlation between atrial (faster) and ventricular (slower) rhythms; P waves "march through" the rhythm strip ignoring the QRS complexes.

Type II second-degree block has a worse prognosis than type I.

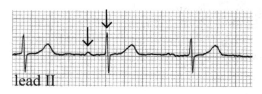

FIGURE 7-5. First-degree AV block. PR interval >0.2.

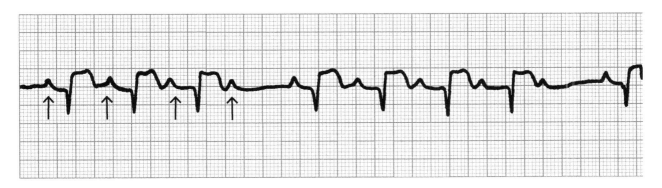

FIGURE 7-6. Mobitz I (Wenckebach) second-degree AV block.

TREATMENT

- ABCs, IV access, O₂, monitor.
- Immediate transcutaneous or transvenous pacemaker.
- Eventual implantable pacemaker if no reversible cause found.
- Treat underlying cause if possible.

Left Anterior Fascicular Block (LAFB)

ECG:

- Left axis deviation (LAD).
- QRS duration 0.10 to 0.12 second.
- Peak of terminal R in aVL precedes peak of terminal R in aVR.
- Deep S waves in II, III, and aVF.
- Lead I R wave > leads II or III.

Left Posterior Fascicular Block (LPFB)

ECG:

- Right axis deviation
- QRS duration 0.10–0.12 second
- Small R and deep S in lead I
- Lead III R wave > lead II
- Small Q in II, III, and aVF

Causes of AV Blocks
- Age
- Ischemia
- Cardiomyopathies
- Myocarditis
- Congenital
- Surgery
- Valvular disease
- Drugs

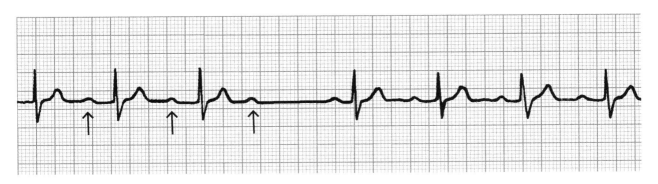

FIGURE 7-7. Mobitz II second-degree AV block.

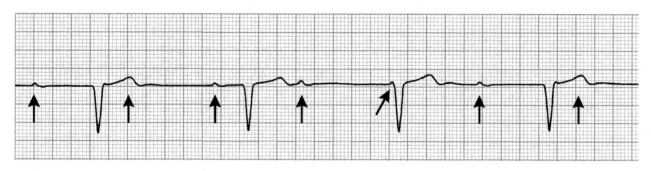

FIGURE 7-8. Third-degree (complete) AV block.

Note the P waves (arrows) "marching through."

Presence of new LBBB may indicate acute MI.

Left Bundle Branch Block (LBBB)

- Conduction blocked before anterior and posterior fascicles split (Figure 7-9).
- Ischemia can be masked with LBBB. Use of Sgarbossa criteria can be helpful.
  1. Point system for determining acute ischemic change in the presence of LBBB (the more points, the more likely is ischemia):
  2. ST segment elevation ≥ 1 mm concordant (in the same direction) with its QRS axis = 5 points.
  3. ST segment elevation ≥ 1 mm in V_1–V_3 = 3 points.
  4. ST segment elevation ≥ 5 mm, discordant with QRS = 2 points.
  5. Score ≥ 3 predicts MI.
- ECG:
  - QRS duration > 0.12 second.
  - ST and T waves directed opposite to terminal 0.04-second QRS.
  - No Q waves in I, aVF, V_5, V_6.
  - Large wide R waves in I, aVL, V_5, V_6.

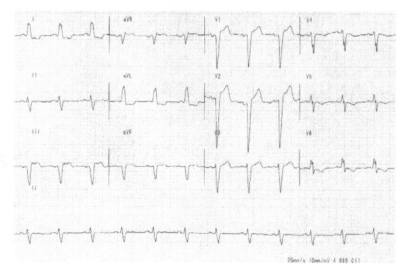

FIGURE 7-9. Left bundle branch block.

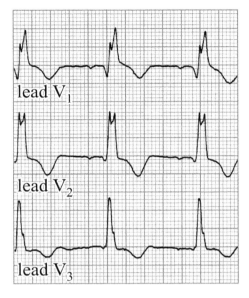

FIGURE 7-10. Right bundle branch block.

Note the M-shaped QRS complex (R,R').

Right Bundle Branch Block (RBBB)

- Ischemia is not masked with RBBB (see Figure 7-10), except in leads V_1–V_3.
- ECG:
  - QRS duration > 0.12 second.
  - Triphasic QRS complexes.
  - Regular sinus rhythm (RSR) described as "rabbit ears" in morphology in V_1, V_2.
  - Wide S waves in I, aVL, V_5, V_6.

DYSRHYTHMIAS

Prolonged QT Syndrome

DEFINITION

- $QT_c > 430$ msec in men
- $QT_c > 450$ msec in women

SIGNS AND SYMPTOMS

- Syncopal episodes.
- Can predispose to paroxysmal episodes of ventricular tachycardia and torsade de pointes by "R-on-T phenomenon." This is when a premature ventricular complex–QRS fires at the same time as the peak of the T wave or "vulnerable period" in ventricular repolarization (when some but not all myocardial tissue is ready for the signal) inducing ventricular tachycardia or ventricular fibrillation via a ventricular reentry pathway.

Causes of prolonged QT—

QT WIDTH

QT: Prolonged QT syndromes, including Romano-Ward and Jervell and Lange-Nielsen

Wolff-Parkinson-White (WPW) syndrome

Infarction

Drugs

Torsades

Hypocalcemia, hypokalemia, hypomagnesemia

Prolonged QT and hypertrophic cardiomyopathy are causes of sudden death in young people.

If the RR distance is at least one inch, consider —
One INCH
Overmedication
Inferior wall MI, Increased intracranial pressure
Normal variant
Carotid sinus hypersensitivity
Hypothyroidism

Sinus bradycardia is commonly seen in inferior wall MI, but usually resolves within 1–2 days.

DIAGNOSIS

- QT_I (QT interval) = 0.34 to 0.42 second or 40% of RR interval
- QT_c = HR corrected QT = $QT_I \div \sqrt{RR}$

See Diagnostics chapter, Figure 2-1, for ECG of prolonged QT.

TREATMENT

- ABCs, monitor.
- Correct electrolytes.
- Discontinue offending medications (Table 7-2).
- If inherited, beta blockers to ↓ sympathetic stimulus and implantable overdrive pacemaker/defibrillator.
- Magnesium sulfate IV for torsade de pointes.

Sinus Bradycardia

DEFINITION

HR < 60 bpm and regular:

- P wave prior to every QRS complex
- Upright Ps in I and aVF
- Narrow (< 0.12 second) QRS complexes

ETIOLOGY

- Can be normal, especially in athletes
- Hypoxemia
- Hypothyroidism
- Excessive vagal tone
- Hypothermia
- Medication side effects: Beta blockers, digoxin, Ca^{2+} channel blockers, cholinergic toxins

TREATMENT

- Correct underlying problem.
- In code situation, give atropine 0.5–1.0 mg IV followed by epinephrine and transcutaneous pacing.
- May require transvenous pacemaker if severe and there is evidence of cardiac compromise.

Sinus Tachycardia

DEFINITION

- HR > 100 bpm and regular
- Usually < 150 bpm
- P wave prior to every QRS complex
- Upright Ps in I and aVF
- Narrow QRS complexes

ETIOLOGY

- Anemia
- Dehydration/hypovolemia
- Fever
- Sepsis

TABLE 7-2. Drugs That Prolong the QT_c Interval

Antiarrhythmics
- Amiodarone
- Flecainide
- Quinidine (Quinaglute, Cardioquin)
- Procainamide (Pronestyl, Procan)
- Sotalol (Betapace)
- Bepridil (Vasocor)
- Disopyramide (Norpace)
- Dofetilide (Tikosyn)
- Ibutilide (Corvert)

Antimicrobials
- Sparfloxacin (Zagam)
- Pentamidine (Pentam)
- Quinolone antibiotics (eg, levofloxacin)
- Macrolide antibiotics (eg, erythromycin, clarithromycin)
- Fluconazole (Diflucan)
- Chloroquine (Arelan)

Antidepressants
- Fluoxetine (Prozac)
- Quetiapine (Seroquel)
- Sertraline (Zoloft)

Antipsychotics
- Chlorpromazine (Thorazine)
- Haloperidol (Haldol)
- Mesoridazine (Serentil)
- Pimozide (Orap)
- Thioridazine (Mellaril)

Other
- Cisapride (Propulsid)
- Salmeterol (Serevent)
- Arsenic trioxide (Trisenox)

- Drug overdose
- Anxiety
- Hypermetabolic state

TREATMENT

Correct underlying problem.

Atrial Ectopy

- **Premature atrial complexes (PACs):** Abnormal electrical focus triggers an atrial contraction before the sinus node fires, thus triggering a QRS and ventricular contraction. There is a compensatory pause (longer RR interval) before the next sinus beat. Benign and asymptomatic.
- **Wandering atrial pacemaker:** ≥ 3 different P wave morphologies/foci in a normal 12-lead ECG rhythm strip with an HR between 60 and 100 bpm. QRS follows each P wave. Usually asymptomatic; patient may complain of palpitations or anxiety.
- **Multifocal atrial tachycardia (MAT):** Wandering atrial pacemaker with a rate > 100 bpm. Patient is usually symptomatic (dyspnea, diaphoresis, ± angina). Associated with COPD and theophylline overdose. Rate is often difficult to control.

Atrial Flutter

- Rapid atrial depolarization (240–350 bpm) from an abnormal focus within the atria and variable ventricular conduction described as block (ie, 2:1–4:1 flutter [see Figure 7-11]).

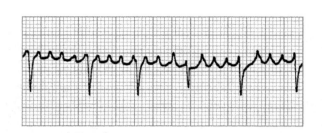

FIGURE 7-11. Atrial flutter.

- Can be considered a transitional dysrhythmia between normal sinus and atrial fibrillation.
- Causes are same as for atrial fibrillation.

Atrial Fibrillation

DEFINITION

Very rapid atrial depolarization (350–600 bpm) from many ectopic atrial foci, usually with ineffective conduction to ventricles.

ETIOLOGY

- Hypertensive heart disease
- Ischemic heart disease
- Valvular heart disease
- Alcohol
- Thyrotoxicosis
- Lung disease
- Fever

EPIDEMIOLOGY

- Most common sustained cardiac dysrhythmia, very frequently seen in the ED.
- Lifetime risk for developing atrial fibrillation is 25% for men and women over age 40 (Framingham Heart Study).

PATHOPHYSIOLOGY

- Rapid ventricular response gives ineffective systole (from poor filling) and subsequent heart failure/pulmonary edema, palpitations, or angina.
- Presence of atrial fibrillation predisposes to atrial blood stasis and subsequent clotting, which can embolize and cause stroke.
- Ineffective atrial contraction results in complete loss of atrial kick and its contribution to cardiac output, most relevant to those with heart failure.

DIAGNOSIS

- ECG (see Figure 7-12):
  - Irregularly irregular ventricular rhythm.
  - Narrow QRS complexes (unless coexistent bundle branch block or aberrant ventricular conduction).
  - Ventricular rate can be rapid (uncontrolled) or controlled (with medications).

Causes of atrial fibrillation—
PIRATES
Pulmonary disease
Ischemia
Rheumatic heart disease
Anemia, atrial myxoma
Thyrotoxicosis
Ethanol
Sepsis

Atrial fibrillation and stroke: Atrial fibrillation ↑ the risk of acute ischemic stroke (AIS) fivefold. It is responsible for 15–20% of all AIS.

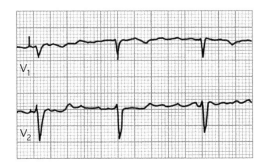

FIGURE 7-12. Atrial fibrillation.

Note lack of distinct P waves.

- Echocardiography should be done to identify structural heart disease and rule out atrial thrombi prior to electrical cardioversion (transesophageal).
- Labs: Check CBC, cardiac enzymes, thyroid function tests (TFTs), and ethanol level to look for underlying cause.

TREATMENT

- ABCs, IV, O_2, monitor.
- Control ventricular response rate to between 60 and 100 with AV nodal blocking drug (Ca^{2+} channel blocker or beta blocker acutely, and digoxin long term).
- Consider elective cardioversion (see Procedures chapter) if < 48 hours duration. If > 48 hours, anticoagulate for 4 weeks prior to cardioversion (or until transesophageal echo demonstrates no atrial clot). Emergency cardioversion if severe compromise refractory to medications, regardless of duration (rare).
- Anticoagulation in new-onset atrial fibrillation is mandatory because of the significant risk for embolization, which can result in stroke, ischemic bowel, and deep venous thrombosis.
- Consider and treat for ACS as appropriate.

Supraventricular Tachycardia (SVT)

DEFINITION

Narrow QRS complex tachycardia with regular RR intervals at a rate of 150–250 bpm.

ETIOLOGY

- Due to either ↑ atrial automaticity or reentry phenomenon.
- Etiologies similar to atrial fibrillation.

SIGNS AND SYMPTOMS

- Dyspnea
- Palpitations
- Angina
- Diaphoresis
- Varying degrees of hemodynamic stability

SVT is the most common pediatric dysrhythmia.

HIGH-YIELD FACTS

Cardiovascular Emergencies

- Weak or nonpalpable pulses
- CHF
- Shock

DIAGNOSIS

- Chest x-ray (CXR): Most often normal
- ECG:
  - Narrow QRS complex.
  - Tachycardia at a rate > 150 bpm.
  - Typically **regular,** P waves may or may not be visible.

TREATMENT

- ABCs, IV, O_2, monitor.
- Immediate synchronized cardioversion (50 J) if hemodynamically unstable, in CHF or ACS.
- Vagal maneuvers or adenosine (6-mg rapid IV push followed by 20 mL flush, repeat as needed × 2 with 12 mg each time) to block AV nodal conduction.
- Diltiazem (0.25 mg/kg IV over 2 minutes) or verapamil (0.15 mg/kg IV over 1 minute) or beta blocker to control rate: Watch out for hypotension.

Vagal maneuvers:
- Carotid massage (check carotids for bruits prior to massage; never massage both sides simultaneously)
- Diving reflex (cold water immersion of head)
- Valsalva maneuver

Wolff-Parkinson-White (WPW) Syndrome

DEFINITION

- A syndrome in which there is an accessory electrical pathway that causes SVT in older children and adults.
- Heart beats too fast for adequate filling and may → shock.

SIGNS AND SYMPTOMS

- Palpitations
- Diaphoresis
- Tachypnea
- Variable degrees of hemodynamic stability
- Weak to no pulses
- CHF
- Shock

Features of WPW:
- Short PR interval
- Widened QRS interval
- Delta wave slurring QRS upswing

DIAGNOSIS

ECG (see Figure 7-13):

- Narrow QRS complex.
- HR > 200 bpm.
- P waves present.
- Slurred upstroke of QRS (delta wave)—may not be evident during tachyarrhythmia.

TREATMENT

- ABCs, monitor, IV access, O_2.
- Patients with WPW, and rapid atrial fibrillation, with rapid ventricular response require emergent cardioversion.

Don't give ABCD (adenosine, beta blockers, calcium channel blockers, or digoxin) to someone with WPW.

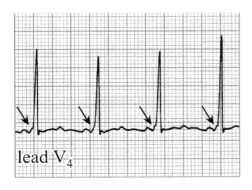

FIGURE 7-13. WPW syndrome.

Arrows indicate pathognomonic delta waves.

- Stable patients with WPW and atrial fibrillation are treated with amiodarone, flecainide, procainamide, propafenone, or sotalol.
- Adenosine, beta blockers, calcium channel blockers, and digoxin are *contraindicated* because they preferentially block conduction at the AV node, allowing unopposed conduction down the accessory bypass tract.

Sick Sinus Syndrome (SSS)

DEFINITION

- Sinus arrest: Also known as "pause" of sinoatrial node signal that usually results in "ectopic" or "escape" beats and rhythms that take over as source for ventricular impulse.
- Also called tachy-brady syndrome: Any combination of intermittent fast and slow rhythms with associated AV block and inadequate escape rhythm:
  - Fast: A-fib, atrial flutter, SVT, junctional tachycardia
  - Slow: Sinus brady, varying sinus pauses, escapes

SIGNS AND SYMPTOMS

Reflect fast or slow HR:

- Palpitations
- Syncope
- Dyspnea
- Angina
- Embolic events

DIAGNOSIS

ECG: Any of above rhythms (see definition).

TREATMENT

- ABCs, IV, O$_2$, monitor
- Follow ACLS protocols
- Pacemaker

Junctional Ectopy

- Ectopic beats that originate from the junction of atria and ventricle.
- Normal ventricular depolarization and repolarization.
- Narrow QRS complexes.
- Absent or late, retrograde P waves coming on or after the QRS.

Ventricular Ectopy

DEFINITION

Ectopic beats that originate from below the AV node.

ETIOLOGY

- Normal
- Ischemia
- Electrolyte abnormality
- Medications (digoxin, beta blockers, Ca^{2+} channel blockers)
- Caffeine, alcohol

DIAGNOSIS

ECG (see Figure 7-14):

- Wide QRS
- No preceding P wave

TREATMENT

None; treat underlying cause.

Torsades de Pointes

- French: "Twisting of the points."
- Refers to a ventricular tachycardia variation in which QRS axis swings from positive to a negative in a single lead (see Figure 7-15).
- Can be caused by R-on-T phenomenon.
- Treatment: IV magnesium sulfate, cardioversion if unstable.

Causes of torsades:
POINTES
Phenothiazines
Other medications (tricyclic antidepressants)
Intracranial bleed
No known cause (idiopathic)
Type I antidysrhythmics
Electrolyte abnormalities
Syndrome of prolonged QT

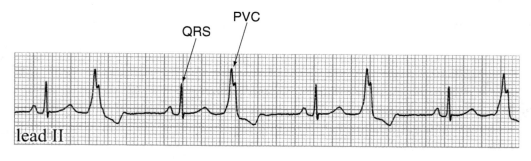

FIGURE 7-14. Ventricular bigeminy.

Note the premature ventricular complex (PVC) that regularly follows the QRS complex.

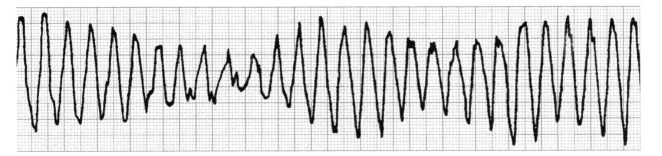

FIGURE 7-15. Torsade de pointes.

Ventricular Tachycardia

- ≥ 3 ectopic ventricular beats in a row.
- See the Resuscitation chapter.

Ventricular Fibrillation

See the Resuscitation chapter.

CARDIOMYOPATHIES

There are three types of cardiomyopathies: dilated, restrictive, and hypertrophic. The end stages of dilated and restrictive cardiomyopathies ultimately result in heart failure, and thus ED management of these conditions is the same as for decompensated heart failure from any other cause. More details on these cardiomyopathies are not immediately relevant to emergency medicine. Hypertrophic cardiomyopathy, however, does have special relevance to emergency medicine and is thus discussed in detail here.

Hypertrophic Cardiomyopathy

A 25-year-old man presents to the ED with syncope and chest pain. On physical exam, he has loud systolic murmur. What is the diagnosis?
The patient is presenting with hypertrophic cardiomyopathy (HCM) or idiopathic hypertrophic subaortic stenosis (IHSS). Symptoms include chest pain, dizziness, and syncope. Physical exam will often reveal a murmur. *Syncope + murmur: Think HCM.* Brugada syndrome is another cause of sudden death in young adults. The classic ECG finding of Brugada is an RBBB with anterior ST elevations.

Hypertrophic cardiomyopathy: Symptoms prior to 30 years correlates with ↑ risk of sudden death, but severity of symptoms (whenever they occur) does not.

DEFINITION

- Hypertrophied, nondilated, often asymmetric left ventricle (septum > free wall) with second-degree atrial dilation.
- Also known as idiopathic hypertrophic subaortic stenosis, or IHSS.

PATHOPHYSIOLOGY

Results in:

- Systolic dysfunction (end-stage dilation)
- Diastolic dysfunction (poor filling and relaxation)
- Myocardial ischemia ($\uparrow$ O_2 demand because of $\uparrow$ myocardial mass)

ETIOLOGY

- Idiopathic or inherited (50%)
- HTN
- Aortic or pulmonic stenosis

SIGNS AND SYMPTOMS

- Angina:
  - Not well understood in terms of known pathophysiology.
  - Occurs at rest and during exercise.
  - Frequently unresponsive to nitroglycerin.
  - May respond to recumbent position (pathognomonic but rare).
- Syncope: Most often occurs following exercise—$\downarrow$ *afterload* due to peripheral vasodilation resulting in peripheral pooling since muscular contractions no longer enhance return to heart, causing $\downarrow$ *preload*.
- Arrhythmias: atrial fibrillation, ventricular tachycardia.
- Palpitations due to arrhythmias.
- Signs of CHF.
- Pulsus bisferiens (rapid biphasic carotid pulse).
- S4 gallop.
- Systolic ejection murmur heard best along the left sternal border, $\downarrow$ with $\uparrow$ LV blood volume (squatting), $\uparrow$ with $\uparrow$ blood velocities (exercise), and $\downarrow$ LV end-diastolic volume (Valsalva).
- Paradoxical splitting of S2.
- Sudden death is usually due to an arrhythmia rather than obstruction.

DIAGNOSIS

- ECG: Left ventricular hypertrophy (LVH), premature ventricular contractions (PVCs), A-fib, septal Q waves, nonspecific ST segment and T wave abnormalities.
- Echocardiography: Septal hypertrophy, LVH but small LV size, atrial dilatation, mitral regurgitation with systolic anterior motion of mitral valve leaflets.

TREATMENT

- Beta blockers to reduce HR, increasing LV filling time and decreasing inotropy are first line; calcium channel blockers considered second line.
- Anticoagulation for A-fib or signs of peripheral embolization.
- Septal myomectomy or transcatheter alcohol septal ablation for severely symptomatic patients.
- Permanent pacemaker to change pattern of ventricular contraction, reducing obstruction.
- Implanted automatic defibrillator should be considered.
- Bacterial endocarditis prophylaxis for dental, gastrointestinal, and genitourinary procedures.
- Vigorous exercise should be discouraged.

Hypertrophic cardiomyopathy: Very few murmurs $\downarrow$ with squatting (this one does).

Causes of paradoxical splitting of S2:
- Hypertrophic cardiomyopathy
- Aortic stenosis
- LBBB

Hypertrophic cardiomyopathy: Digitalis and other positive inotropic agents are contraindicated even if presenting symptoms are those of CHF (because they $\uparrow$ outflow obstruction).

A 28-year-old man presents with a fever. He reports frequent use of IV heroin. He has a temperature of 103.1°F (39.6°C). His physical exam reveals a loud systolic ejection murmur. What is the diagnosis?

The patient has bacterial endocarditis until proven otherwise. IV drug abusers with a fever and murmur should be started on broad-spectrum antibiotics that include coverage for *S aureus*. Three sets of blood cultures should be obtained. An echo is needed to visualize vegetations on the valve leaflets. Bacterial endocarditis should also be suspected in patients with prosthetic valves that presents with fever.

DEFINITION

Bacterial infection of endocardium.

ETIOLOGY

Duke criteria:

1. Positive blood culture for infective endocarditis (IE):
   - Isolation of typical organisms from two positive cultures of blood samples drawn > 12 hours apart, or all of three or a majority of four separate cultures of blood (with first and last sample drawn 1 hour apart).
   - Typical microorganisms consistent with IE include viridans streptococci, *Streptococcus bovis*, HACEK (*Haemophilus aphrophilus*, *Actinobacillus actinomycetemcomitans*, *Cardiobacterium hominis*, *Eikenella corrodens*, and *Kingella kingae*) group, or community-acquired *Staphylococcus aureus* or enterococci, in the absence of a primary focus.
2. Endocardial involvement as evidenced by positive echocardiogram for IE defined as:
   - Oscillating intracardiac mass on valve or supporting structures, in the path of regurgitant jets, or on implanted material in the absence of an alternative anatomic explanation, or
   - Abscess, or
   - New partial dehiscence of prosthetic valve

Frequency of valves affected in ABE: aortic > mitral >> tricuspid

RISK FACTORS

- Congenital heart disease
- Valvular heart disease
- Prosthetic valve
- IV drug abuse
- Indwelling venous catheters
- Dialysis
- Previous history of IE

CLINICAL PRESENTATION

- Fever: temperature > 38.0°C (100.4°F).
- Arthralgias.
- Pleuritic chest pain.

Echo for ABE:
Transesophageal
  echocardiography :
  90–100% sensitive
Transthoracic
  echocardiography:
  28–63% sensitive

- Vascular phenomena: Major arterial emboli, septic pulmonary infarcts, mycotic aneurysm, intracranial hemorrhage, conjunctival hemorrhages, splinter hemorrhages, and **Janeway lesions** (nontender palmar plaques).
- Immunologic phenomena: Glomerulonephritis, **Osler's nodes** (tender fingertip nodules), **Roth spots** (retinal hemorrhages).

TREATMENT

First-line treatment is vancomycin; therapy can be narrowed with blood culture results.

HEART FAILURE

DEFINITION

- Condition characterized by inadequate systemic perfusion to meet body's metabolic demands due to "failure" of the heart's pump function. Also known as congestive heart failure (CHF).
- Systolic failure: Reduced cardiac contractility.
- Diastolic failure: Impaired cardiac relaxation and abnormal ventricular filling.

EPIDEMIOLOGY

- **United States:**
  - Prevalence is 4.7 million (~ 1.5% of the population).
  - There are 1 million hospital admissions per year in which CHF is the primary diagnosis, and another 2 million hospitalizations with heart failure as a secondary diagnosis.
  - One-third of these patients are readmitted within 90 days for recurrent decompensation (see next section).
- **Worldwide:**
  - It is estimated that there are 15 million new cases of CHF per year.
  - Aging population contributes to the increasing incidence.

PATHOPHYSIOLOGY

- **Systolic dysfunction:**
  1. Cardiac output is low, pulmonary pressures are high.
  2. This leads to pulmonary congestion and systemic hypoperfusion.
  3. Neurohormonal pathways activated to ↑ circulating blood volume.
  4. Sympathetic nervous system ↑ heart rate and contractility, → ↑ cardiac output.
  5. Catecholamine release also aggravates ischemia; can potentiate arrhythmias; promotes cardiac remodeling (LV dilation and hypertrophy); and stimulates renin-angiotensin system, which exacerbates arteriolar vasoconstriction, causing retention of sodium and water.
  6. Clinical symptoms of CHF appear when these mechanisms can no longer compensate.
- **Diastolic dysfunction:**
  1. Main problem is impaired LV relaxation. This causes high diastolic pressures and poor filling of the ventricles.
  2. In order to ↑ diastolic filling, left atrial pressure ↑ until it exceeds the hydrostatic and oncotic pressures in the pulmonary capillaries.

3. Pulmonary edema results.
4. Patients are therefore symptomatic with exertion when ↑ HR reduces LV filling time.
5. Circulating catecholamines worsen diastolic dysfunction.
6. Clinical symptoms of CHF appear when these mechanisms can no longer compensate.

ETIOLOGY

- LV **systolic** dysfunction:
  - Most common cause (~60%)
  - History of MIs and chronic underperfusion
  - Valvular heart disease
  - HTN
  - Dilated cardiomyopathy
  - Toxins (eg, alcohol, doxorubicin, lithium, cocaine)
  - Heavy metals (lead, arsenic, mercury)
  - Viral (eg, coxsackie)
  - Familial predisposition/congenital disease
  - Neuromuscular disease
- Right ventricular (RV) **systolic** dysfunction:
  - LV systolic dysfunction
  - RV infarction
  - Pulmonary HTN
  - Chronic severe tricuspid regurgitation
  - Arrhythmogenic RV dysplasia
- LV **diastolic** dysfunction:
  - Restrictive cardiomyopathy
  - Hemochromatosis
  - Sarcoidosis
  - Carcinoid heart disease (eg, Gaucher, Hurler, glycogen storage diseases)
  - Hypertrophic cardiomyopathy
  - Infiltrative cardiomyopathy (eg, amyloidosis)
  - Pericardial constriction
  - Cardiac tamponade
  - High-output states: Pregnancy, thyrotoxicosis, wet beriberi, arteriovenous fistulae, Paget disease, severe chronic anemia

SIGNS AND SYMPTOMS

Left Heart Failure	Right Heart Failure
Orthopnea	RUQ pain (due to hepatic congestion
Paroxysmal nocturnal dyspnea	Hepatomegaly with mild jaundice
Dyspnea on exertion	Hepatojugular reflex
Rales	Jugular venous distention (JVD)
Cough (sometimes frothy pink); hemoptysis; wheezing ("cardiac asthma")	Ascites
	Peripheral cyanosis
S3 and/or S4 heart sound	Peripheral edema (pitting)
Tachycardia	Nausea
Diaphoresis	Wasting
	Oliguria and nocturia

RV failure manifests as peripheral vascular congestion (pedal edema, JVD, hepatomegaly).

LV failure manifests as pulmonary edema or shock (dyspnea, orthopnea, hypotension).

DIAGNOSIS

- ECG:
  - Pattern may reveal normal sinus, sinus tachycardia, or A-fib.
  - Findings commonly seen in CHF include LV hypertrophy, LBBB, intraventricular conduction delay, and nonspecific ST segment and T wave changes. Presence of Q waves suggest old MI.
- CXR: Often reveals cardiomegaly, pulmonary vascular redistribution, pulmonary venous congestion, Kerley B lines, alveolar edema, and pleural effusions.
- Echocardiogram:
  - Most useful to distinguish between systolic and diastolic dysfunction.
  - Can discern regional wall motion abnormalities, LV aneurysm, ejection fraction, diastolic function, valvular problems.
  - Plasma brain natriuretic peptide (BNP): BNP is available as a rapid bedside test and is elevated in decompensated CHF, and can be useful in new diagnoses, before compensated state occurs.

CLASSIFICATION

See Table 7-3.

TREATMENT

- Patients are maintained on a variety of cardiac drugs to optimize cardiac output; scope is beyond this book.
- Ultimately, patients with end-stage heart failure will require heart transplantation.
- Circulatory assist devices can provide a bridge to heart transplantation.

PROGNOSIS

- Poor prognosis is associated with ventricular arrhythmias, NYHA Class III or IV, lower LV ejection fraction, marked LV dilatation, high catecholamine and BNP levels, low serum sodium, and hypocholesterolemia.
- Patients with combined systolic and diastolic LV dysfunction also have a worse prognosis than patients with either in isolation.

TABLE 7-3. New York Heart Association (NYHA) Heart Failure Symptom Classification System

NYHA CLASS	LEVEL OF IMPAIRMENT
I	No symptom limitation with ordinary physical activity
II	Ordinary physical activity somewhat limited by dyspnea (ie, long-distance walking, climbing two flights of stairs)
III	Exercise limited by dyspnea at mild workloads (ie, short-distance walking, climbing one flight of stairs)
IV	Dyspnea at rest or with very little exertion

Circulatory Assist Devices

Circulatory assist devices are mechanical devices that allow an ↑ in myocardial oxygen supply and ↓ the workload of the left ventricle, thereby increasing cardiac output and perfusion to vital organs. There are three main types of circulatory assist devices:

- Counterpulsation devices such as intra-aortic balloon pump (IABP):
  - Most commonly used.
  - Percutaneous insertion (most often through femoral artery).
  - Balloon is placed within the descending aorta.
  - Device is designed to inflate during diastole and deflate during systole, synchronized with native heartbeat.
- Cardiopulmonary assist devices.
- LV assist devices:
  - Centrifugal pumps: Limits ambulation.
  - Extracorporeal pumps: Require heparinization.

INDICATIONS

- Cardiogenic shock
- Intractable angina
- Weaning from cardiopulmonary bypass
- As adjunctive therapy after thrombolysis in patients at high risk for stenosis
- As prophylactic therapy in patients with severe left main coronary arterial stenosis or critical aortic stenosis in whom surgery is pending

CONTRAINDICATIONS

- Aortic valve regurgitation
- Aortic aneurysm
- Severe peripheral vascular disease
- Coagulopathy
- Uncontrolled sepsis
- Aortic stenosis or prosthetic aortic valve (LV assist device only)

Acute Decompensated Heart Failure (Cardiogenic Pulmonary Edema)

A 55-year-old woman presents to the ED with severe respiratory distress at 4 A.M. She has past medical history of end-stage renal disease (ESRD) and is due for dialysis in a few hours. Her vital signs are pulse 130 bpm, BP 205/104 mm Hg, RR 34 bpm, pulse oximetry 91%. Her chest exam reveals crackles throughout. What are the treatment options?

The patient is presenting with acute pulmonary edema secondary to volume overload. Therapy should be directed at improving oxygenation and decreasing afterload. Noninvasive positive pressure ventilation such as BiPAP would be a good choice in this setting. Nitrates could be used to reduce preload, or an angiotensin-converting enzyme (ACE) inhibitor can be used to reduce afterload. The use of sublingual captopril has been well described in the setting of acute pulmonary edema in ESRD.

DEFINITION

Also known as acute cardiogenic pulmonary edema.

ETIOLOGY

- Most common reason is noncompliance with medications
- Dietary indiscretion (excess salt intake)
- Acute MI
- Sepsis

DIAGNOSIS

- CXR: Cardiomegaly, bilateral interstitial infiltrates ("hazy" appearance).
- ECG: Often sinus tachycardia or atrial fibrillation.
- Laboratory studies: Obtain CBC, electrolytes, cardiac biomarkers (elevated in acute MI) and BNP (elevated in acute decompensated CHF).

TREATMENT

- First line:
  - Oxygen: 100% O_2 by face mask to maintain O_2 saturation above 90%. In patients for whom this is inadequate, bilevel positive airway pressure (BiPAP) is an excellent option. Often, use of BiPAP will obviate the need for endotracheal intubation, and is considered first line where available.
  - Aspirin: Given as part of protocol to rule out acute coronary syndrome, 162–325 mg PO.
  - Nitroglycerin: Reduces preload and thus pulmonary capillary wedge pressure. Can be given in the transdermal (nitropaste 1–2 inches), SL (0.4 mg q 5 minutes) or IV form (5 μg/min, titrated to effect).
  - Diuretics: Loop diuretics (eg, furosemide, bumetanide) are used to produce venodilation, which reduces pulmonary capillary pressure by causing diuresis. With furosemide (40–80 mg IV), peak onset of diuresis occurs in about 30 minutes and lasts about 6 hours.
  - Noninvasive positive pressure ventilation can be used in severe CHF as temporizing measure until pharmacological therapy can take effect
- Second line: If the above modalities do not reslve the pulmonary edema, then the following agents can be used to boost inotropic support:
  - Dobutamine: ↑ stroke volume and cardiac output by mainly working on β_1 receptors with minimal effect on α_1 receptors. Initial dose is 2.5 μg/min, gradually ↑ to 7–20 μg/kg/min.
  - Dopamine: Reserved for hypotensive patients in whom arterial pressure ↑ is required, due to stimulation of α_1-adrenergic receptors in addition to β_1 (cardiac) receptors. "Cardiac dosing" is 3–10 μg/min.
- Other pharmacologic therapy: Nesiritide is recombinant human B-type (brain) natriuretic peptide. It produces vasodilatory, natriuretic, and diuretic effects, primarily mediated via natriuretic peptide receptor A on vascular smooth muscle, endothelium, kidneys, and adrenals. It has no direct inotropic effect. Its use is limited to those who are hospitalized for severe CHF, who are not in cardiogenic shock, in whom first-line therapy in inadequate. Use is controversial.

Treatment of acute pulmonary edema (APE) —
NOt BAD
Nitroglycerin
Oxygen therapy
BiPAP (or CPAP)
Aspirin
Diuretics

DEFINITION

Inflammatory damage of myocardium.

PATHOPHYSIOLOGY

- Myocyte necrosis/degeneration and correlating inflammatory infiltrate due to infectious and inflammatory etiologies.
- Some infectious agents cause an autoimmune response to cardiac myocytes by molecular mimicry.
- Some cases spontaneously resolve.
- Some cases progress to end-stage dilated cardiomyopathy.

ETIOLOGIES

- Viral (coxsackie B4, adenovirus, influenza A and B, varicella-zoster virus, HIV, cytomegalovirus, hepatitis A and B, Epstein-Barr virus)
- Vaccine related
- Bacterial (*Mycoplasma, Streptococcus, Chlamydia*)
- Lyme disease *(Borrelia burgdorferi)*
- Chagas disease *(Trypanosoma cruzi)*
- Kawasaki disease
- Steroid abuse

CLINICAL FINDINGS

- Fever
- Chest pain
- Tachycardia out of proportion to fever
- Syncope
- Dyspnea
- Fatigue
- Palpitations
- Soft S1
- S3 or S4 gallop
- Mitral or tricuspid regurgitation murmur

DIAGNOSIS

- CXR: ± Cardiomegaly/pulmonary edema.
- ECG: Sinus tachycardia, low voltage, long QT/PR/QRS, AV blocks, ↑ or ↓ STs, ↓ Ts. Diffuse changes, not localized to one anatomic distribution.
- Labs: ↑ ESR, ↑ WBC count, ↑ creatine kinase myocardial band (CK-MB), ↑ troponin.
- Echocardiography: Multichamber dysfunction, ↓ LV ejection fraction, global hypokinesis, focal wall motion abnormality.

TREATMENT

- Intensive care unit admission
- Bed rest, supportive care, vital signs
- Antibiotics for bacterial and parasitic causes
- ASA and gamma globulin for Kawasaki disease
- ACE inhibitors for CHF associated with myocarditis

A 29-year-old man presents with fever and retrosternal chest pain. He had "the flu bug" 2 weeks ago. He is tachycardic. *Think: Myocarditis.*

In new diagnosis of refractory asthma in a young adult, consider myocarditis.

A 31-year-old woman presents with pleuritic chest pain that improves with leaning forward. Cardiac auscultation reveals a pericardial friction rub. ECG demonstrates diffuse PR depression. *Think: Pericarditis.*

Constrictive

- Fibrous reparative thickening of pericardial layers (sometimes calcified) that restricts diastolic ventricular filling.
- Caused by trauma, uremia, tuberculosis (TB), radiation.

Acute Inflammatory

Inflammation of pericardial tissue resulting in pain and effusion. Causes include:

- Trauma
- Uremia
- Infectious (viral > bacterial > parasitic > fungal)
- Post irradiation
- Post MI
- Aortic dissection
- Tumors

CLINICAL FINDINGS

- Fever
- Pleuritic and positional chest pain
- Tachycardia
- Myalgias
- Shallow breathing
- Anxiety
- Pericardial friction rub
- Distant heart sounds.
- Pulsus paradoxus: Exaggeration of more than 10 torr of the normal variation during the inspiratory phase of respiration, in which the blood pressure declines as one inhales and increases as one exhales.

DIAGNOSIS

- CXR: May see cardiomegaly if effusion present.
- ECG (see Figure 7-16):
  - Stage 1 (first few hours/days): Diffuse ST elevations with PR depression
  - Stage 2: Normalization of STs and PRs
  - Stage 3: Diffuse T wave inversions
  - Stage 4: Normalization of T waves
- Labs: ↑ ESR and WBC counts, + CK and troponin if concomitant myocarditis or endocarditis; check blood urea nitrogen (BUN)/creatinine (Cr), blood cultures.
- Echocardiography: Normal global cardiac function unless an effusion is present.

TREATMENT

- Rule out ACS.
- Nonsteroidal anti-inflammatories (NSAIDs) for viral, post MI, and idiopathic causes.
- Antimicrobials for bacterial, fungal, TB, and parasitic causes.
- Surgical pericardiectomy for purulent pericarditis.
- Dialysis for uremic pericarditis.

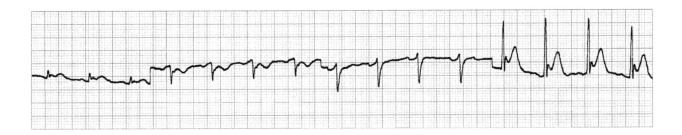

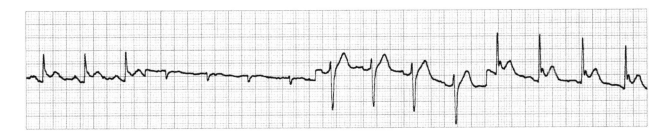

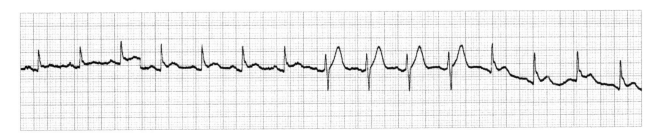

FIGURE 7-16. ECG in pericarditis.

Note diffuse ST elevations with PR depression, early stage of pericarditis. ECG will change and normalize as disease progresses and resolves.

PERICARDIAL EFFUSIONS

DEFINITIONS

- **Pericardial effusion:** Excessive fluid in pericardial space.
- **Cardiac tamponade:** Pericardial effusion that restricts ventricular filling and eventually stroke volume, → systemic hypotension, shock, pulseless electrical activity (PEA), and death.

ETIOLOGIES

Same as pericarditis.

CLINICAL FINDINGS

- Same as pericarditis, but alterations in vital signs may be more pronounced and shock state may exist.
- Often asymptomatic when small.
- Beck's triad for cardiac tamponade.

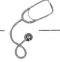

Always rule out ACS in a patient presenting with classical signs of pericarditis.

195

Cardiac tamponade is one of the reversible causes of PEA. Either a bedside ultrasound or pericardiocentesis should be performed in patient with PEA.

Beck's triad:
- Hypotension
- JVD
- Muffled heart sounds

DIAGNOSIS

- CXR: Cardiomegaly (see Figure 7-17).
- ECG: Differing QRS amplitudes ("alternans," Figure 7-18) and axes caused by ventricle swaying within fluid-filled pericardial sac with each beat.
- Echocardiography: Effusion, ↓ systolic and diastolic function, collapse of RV/right atrial free walls in diastole.

TREATMENT

- ABCs, IV, O$_2$, monitor.
- Pericardiocentesis immediately if hemodynamically unstable or pulseless (see Procedures chapter).
- If more stable, a pericardial window can be created in the operating room (OR) to prevent reaccumulation of effusion.

VALVULAR LESIONS

Aortic Stenosis

DEFINITION

Valve hardening obstructs blood flow from left ventricle. Results in progressive LVH, ↓ cardiac output, hypertrophic and later dilated cardiomyopathy. Predisposes to endocarditis.

ETIOLOGY

- Congenital
- Rheumatic fever
- Degenerative calcification

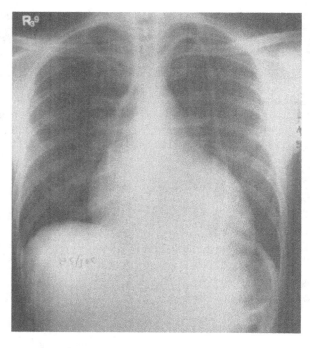

FIGURE 7-17. CXR demonstrating cardiomegaly secondary to pericardial effusion.

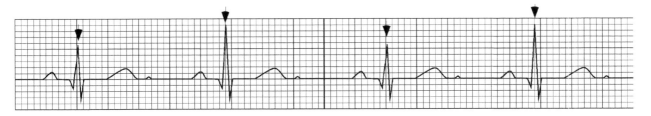

FIGURE 7-18. **ECG demonstrating electrical alternans. Note alternating heights in the R (arrow) in the QRS complexes.**

SIGNS AND SYMPTOMS

Dyspnea on exertion, angina, syncope on exertion, sudden death, low-pitched crescendo-decrescendo murmur at the base radiating to carotids, carotid pulse weak (parvus) and slow-rising (tardus), S3, S4.

DIAGNOSIS

- CXR: Cardiomegaly ± pulmonary edema.
- ECG: LVH ± ischemic change.
- Echocardiography: Can estimate severity of obstruction and LV systolic function, and may identify cause (eg, calcified bicuspid valve).

TREATMENT

- Definitive treatment is valve replacement.
- Acute presentation warrants ruling out ACS, CHF, and other etiologies.
- ABCs, IV, O₂, monitor.
- Gentle hydration if hypotensive.

Aortic Insufficiency

DEFINITION

Regurgitation of blood flow back into the ventricle, → dilated cardiomyopathy and failure.

ETIOLOGY

- **Acute causes:**
  - Infective endocarditis
  - Aortic root dissection
- **Chronic causes:**
  - Rheumatic fever
  - Congenital
  - Ankylosing spondylitis
  - Syphilis
  - Carcinoid
  - Reiter's syndrome
  - Fen-Phen (fenfluramine and phentermine) use

SIGNS AND SYMPTOMS

- Dyspnea
- Angina
- Presence of S3 heart sound

Prognosis: *Mean survival for patients with AS and:*
Angina = 5 years
Syncope = 2–3 years
Heart failure = 1–2 years

Any change in preload *or* afterload can cause acute decompensation in AS.

In patients with AS presenting with angina, rule out ACS.

- High-pitched blowing diastolic murmur at base, ± systolic flow murmur.
- "Water-hammer" pulse: Peripheral pulse with quick upstroke and then collapse.
- Wide pulse pressure.
- Bounding "Corrigan" pulse, "pistol shot" femorals, pulsus bisferiens (dicrotic pulse with two palpable waves in systole).
- Duroziez sign: Presence of diastolic femoral bruit when femoral artery is compressed enough to hear a systolic bruit.
- Hill's sign: Systolic pressure in the legs 20 mm Hg higher than in the arms.
- Quincke's sign: Visible capillary pulse in nails.
- De Musset's sign: Bobbing of head with heartbeat.

DIAGNOSIS

- CXR:
  - Chronic: Cardiomegaly ± pulmonary edema.
  - Acute: Pulmonary edema without cardiomegaly.
- ECG:
  - Chronic: LVH ± strain pattern.
  - Acute: ± ischemic change (especially inferior leads), low voltage, if dissection—tachycardia.
- Echocardiography: Will diagnose disease by visualizing regurgitant flow, may identify cause (eg, vegetations), and facilitates assessment of LV systolic function and chamber size.

TREATMENT

- ABCs, IV, O$_2$, monitor.
- In acute and chronic cases of pulmonary edema, reduce afterload with nitrates and diuretics.
- Treat endocarditis as indicated.
- Dissection treated with surgical repair.
- Valve replacement is indicated once LV becomes enlarged or systolic function is impaired.

Mitral Stenosis

DEFINITION

↓ in cross-sectional area for blood flow from left atrium to left ventricle, resulting in atrial dilatation, atrial fibrillation, left heart failure, progressive pulmonary HTN, pulmonic and tricuspid valve regurgitation, and right heart failure.

ETIOLOGY

- Rheumatic fever
- Atrial myxomas
- Congenital
- Degenerative calcification

SIGNS AND SYMPTOMS

- Dyspnea on exertion
- Orthopnea
- Early diastolic opening snap followed by diastolic rumble at the apex

A 70-year-old man presents with angina. Physical exam reveals bounding pulses and there is an SBP difference of 25 mm Hg between the upper and lower extremities. *Think: Aortic insufficiency.*

- CXR: Can be normal; severe disease can show a straightening of the LV border ± pulmonary edema. It may reveal double-density sign, straightening and lifting of carina.
- ECG: Left atrial enlargement ± atrial fibrillation, right axis deviation.
- Echocardiography: Will diagnose disease by showing thickened valve leaflets, ↓ valve movement, and commissural fusion.

TREATMENT

- ABCs, IV, O_2, monitor.
- Acute atrial fibrillation: See above.
- Pulmonary edema: Nitrates, diuretics, oxygen, and morphine.
- Surgical valvulotomy or valve replacement is indicated when significant symptoms develop despite medical treatment or if pulmonary hypertension develops.

Mitral Regurgitation

DEFINITION

Regurgitation from left ventricle to left atrium during systole, results in ↑ LV stroke volume with eventual LV dilatation and dysfunction.

ETIOLOGY

- **Acute causes:**
  - MI with ischemic necrosis and subsequent rupture of papillary muscle or chordae tendineae usually from right coronary infarct.
  - Infective endocarditis.
  - Trauma.
- **Chronic causes:**
  - Rheumatic fever heart damage.
  - Appetite suppressant drugs (Fen-Phen).
  - Mitral valve prolapse.
  - Carcinoid tumor syndrome.
  - Marfan syndrome.
  - Any cause of LV dilatation can cause *secondary* MR.

SIGNS AND SYMPTOMS

- Dyspnea
- Tachycardia and tachypnea
- Angina
- Presence of S3 and S4 heart sounds
- Loud crescendo-decrescendo murmur between S1 and S2 at the apex radiating to axilla
- Rales
- Rapidly rising and poorly sustained carotid pulse

DIAGNOSIS

- CXR:
  - Chronic: Cardiomegaly ± pulmonary edema.
  - Acute: Pulmonary edema without cardiomegaly.
- ECG:
  - Chronic: LVH, atrial enlargement, A-fib.
  - Acute: ± Ischemic change, tachycardia without chronic changes.

- Echocardiography: Can diagnose acute and chronic cases by visualizing chordae tendineae, vegetations, wall motion abnormality, and estimating severity of disease (volume of MR jet, LV size and function).
- Cardiac catheterization: Indicated in acute cases to evaluate and treat ACS.

TREATMENT

- ABCs, IV, O_2, monitor
- Nitrates, morphine, and diuretics for pulmonary edema, reducing afterload and regurgitant flow
- Antibiotics for IE
- Catheterization and emergency mitral valve reconstruction for ischemic rupture
- ACE inhibitors, long-acting nitrates, and salt restriction for chronic disease

Loss of the click of the mechanical valve may indicate valvular dysfunction, infection, dehiscence, or abscess formation.

Artificial Valves

- Mechanical: Bileaflet hinged disk, tilting disk, or caged-ball prostheses:
  - Patients require lifelong anticoagulation (warfarin).
  - Monitor INR (usual range 2–3).
  - "Mechanical murmur" systolic with loud, closing machine-like sound.
  - Complications: Chronic low-grade hemolysis from turbulent flow and subsequent anemia, valve failure, thrombosis, systemic emboli, bleeding from high INR, risk for IE (contamination and bacteremic).
- Bioprosthetic: Bovine or porcine:
  - ASA only anticoagulation.
  - Mitral bioprosthesis has diastolic rumble.
  - Complications: 30–70% failure rate at 10 years, risk for IE (contamination and bacteremic), valve failure, thrombosis, systemic emboli.

HEART TRANSPLANT

- Denervated hearts have no native sympathetic and parasympathetic tone, responding only to circulating catecholamines and medications, so don't try any vagal maneuvers or atropine (which inhibits vagal tone).
- All transplant patients are immunocompromised. If they present with fever, diagnose and treat aggressively with broad-spectrum antibiotics.
- With piggyback heart transplant, you may see two separate independent P waves in the ECG, one from the old heart and one from the new heart.
- Before prescribing anything for the transplant patient as an outpatient, find out if it will interact with his or her immunosuppressant medication.
- Dysrhythmias, atypical fatigability, and exertion intolerance should be treated as acute rejection until proven otherwise. If hemodynamically unstable because of the dysrhythmias, acute rejection regimen should be instituted (methylprednisolone 1 g IV), and modified ACLS protocols should be followed.

Abdominal Aortic Aneurysm (AAA)

Abdominal aneurysms **rupture;** thoracic aneurysms **dissect.**

A 73-year-old man who is a 2-pack-per-day smoker with HTN and peripheral vascular disease presents with severe midabdominal and left flank pain. He states he had this same pain 1 week ago, and that it got so bad he passed out. Physical exam reveals bruits over the abdominal aorta and a tender pulsatile mass. What is the diagnosis?

This is the classic presentation of abdominal pain with pulsatile mass. Many patients with AAA will not have a pulsatile mass. AAA is one of the true life threats that needs to ruled out in every patient with abdominal or back pain. It is often misdiagnosed as renal colic or musculoskeletal back pain.

PATHOPHYSIOLOGY

- Atherosclerotic, thinned tunica media has ↓ elastin fibers and forms aneurysm from HTN.
- The larger the aneurysm, the weaker the wall, and therefore gradual enlargement of AAA.

RISK FACTORS

- Age > 60 years
- Male gender
- HTN
- Cigarette smoking
- Coronary artery disease
- Peripheral vascular disease
- Family history of AAA in first-degree relative

SIGNS AND SYMPTOMS

- Abdominal pain (77%)
- Pulsatile abdominal mass (70%)
- Back/flank pain (60%)
- Tender abdomen (41%)
- Nausea/vomiting (25%) with blood (5%)
- Syncope (18%)
- Nonpalpable distal pulses (6%)
- Known history of AAA (5%)

AAA is most frequently misdiagnosed as renal colic.

The mortality is 50% for those who rupture and get to the OR.

DIAGNOSIS

- CXR: Can be normal.
- Abdominal x-ray: May see calcified outline of AAA.
- ECG: Tachycardia ± ischemic changes.
- Ultrasound: Ideal for the unstable patient because of machine portability; however, bowel gas and obesity may obscure visualization.
- Computed tomography (CT) scan: Only for hemodynamically stable patients. Contrast allows full evaluation for both aneurysmal size and possible dissection.

- Magnetic resonance imaging (MRI)/magnetic resonance angiography (MRA): Best for the asymptomatic patient. Useful in evaluation of patients in whom IV contrast is contraindicated.

TREATMENT

- ABCs, IV access (two large bore), O_2, monitor
- IV fluid if in a shock state
- In unstable patients, rapid transport to OR with vascular surgeon

Aortic Dissection

A 67-year-old man with a history of HTN presents with a sudden-onset tearing chest pain radiating to back. Physical exam reveals a BP of 130/64 mm Hg in the right arm and 217/110 mm Hg in the left arm. CXR reveals a widened mediastinum. What is the diagnosis?

The tearing chest pain radiating to the back combined with unequal blood pressures is highly suggestive of an aortic dissection. A CT scan should be obtained to confirm the diagnosis. BP should be controlled, and a beta blocker should be administered to ↓ wall stress.

DEFINITION

A tearing of the aorta due to hypertensive "shearing forces" on an atherosclerotic vessel that infiltrate through the intima and track or "dissect" between the intima and adventitial layers. Dissection can occur proximally or distally and can involve other vessels (carotids, renals, iliacs, pericardium).

CLASSIFICATION

- DeBakey classification (anatomic):
  - Type I: Ascending and descending
  - Type II: Ascending only
  - Type III: Descending only
- Stanford classification (more widely used clinically):
  - Type A: Ascending aorta
  - Type B: Descending aorta

RISK FACTORS

- HTN
- Connective tissue disease (Marfan, Ehlers-Danlos)
- Male gender (three times more affected than women)
- Congenital heart disease
- Third-trimester pregnancy
- Turner syndrome
- Cocaine use

SIGNS AND SYMPTOMS

- Abrupt onset of pain that is maximal at onset and migrates:
  - Type I: Pain begins in anterior chest and radiates to jaw, neck, or arms.

- Type II: Pain begins between the scapulae and radiates to the abdomen and lumbar area.
- Elevated BP.
- Tachycardia.
- Shock.
- Focal neurological deficits:
  - Stroke like syndrome if carotid involvement.
  - Hoarse voice if there is compression of recurrent laryngeal nerve.
  - Horner syndrome if superior cervical sympathetic ganglion is compressed.
  - ≥ 20 mm Hg BP difference between upper and lower extremities.
  - Aortic insufficiency murmur.
  - May present with cold pulseless extremity.

DIAGNOSIS

- ECG: LVH with strain pattern, ± ischemic change if dissection into coronaries or if MI, low voltage if effusion, electrical alternans if tamponade.
- CXR/CT scan: Mediastinal widening (75%) (see Figure 7-19), calcification of aortic arch, displacement of trachea and/or nasogastric tube to one side.
- Transesophageal echocardiography (TEE): Diagnostic study of choice with almost 100% sensitivity and specificity. Can differentiate between true and false lumens. Does not require IV contrast. May not, however, be readily available. Other limitations include difficult positioning and poor and incomplete visualization in certain patients.
- MRI/MRA: Also close to 100% sensitivity and specificity, but time consuming and allows limited access to patient during scan. Use Gadolillium. Good people with CT contrast allergy. Time consuming.
- CT scan: Rapid dynamic scans of multiple levels of chest immediately following IV bolus of contrast (67–85% sensitivity). May not always readily detect communication between true and false lumen.

Thoracic dissections are most frequently misdiagnosed as AMIs.

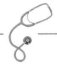

Always get at least a chest film when you suspect MI: Some of these patients will have aortic dissection, and thrombolysis may kill them.

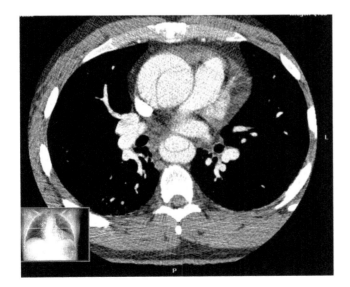

FIGURE 7-19. **CT chest demonstrates aortic dissection involving ascending and descending aorta (Stanford A).**

- Aortography: Used to be gold standard. Invasive, requires contrast dye. About 90% sensitive and specific. Can miss thrombosed false lumens. Time consuming, takes patient out of ED suite.

TREATMENT

- ABCs, IV access (two large bore), O_2, monitor.
- Antihypertensive medications ($\downarrow$ shearing force), labetalol IV 0.25 mg/kg (or 20 mg) over 2 minutes and then nitroprusside 0.3 to 10 µg/kg/min.
- Immediate surgical consultation: Go to OR for repair if patient is unstable or hypotensive.
- Ascending involvement = repair.
- Descending involvement unless medical management.

The most specific CXR sign for thoracic dissection is extension of the aortic shadow by more than 5 mm beyond its calcified aortic wall.

PERIPHERAL ARTERIAL OCCLUSION

PATHOPHYSIOLOGY

- A blockage in arterial flow compromises tissue distally, resulting in irreversible cell death within 4–6 hours.
- Without rapid aggressive treatment, it can → gangrene, limb amputation, and death.
- Embolic sources (eg, thrombus of cardiac origin breaks off and travels distally) and nonembolic sources (eg, atherosclerosis and plaque rupture with thrombus occlusion, vasospasm, and/or arteritis).

RISK FACTORS

- HTN
- Smoking
- High cholesterol
- Diabetes
- Recent MI or atrial fibrillation
- Aortic aneurysm

The **6 Ps** of peripheral artery occlusion:
Pain
Pallor
Polar (coldness)
Pulselessness
Paresthesias
Paralysis

CLINICAL FINDINGS

- Abrupt onset of pain in leg, which may be known to have poor circulation.
- The 6 Ps may not all be present.
- Use handheld Doppler to try finding nonpalpable pedal pulse.

DIAGNOSIS

- ECG: Atrial fibrillation or atrial flutter, or sinus rhythm, LVH
- CXR: ± Cardiomegaly
- Lower limb vascular imaging (femoral angiogram, MRA)

TREATMENT

- ABCs.
- Immediate vascular surgery consult for consideration of thrombectomy.
- IV heparinization if no contraindications.

Hypertensive Urgency

- SBP ≥ 180 mm Hg, DBP ≥ 110 mm Hg without evidence of end-organ damage.
- Most common cause is noncompliance with medications.
- Treatment: Oral agents.

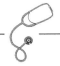

The *mean arterial pressure* is: (2DBP + SBP)/3

Hypertensive Emergency

DEFINITION

HTN that causes end-organ damage.

SIGNS AND SYMPTOMS

Signs of end-organ damage:
- Brain:
  - Hypertensive encephalopathy: Loss of integrity of the blood-brain barrier and resulting cerebral edema.
  - Intracerebral hemorrhage: A result of long-standing HTN, vascular disease, or aneurysm rupture.
- Eye: Hypertensive retinopathy: "Cotton-wool" spots (focal ischemia), hemorrhage, and papilledema (optic disc edema from hypoxia).
- Heart: LV failure and pulmonary edema due to ↑ afterload.
- Kidney: Acute renal failure—causes and is caused by HTN.
- Pregnancy: Eclampsia (see obstetrics section).
- Vascular: Aortic dissection (see above).

Nitroprusside can cause cyanide toxicity.

DIAGNOSIS

- Labs: Elevated BUN and Cr, urinalysis (for red blood cells [RBCs], protein, and casts), cardiac enzymes if chest pain or pulmonary edema, CBC, electrolytes
- CXR: ± Pulmonary edema, ± cardiomegaly
- ECG: LVH, ischemic change
- CT head: ± Bleed/edema

A 47-year-old woman presents with BP of 200/130 mm Hg. She is a known hypertensive but admits to being noncompliant with her medications. Physical examination is unremarkable. *Think: Hypertensive urgency.*

TREATMENT

- Reduce the mean arterial pressure by no more than 25% within minutes to 1 hour.
- For stable patients, initial reduction should be followed by further reduction toward a goal of 160/110 mm Hg within 2–6 hours.
- Parenteral therapy is preferred because of rapidity of action and ease of titration. Also, the treatment can be stopped if the patient becomes hypotensive.
- Common intravenous agents: Vasodilators (nitroprusside, nicardipine, hydralazine, enalapril, fenoldopam); adrenergic inhibitors (labetalol, esmolol, phentolamine).
- Nitroprusside: A powerful direct vasodilator. Prolonged use may cause cyanide toxicity.
- Nicardipine: Antihypertensive response is comparable to nitroprusside, with much fewer side effects.
- Labetalol: A combined alpha and beta blocker—an excellent agent of choice. The main drawback is prolonged duration of action.

- Remember, hypertensive emergency is a state of volume depletion, so diuretics should be avoided unless specifically indicated.

VENOUS INSUFFICIENCY

PATHOPHYSIOLOGY

- Incompetent valves in peripheral venous system (~90% lower extremities) cause "venous stasis" of peripheral blood, microextravasation of RBCs, and fluid causing pigment (hemosiderin) deposition in local tissues (stasis dermatitis) and pitting edema.
- Stasis in turn can → poor wound healing and intravascular thrombosis (see below).

TREATMENT

- Advise avoidance of prolonged periods of standing/working on feet.
- Elevate legs when resting.
- Wear gradient compression hose.
- A mild diuretic in a low dose may be helpful.

DEEP VENOUS THROMBOSIS

DEFINITIONS

- Deep venous thrombosis (DVT): Involves the deep venous system, typically calf, popliteal, femoral, common femoral, and iliac.
- Superficial thrombophlebitis can be present at the same time as DVT and can occur in any superficial vein. Varicose veins are a predisposing factor.

PATHOPHYSIOLOGY

- Intravascular (intravenous) spontaneous clot (thrombosis) and concurrent surrounding inflammatory response to that clot.
- Clot can dissolve, propagate, or embolize to a distal site (creating pulmonary embolus or a paradoxic cerebrovascular accident [CVA] through ASD/VSD).

RISK FACTORS

- Prior DVT
- Pregnancy or postpartum state
- Malignancy
- Prolonged immobility
- IV drug abuse
- Recent trauma or burns
- Coronary artery disease
- Polycythemia vera
- Thrombocytosis
- Antithrombin III, protein C or S deficiency
- Aquired immune deficiency syndrome
- Autoimmune disease (eg, systemic lupus erythematosus)
- Indwelling catheter

A 39-year-old woman who arrived home from her 18-hour car ride the previous evening presents with right calf swelling and pain. Physical exam reveals the right calf to be 4 cm larger than the left, and it is warm to the touch. *Think: DVT.*

HIGH-YIELD FACTS

Cardiovascular Emergencies

CLINICAL FINDINGS

- Unilateral swelling and pitting edema of a lower extremity.
- Redness, pain, heat (very similar to cellulitis in appearance).
- Palpable pulses in extremity.
- Palpable cord if superficial enough.

DIAGNOSIS

- Labs: Prothrombin time (PT) and partial thromboplastin time (PTT) should be normal. D-Dimer may be elevated but is nonspecific.
- Ultrasound of affected lower extremity: Looking at venous system and its compressibility is the most readily available imaging study, while venography is the gold standard.

TREATMENT

- Anticoagulation with heparin if DVT or PE present: 80 U/kg IV bolus followed by 18 U/kg/h infusion. Low-molecular-weight heparin can be used for DVT without PE.
- Inferior vena caval filter (Greenfield) for patients with malignancy, already on oral anticoagulation, or who have a contraindication to anticoagulation (frequent falls in elderly).
- Consider thrombolytics for massive iliofemoral thrombosis.

Gastrointestinal Emergencies

A 26-year-old woman complains of severe left lower quadrant (LLQ) pain, vaginal bleeding, weakness, and light-headedness. Her last menstrual period was 6 weeks ago. Her abdominal exam reveal LLQ tenderness with rebound. Her urine human chorionic gonadotropin (hCG) is positive. What diagnosis must be ruled out?

Ectopic pregnancy needs to be considered and excluded in all women with abdominal pain. Ectopic pregnancy is a life-threatening diagnosis that presents with abdominal pain and/or vaginal bleeding.

Visceral Pain

- Vague, dull, and poorly localized pain.
- Midline location due to bilateral innervation of organs based on their embryological origin.
- Associated with stretching, inflammation, or ischemia, involving bowel walls or organ capsules.

V is for Vague. **Example:** Early appendicitis; initially dull periumbilical pain.

Parietal Pain

- Sharp, well-localized pain; peritonitis associated with rebound and involuntary guarding.
- Pain location correlates with associated dermatomes: Occurs commonly with inflammation, frank pus, blood, or bile in or adjacent to the peritoneum.
- *Peritonitis is associated with rebound tenderness and involuntary guarding.*

P is for Pinpoint. **Example:** Late appendicitis; local inflammation → tenderness in the RLQ.

Referred Pain

- Pain stimuli generated at an afflicted location are perceived as originating from a site in which there is no current pathology.
- These sites are usually related by a common embryological origin.
- The pain can sometimes be perceived in both locations.

Example: Ureteral obstruction can produce pain in the ipsilateral testicle.

HIGH-YIELD FACTS

Gastrointestinal Emergencies

CAUSES OF ABDOMINAL PAIN (BY QUADRANTS)

Right Upper Quadrant
Gastric ulcer
Peptic ulcer
Biliary disease
Hepatitis
Pancreatitis
Retrocecal appendicitis
Renal stone
Pyelonephritis
MI
Pulmonary embolus
Pneumonia

Left Upper Quadrant
Gastric ulcer
Gastritis
Pancreatitis
Splenic injury
Renal stone
Pyelonephritis
MI
Pulmonary embolus
Pneumonia

Right Lower Quadrant
Appendicitis
Ovarian cyst
Mittelschmerz
Pregnancy (ectopic or normal)
Tubo-ovarian abscess
Pelvic inflammatory disease
Ovarian torsion
Cystitis
Prostatitis
Ureteral stone
Testicular torsion
Epididymitis
Diverticulitis
Abdominal aortic aneurysm

Left Lower Quadrant
Diverticulitis
Ovarian cyst
Mittelschmerz
Pregnancy (ectopic or normal)
Tubo-ovarian abscess
Pelvic inflammatory disease
Ovarian torsion
Cystitis
Prostatitis
Ureteral stone
Testicular torsion
Epididymitis
Diverticulitis
Abdominal aortic aneurysm

Note: *All premenopausal women with abdominal pain must have a pregnancy test, even if they say they are not sexually active.*

OTHER CAUSES OF ABDOMINAL PAIN

A 28-year-old woman presents with diffuse abdominal pain, nausea, and confusion. She is not pregnant. She currently takes a stained-glass class. Her abdominal exam is diffuse mild tenderness without rebound or guarding. In addition to routine blood work, what other test should be considered?

Lead poisoning can present with nausea, vomiting, altered mental status, and abdominal pain. A lead level should be checked.

- **Abdominal wall:**
  - Hernia
  - Rectus sheath hematoma
- **Metabolic:**
  - Diabetic ketoacidosis
  - Acute intermittent porphyria
  - Hypercalcemia

- **Infectious:**
  - Herpes zoster
  - Mononucleosis
  - Human immunodeficiency virus (HIV)
- **Drugs/toxins:**
  - Heavy metal poisoning (lead)
  - Black widow spider envenomation
- **Other:**
  - Sickle cell anemia
  - Mesenteric ischemia

Abdominal Pain in the Elderly

Elderly patients who present with abdominal pain must be treated with particular caution. Common problems that complicate the diagnosis include:

- Difficulty communicating
- Comorbid disease
- Inability to tolerate intravascular volume loss
- Unusual presentation of common disease
- May not mount a WBC count or a fever
- Complaint often incommensurate with severity of disease

Note: Up to 10% of elderly patients with an MI will present with abdominal pain.

In elderly patients with abdominal pain, always consider vascular causes, including:
- Abdominal aortic aneurysm
- Mesenteric ischemia
- MI

ESOPHAGUS

Varices

DEFINITION

Dilated submucosal veins.

EPIDEMIOLOGY

- Found in 25–40% of patients with cirrhosis.
- Usually develop due to portal hypertension.
- Thirty percent of patients with varices develop upper gastrointestinal (GI) bleeds.

Higher morbidity and mortality rate than any other source of upper GI bleed.

CLINICAL FINDINGS

- Asymptomatic until rupture.
- Bleeding is usually massive.
- Present with spontaneous emesis of either bright red blood or coffee ground material.

Many patients with varices have coagulopathy due to underlying cirrhosis.

TREATMENT

- Two large-bore IVs.
- Volume replacement with normal saline (NS) and packed red blood cells.
- Nasogastric (NG) lavage.
- IV proton pump inhibitor (PPI).
- IV vasopressin or octreotide to control bleeding.
- GI consult.

- Emergent endoscopy to localize bleeding for possible sclerotherapy or rubber band ligation of varices.
- Consider tamponade with Sengstaken-Blakemore tube for persistent bleeding.
- Hospital admission for all unstable cases.

Esophageal Foreign Body (FB) Ingestion

SITES OF IMPACTION

- The most common site in children is at the cricopharyngeus muscle (C5).
- The most common site in adults is at the lower esophageal sphincter (LES) (T10).
- Physiologic narrowings of the esophagus:
  - Proximal esophagus—at level of thoracic inlet
  - Mid esophagus—level of carina and aortic arch
  - Distal esophagus—level just proximal to gastroesophageal junction

EPIDEMIOLOGY

- Eighty percent of obstructions occur in children and are due to coins, marbles, buttons, etc.
- Twenty percent of obstructions occur in adults and are due to meat impaction.

SIGNS AND SYMPTOMS

- Dysphagia
- Gagging
- Throat pain
- FB sensation
- Vomiting
- Anorexia
- Anxiety

DIAGNOSIS

- Chest x-ray (CXR) and soft-tissue films of the neck to look for:
  - The flat surface of a coin or other such FB will be seen when it is lodged in the esophagus (see Figure 8-1).
  - The edge will be seen when located in the trachea.
- If radiographs do not demonstrate FB, then consider esophagogram with contrast or endoscopy.

TREATMENT

- Eighty percent of ingested FBs pass spontaneously; no treatment is required in these cases, except observation of stool for 3–5 days. Patients unable to swallow liquids require emergent endoscopy because of complete obstruction.
- If FB is in the upper third of the esophagus (cervical esophagus, top 5 cm), it can be removed with a Magill forceps and a laryngoscope.
- For meat impactions in the distal (last 3 cm) esophagus:
  - IV glucagon or sublingual nitroglycerin can be used to relax smooth muscle and ↓ LES tone.
  - Carbonated beverages and other gas-forming agents may be useful to push the meat impaction down into the stomach by raising the intraluminal pressure; however, there is risk of aspiration and perforation.

Adults with esophageal meat impactions almost always have underlying pathology such as carcinoma or strictures.

Endoscopy offers the advantage of being able to visualize and *remove* FB.

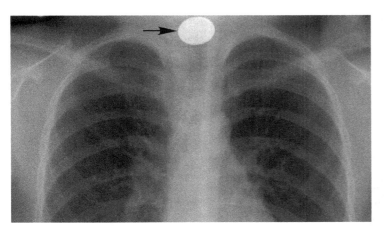
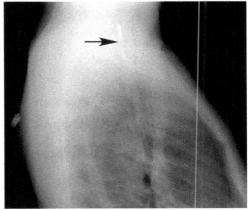

FIGURE 8-1. AP and lateral views demonstrating a coin in the esophagus.

A coin in the trachea would present in the opposite manner—the coin would be seen on edge on the AP view, and flat on the lateral view.

- Endoscopic removal is required for sharp objects and objects larger than 2 cm wide or 5 cm long.
- Removal of these objects before they pass the pylorus ↓ chance of perforation.
- Approximately 1% of impacted FBs cannot be removed by direct visualization or do not pass into the stomach and must be removed surgically.

Gastroesophageal Reflux Disease (GERD)

DEFINITION

Reflux of acidic gastric contents into the esophagus.

CAUSES

- Relaxed or incompetent LES
- Hiatal hernia
- ↓ esophageal motility
- Delayed gastric emptying
- Diabetes mellitus
- Gastroparesis
- Gastric outlet obstruction
- Anticholinergic use
- Fatty foods

CAUSES OF LOWERED LES TONE

- Coffee
- Cigarettes
- Alcohol
- Chocolate
- Peppermint
- Anticholinergics
- Progesterone
- Estrogen
- Nitrates
- Calcium channel blockers

> Most alkaline batteries will pass into the stomach and can be managed expectantly. However, 10% of button batteries will lodge in the esophagus, and these must be removed because they are highly corrosive (alkali causes liquefaction necrosis).

A majority of patients with asthma have associated GERD.

SIGNS AND SYMPTOMS

- Substernal burning pain
- Dysphagia
- Hypersalivation (water brash)
- Cough

DIAGNOSIS

Barium swallow, endoscopy, mucosal biopsy.

TREATMENT

- Elevate head of bed.
- Discontinue foods that ↓ LES tone.
- Oral antacids.
- H_2 blocker or PPI.
- Patients with hiatal hernia may be candidates for Nissen fundoplication (the stomach is wrapped around the distal esophagus to create a "new sphincter").

COMPLICATIONS OF GERD

- **Esophagitis:** Esophageal damage, bleeding, and friability due to prolonged exposure to gastric contents.
- **Peptic stricture:** Occurs in about 10% of patients with GERD.
- **Barrett's esophagus:** Transformation of normal squamous epithelium to columnar epithelium, sometimes accompanied by an ulcer or stricture.
- **Esophageal cancer:** Upper two-thirds squamous, lower one-third adenocarcinoma.

Barrett's esophagus carries a 2–5% risk of development of esophageal adenocarcinoma, which carries a < 5% chance of 5-year survival.

Boerhaave Syndrome

- Spontaneous rupture of the esophagus that typically occurs after forceful emesis.
- Most lethal perforation of the GI tract, with mortality ~35%.

RISK FACTORS

Alcohol ingestion.

CLINICAL FINDINGS

- The Mackler triad: Vomiting, lower thoracic pain, and subcutaneous emphysema.
- Pneumomediastinum.
- Crackling sound on chest auscultation ("Hamman's crunch").

Boerhaave syndrome is a transmural perforation of the esophagus to be distinguished from Mallory-Weiss syndrome, a nontransmural esophageal tear also associated with vomiting.

DIAGNOSIS

- CXR in 90% of patients shows abnormal findings after perforation.
- The most common findings on CXR are pleural effusion (usually left), pneumothorax, hydropneumothorax, pneumomediastinum, subcutaneous emphysema, or mediastinal widening.
- Water-soluble contrast esophagram helps confirm the diagnosis.

TREATMENT

- IV volume resuscitation.
- Administration of broad-spectrum antibiotics.

Mallory-Weiss syndrome: Upper GI bleeding secondary to longitudinal mucosal lacerations at the gastroesophageal junction or gastric cardia.

Mallory-Weiss Tear

DEFINITION

A **partial-thickness** tear at the gastroesophageal junction associated with hematemesis, usually self-limited.

RISK FACTORS

- Alcoholism
- Hiatal hernia
- Gastritis

CLINICAL FINDINGS

- Prior history of vomiting, retching, or straining.
- Endoscopy establishes diagnosis.

TREATMENT

- Usually self-limited.
- Actively bleeding Mallory-Weiss tears can be treated with multipolar electrocoagulation with or without epinephrine injection, polydocanol injection (sclerosant), or endoscopic hemoclipping.
- Remember: Balloon tamponade is not an option here. It recreates the force leading up to the tear, and can make things worse.
- PPIs, mucosal protectants like sucralfate, and antiemetics are important cotherapies.

Acute Gastritis

DEFINITION

Inflammation of the stomach.

ETIOLOGIES

- Stress gastritis is due to severe medical or surgical illness including trauma, burns, hypotension, sepsis, central nervous system (CNS) injury (Cushing ulcer), mechanical respiration, and multiorgan failure.
- Corrosive gastritis is most commonly seen with alcohol.
- Often associated with *Helicobacter pylori* infection.

CLINICAL FINDINGS

- Most asymptomatic unless ulcers or other complications develop.
- Symptomatic: Abdominal pain, nausea/vomiting, GI bleed.
- Typically diagnosed at endoscopy for complaints of dyspepsia or upper GI bleed.

Things that cause gastritis—
SPIT BANDS
Shock states
Pancreatic juice
Infection with *Helicobacter pylori*
Tobacco
Bile
Alcohol
Nonsteroidal anti-inflammatory drugs (NSAIDs)
Drug-induced
Steroids/Stress

The most common cause of gastritis is chronic use of NSAIDs.

TREATMENT

- Avoid alcohol, cigarettes, caffeine, and citrus and spicy foods for 6 weeks.
- Prophylaxis with H_2 blocker.

Upper GI Bleed

DEFINITION

Bleeding that is proximal to ligament of Treitz.

ETIOLOGY (IN ORDER OF DECREASING FREQUENCY)

- Peptic ulcer (accounts for > 50%)
- Gastric erosions
- Varices
- Mallory-Weiss tear
- Esophagitis
- Duodenitis

CLINICAL FINDINGS

- Most common presentation is hematemesis (bright red blood or "coffee grounds") or melena (dark tarry stool) with or without abdominal pain.
- Hematochezia (bright red bloody stool) usually indicates lower GI bleed, but may also be present in massive upper GI bleeds.
- Check for hypotension, tachycardia, weakness, pallor, syncope, and diaphoresis.
- Ear, nose, and throat exam should be done to rule out nosebleeds, which can mimic upper GI bleed (swallowed blood).

DIAGNOSIS

- Routine labs: Complete blood count (CBC), prothrombin time (PT), partial thromboplastin time (PTT), type and crossmatch 4–6 units, electrolytes, liver function tests (LFTs).
- Abdominal radiograph (AXR): Usefulness very limited but may rule out free air caused by perforated ulcers.

TREATMENT

- Rapid assessment and management with ABCs (airway, breathing, and circulation), supporting airway, IV (NS or lactated Ringer's solution), O_2, and monitor.
- Blood products for continued active bleeding or failure to improve vitals. Consider use of IV vasopressin or octreotide.
- NG lavage looking for coffee grounds or fresh blood.
- GI consult for identification of bleeding sites with endoscopy.
- Surgical consultation and intervention is indicated if patient does not respond to medical or endoscopic treatment.
- Admit all unstable patients.

Crossmatching blood takes ~45–60 minutes. Use O negative if type-specific blood is not ready and patient unstable.

Chronic liver disease: *Think: Esophageal varices or portal hypertension.*

Heavy alcohol ingestion or retching: *Think: Mallory-Weiss tear.*

Peptic Ulcer Disease (PUD)

DEFINITION

Disruption of the mucosal defensive factors by acid and pepsin, which causes ulceration of the mucosa beyond the muscularis.

RISK FACTORS

- Infection with *H pylori*.
- Cigarette use.
- Ethanol use.
- NSAIDs (prostaglandin depletion).
- Others: Steroids, hepatic cirrhosis, renal failure, familial predisposition.
- Hypersecretory states; Zollinger-Ellison syndrome, antral G cell hyperplasia, systemic mastocytosis, basophilic leukemias.
- Chemotherapy.
- Cocaine/crack usage.

CLINICAL FINDINGS

- Classically, the pain is described as burning, gnawing, dull, or hunger-like.
- Gastric ulcer (GU) pain begins shortly after eating.
- Duodenal ulcer (DU) pain occurs 2–3 hours after meal and is relieved by food or antacids.
- Ulcers are most commonly located along the lesser curvature of the stomach or the first portion of duodenum.
- Simple bleeding (most common cause of upper GI bleed):
  - Most stop spontaneously.
  - Posterior ulcer erodes into the gastroduodenal artery.

DIAGNOSIS

- Most PUD is not definitively diagnosed in the ED, but rather treated empirically.
- Endoscopy is 95% accurate for diagnosis.

TREATMENT

- Treatment is primarily outpatient unless complications occur.
- Advise patient to avoid substances that exacerbate ulcers.
- Eradicate *H pylori* disease.
- Pain relief with antacids given 1 hour before and 3 hours after meal (poor compliance due to frequency of therapy).
- H_2 receptor antagonists (cimetidine, ranitidine, famotidine, or nizatidine) and PPIs (eg, omeprazole, lansoprazole) are mainstay of therapy in noninfected individuals.
- Patients who demonstrate any complication should be stabilized and admitted.

NSAID use, steroids, or dyspepsia: *Think: Peptic ulcer disease (PUD).*

H pylori is associated with 80% of GUs and 95% of DUs.

Pain is visceral in nature and is therefore vague and midline.

First-line therapy for *H pylori:*
PPI + amoxicillin 1 g + clarithromycin 500 mg all twice daily for 7–14 days

Adverse effects of cimetidine:
- ↑ levels of drugs cleared via P450 system (eg, warfarin, phenytoin, diazepam, propranolol, lidocaine, theophylline, tricyclic antidepressants)
- Central nervous system dysfunction in the elderly
- Thrombocytopenia
- Painful gynecomastia

COMPLICATIONS OF PUD

Perforation

A 45-year-old man presents with sudden onset of severe epigastric pain. He has a history of PUD but has stopped taking his H$_2$ blocker. On exam, he is hypotensive with a rigid abdomen. What service should be consulted?

The patient is presenting with a surgical abdomen most likely due to a perforated ulcer.

SIGNS AND SYMPTOMS
- Sudden onset of generalized abdominal pain associated with a rigid abdomen often radiating to back.
- Vomiting involved in 50%.

DIAGNOSIS
- Upright CXR to look for free air: Useful for 70% of anterior perforations (most common type). Does not pick up posterior perforations because the posterior duodenum is retroperitoneal.
- Posterior perforations may → pancreatitis.

TREATMENT
IV fluids, NG drainage, antibiotics, immediate surgery.

Gastric Outlet Obstruction

PATHOPHYSIOLOGY
Healing ulcer may scar and block the antral or pyloric outlet.

SIGNS AND SYMPTOMS
- History of vomiting undigested food shortly after eating
- Succussion splash: Splashing sound made when abdomen is gently rocked
- Early satiety
- Weight loss

DIAGNOSIS
- Characteristic electrolyte abnormalities (hypokalemia, hypochloremia, and metabolic alkalosis).
- AXR will show dilated stomach with large air-fluid level.

TREATMENT
- NG suctioning
- Correction of electrolyte abnormalities
- Hospital admission

Inflammatory Bowel Disease (IBD)

DEFINITION

A chronic, inflammatory disease affecting GI tract. Two major types are Crohn disease (CD) and ulcerative colitis (UC).

Crohn: Lower incidence, lower risk of cancer, more common in women.

EPIDEMIOLOGY

* More common in people of Caucasian and Jewish background
* Peak incidence in ages 15–35 years
* Occurs with familial clustering
* Incidence: UC = 2–10/100,000; CD = 1–6/100,000
* UC more common in men
* CD more common in women
* Associated risk of colon cancer is 10–30 times for UC and 3 times for CD

CLINICAL PRESENTATION AND DIAGNOSIS

See Tables 8-1 and 8-2.

Early institution of NG suction, IV fluids, and steroids to reduce inflammation in suspected bowel obstruction.

TREATMENT

* Supportive care.
* Antidiarrheals:
  * ↓ frequency of stool.
  * Loperamide and diphenoxylate are used for patients with fatty acid–induced diarrhea.
* Cholestyramine:
  * Used for patients without fatty acid–induced diarrhea.
  * Contraindicated in severe colitis due to risk of toxic megacolon.

TABLE 8-1. Clinical Presentation and Diagnosis of Ulcerative Colitis (UC) and Crohn Disease (CD)

	ULCERATIVE COLITIS	CROHN DISEASE
Signs and symptoms	• Bloody diarrhea • Rectal pain	• Crampy abdominal pain, typically in RLQ • Fatigue, malaise (due to chronic anemia)
Location	• Limited to rectum and colon	• Can affect any part of GI tract
Pathology	• Inflammation of mucosa only (exudates of pus, blood, and mucus from the "crypt abscess")	• Inflammation involves all bowel wall layers, which may → fistulas and abscesses • Rectal sparing in 50%
Colonoscopy findings	• Continuous lesions • Lead pipe colon apperance due to chronic scarring and subsequent retraction and loss of haustra	• Skip lesions • Aphthous ulcers • Cobblestone apperance from submucosal thickening interspersed with mucosal alteration
Complications	• Perforation • Stricture • Megacolon	• Abscesses • Fistulas • Obstruction • Perianal lesions

Eye involvement	▪ Uveitis	CD > UC
	▪ Episcleritis	Uveitis, erythema nodosum, and colitic arthritis are commonly seen together
Dermatologic	▪ Erythema nodosum	CD > UC, especially in children
	▪ Pyoderma gangrenosum	Parallels disease course (gets better as IBD improves)
		UC > CD
		May or may not follow disease course
	▪ Aphthous ulcers	CD
Arthritis	▪ Colitic arthritis	CD > UC
	▪ Ankylosing spondylitis	Parallels disease course
		30 times more common in UC
		Unrelated to disease course
Hematologic	▪ Anemia	
	▪ Thromboembolism	
Hepatobiliary	▪ Fatty liver	
	▪ Hepatitis	
	▪ Cholelithiasis	
	▪ Primary sclerosing cholangitis	UC > CD
Renal	▪ Secondary amyloidosis → renal failure	CD
		Unrelated to disease course

▪ Anticholinergics:
  ▪ Reduce abdominal cramping, pain, and urgency.
  ▪ Opium-belladonna combination works well to control diarrhea and pain.

SPECIFIC THERAPY

Sulfasalazine is also used to treat rheumatoid arthritis, but in this case, it is the sulfapyridine component that is the active one.

Drugs with only the 5-ASA component are not effective in IBD.

▪ Sulfasalazine:
  ▪ Consists of 5-acetylsalicylic acid (ASA) (active component) and sulfapyridine (toxic effects are due to this moiety).
  ▪ Side effects include GI distress in one-third of patients (give enteric coated preparation), ↓ folic acid absorption, and male infertility (reversible).
  ▪ Drug appears safe in children and pregnant women.
▪ Corticosteroids:
  ▪ Early phase of action blocks vascular permeability, vasodilation, and infiltration of neutrophils.
  ▪ Late phase of action blocks vascular proliferation, fibroblast activation, and collagen deposition.
  ▪ May be given as enemas (↓ systemic absorption).
▪ Antibiotics (used for CD)
  ▪ Three-week courses of metronidazole and ciprofloxacin have been used to induce disease remission with some success.

- Mechanism of action is unknown because other antibiotics with a similar antimicrobial spectrum have not been shown to be effective.
- Immunomodulators:
  - Used in refractory cases, especially in CD.
  - Include azathioprine, 6-mercaptopurine, and methotrexate.
  - Resistant cases may also benefit from anti–tumor necrosis factor-alpha (TNF-α) antibodies, recombinant anti-TNF cytokines.
- Biologic response modifiers: Monoclonal antibodies that prevent inflammation. Often combined with the above, in unresponsive/progressive disease. They include: infliximab, adalimumab, certolizumab, among others. All of these have serious side effects, and hence should be used only as a last resort.

Mesenteric Ischemia

> An 82-year-old woman with a history of atrial fibrillation presents with sudden-onset severe abdominal pain. She is unable to lie still or get comfortable. On exam, her abdomen is soft, with only mild diffuse tenderness. What is the most likely diagnosis?
> Sudden onset of abdominal pain in a patient with a history of atrial fibrillation is likely to be mesenteric ischemia until proven otherwise.

DEFINITION

- Lack of perfusion to bowel
- High-mortality disease

RISK FACTORS

- Age > 50 years
- Valvular or atherosclerotic heart disease
- Arrhythmias (especially atrial fibrillation)
- Congestive heart failure
- Recent myocardial infarction (MI)
- Critically ill patients with sepsis or hypotension
- Use of diuretics or vasoconstrictive drugs
- Hypercoagulable states
- Low-flow states (hypovolemia, hypotension) can → ischemic colitis

CLINICAL FINDINGS

- Severe acute midabdominal, periumbilical **pain out of proportion to findings** (ie, patient complains of severe pain but is not very tender on exam).
- Sudden onset suggests arterial vascular occlusion by emboli, consistent with acute ischemia.
- Insidious onset suggests venous thrombosis or nonocclusive infarction (intestinal angina), consistent with chronic ischemia.
- As infarct develops, peritoneal signs develop suggestive of necrotic bowel.
- The most common location of mesenteric artery occlusion are:
  - Superior mesenteric artery embolism (50 %)
  - Superior mesenteric artery thrombosis (15–25%)

A diagnosis of mesenteric ischemia requires a high index of suspicion.

- Mesenteric venous thrombosis (5%)
- Nonocclusive ischemia (20–30 %)
- If patient presents with lower abdominal pain associated with hematochezia, consider colonic ischemia.

DIAGNOSIS

Gas in the bowel wall is known as *pneumatosis intestinalis.*

- Laboratory analyses reveal metabolic acidosis, elevated lactate, and elevated phosphorus.
- AXR may reveal dilated loops of bowel, air-fluid level, irregular thickening of the bowel wall (thumbprinting), and gas in the bowel wall or portal system.
- Computed tomography (CT) scan may demonstrate air in the bowel wall, mesenteric portal vein gas, and bowel wall thickening.
- Angiography is the gold standard and should not be delayed.
- Magnetic resonance angiography (MRA) is highly sensitive for mesenteric venous thrombosis.
- Diagnosis can frequently be delayed without high index of suspicion.

TREATMENT

- IV fluid to correct fluid and electrolyte abnormalities.
- Supplemental O_2.
- NG tube to decompress bowel.
- Antibiotics to cover gut flora.
- Selective vasodilator infusion (eg, papaverine) during angiography.
- Surgery to remove emboli or necrotic bowel.
- Patients with mesenteric ischemia often present with hypotension, and if volume resuscitation is unsuccessful, then the vasopressor of choice is dobutamine, low-dose dopamine or milrinone, because these have less effect on the mesenteric circulation.

Hernias

DEFINITIONS

- Protrusion of a structure through an opening that is either congenital or acquired.
- Reducible hernia: Protruding contents can be pushed back to their original location.
- Incarcerated hernia: An irreducible hernia may be acute and painful or chronic and asymptomatic.
- Strangulated hernia: Incarcerated hernia with vascular compromise.

RISK FACTORS

- Obesity
- Chronic cough
- Pregnancy
- Constipation
- Straining on urination
- Ascites
- Previous hernia repair

CLINICAL FINDINGS OF INGUINAL HERNIAS

- **Direct**:
  - Protrudes through floor of Hesselbach's triangle.
  - Frequency ↑ with age.
  - Rarely incarcerates.
- **Indirect**:
  - Protrudes lateral to the inferior epigastric vessels.
  - Most commonly occurring hernia.
  - Frequently incarcerates.
  - History of palpable, soft mass that ↑ with straining (patient bears down and coughs while you pass digit in external canal).
  - Bowel sounds may be heard over hernia if it contains bowel.

DIAGNOSIS

- Can be made from physical exam.
- AXR to look for air-fluid levels (obstruction) or free air under the diaphragm (perforation).

TREATMENT

- May attempt reduction of incarcerated hernia with outpatient referral for surgery. Advise patient to refrain from straining.
- A strangulated hernia requires immediate surgery. Do not attempt to reduce dead bowel into abdomen!

Intussusception

DEFINITION

The telescoping of one segment of bowel into another, the most common being the ileocecal segment.

- Intussusceptum: The segment that telescopes inside.
- Intussuscepiens: The segment that accepts the telescoping segments.

RISK FACTORS

Fifty percent have recent viral infection.

CLINICAL FINDINGS

- Classic triad:
  - Colicky abdominal pain
  - Vomiting
  - Currant jelly stool (late finding)
- Elongated mass may be palpable in right upper quadrant (RUQ).

DIAGNOSIS

Air or barium enema—"coiled spring" appearance of bowel (Figure 8-2).

TREATMENT

Air or barium enema → reduction in 60–70%. Remaining cases require surgery.

Incarcerated hernias are the second most common cause of small bowel obstruction (after adhesions).

Bowel obstruction can be the first presenting sign of a hernia.

Intussusception is the most common cause of bowel obstruction in children ages 2 months to 5 years.

HIGH-YIELD FACTS

Gastrointestinal Emergencies

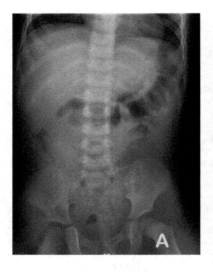
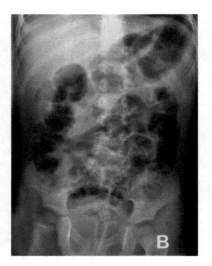
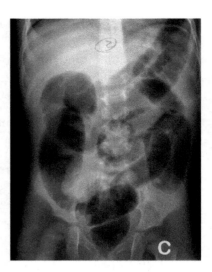

FIGURE 8-2. Intussusception.

Note the paucity of bowel gas in film A. Air enema partially reduces it in film B and further in film C.

Small Bowel Obstruction (SBO)

ETIOLOGIES

Inspect for scars and hernias and ask about past surgical history (risk for adhesions).

- Adhesions (most common)
- Hernia (second most common)
- Neoplasms
- Intussusception
- Gallstones
- Bezoars
- IBD
- Abscess

CLINICAL FINDINGS

- Intermittent crampy abdominal pain
- Vomiting
- Abdominal distention
- Absence of bowel movements or flatulence for several days
- Hyperactive high-pitched bowel sounds (**borborygmi**) (become hypoactive and eventually absent as the obstruction progresses)

DIAGNOSIS

In proximal obstruction, bilious vomiting can occur early with minimal distention.

- AXR may demonstrate stepladder appearance of air-fluid levels (see Figure 8-3), thickening of small bowel wall, or loss of markings (plicae circulares).
- Computed tomography (CT) scan can distinguish partial from complete obstruction.

TREATMENT

- IV fluids, NG suction, and early surgical consult.
- Partial obstructions may be candidates for conservative management.

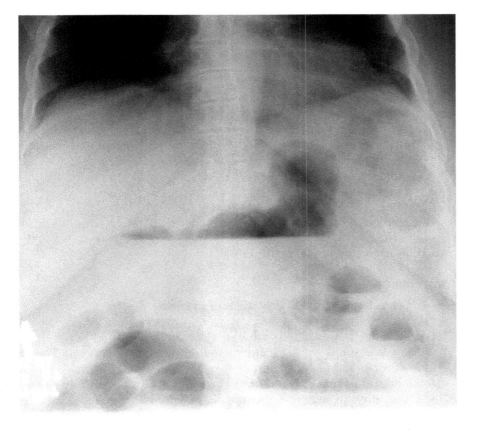

FIGURE 8-3. SBO.

Radiograph of the abdomen demonstrates multiple distended small bowel loops with air-fluid levels throughout abdomen.

Hepatitis

DEFINITION

Inflammation of the liver secondary to a number of causes.

ETIOLOGIES

- Alcohol:
  - Most common precursor to cirrhosis.
  - May develop after several decades of alcohol abuse or within 1 year of heavy drinking.
- Autoimmune: Little is known at this time.
- Toxins: Acetaminophen, carbon tetrachloride, heavy metals, tetracyclines, valproic acid, isoniazid, amiodarone, phenytoin, halothane, methyldopa.
- Viruses:
  - Hepatitis A (HAV): Fecal-oral transmission via contaminated water or food, endemic areas; no carrier state; does not cause chronic liver disease.
  - Hepatitis B (HBV): Sexual and parenteral transmission; has a carrier state and causes chronic disease; effective vaccine available.

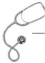

HBV and HCV are more contagious than human immunodeficiency virus (HIV). Always use universal precautions.

Concurrent HBV/HCV infection is common and exacerbates liver disease. Both carry ↑ risk of cirrhosis and hepatocellular carcinoma.

HCV is the most common blood-borne cause of viral hepatitis in the United States.

- Hepatitis C (HCV): Sexual and parenteral transmission; has a carrier state; 85% go on to develop chronic liver disease; no vaccine available.
- Hepatitis D: Sexual and parenteral transmission; incomplete virus—requires coinfection with HBV.
- Hepatitis E (HEV): Similar to HAV but higher incidence of fulminant liver failure; no serologic marker.
- Hepatitis G (HGV): Also known as hepatitis GB virus type C; transmission occurs through blood transfusion and sexual and parenteral transmission.
- Cytomegalovirus.
- Herpes simplex virus.
- Parasites:
  - *Entamoeba histolytica* abscess presents with RUQ pain, fever, and diarrhea.
  - *Clonorchis sinensis* (liver fluke).

CLINICAL FINDINGS

- RUQ tenderness (due to distention of liver capsule).
- Alcoholic:
  - Can range from mild liver disease to acute liver failure.
  - May present with liver enlargement, weakness, anorexia, nausea, abdominal pain, and weight loss.
  - Dark urine, jaundice, and fever are frequent complaints.
  - Physical exam may reveal jaundice, pedal edema, gynecomastia, palmar erythema, and spider angiomata.
  - Complications: Ascites, portal hypertension, esophageal varices, spontaneous bacterial peritonitis (SBP), hepatic abscess, hepatorenal syndrome, hepatic encephalopathy.
- Viral:
  - Prodrome of anorexia, nausea, vomiting, diarrhea, malaise, and flu-like symptoms.
  - History of travel to endemic area for HAV and HEV, IV drug users, homosexuals.
  - Hepatitis B: Arthralgia or arthritis (polyarticular) involving the small joints of hands and the wrists; dermatitis (mainly urticarial).
  - Serologic studies may be ordered in ED, but results are not immediately available.
- Parasites: History of travel to endemic area.

DIAGNOSIS

- Thrombocytopenia.
- Elevated bilirubin.
- Serum glutamate pyruvate transaminase (SGPT) > serum glutamicoxaloacetic transaminase (SGOT) suggestive of viral hepatitis.
- PT usually normal.

In alcoholic hepatitis, the SGOT (AST) is greater than SGPT (ALT) by a factor of 2.

TREATMENT

- Supportive care is the mainstay of therapy; treat complications.
- Alcohol:
  - Hospital admission for all but the mildest cases.
  - Correct electrolyte abnormalities.
  - Supplement thiamine and folate.
  - High-calorie/high-protein diet.

- HBV: Interferon-α_{2b}, ribavirin.
- Acetaminophen poisoning: N-acetylcysteine (best if given within 24 hours of ingestion, but usually no hepatitis by then; can give up to 1 week after ingestion).
- Parasites:
  - Metronidazole/albendazole.
  - Occasionally, needle aspiration and decompression or surgical decontamination.

Hepatic Encephalopathy

DEFINITION

A manifestation of hepatic failure, the final common pathway.

ETIOLOGY

Need to consider what triggered episode:

- Infection: Pneumonia, subacute bacterial peritonitis (SBP)
- GI bleed
- Medication noncompliance
- Alcohol

TREATMENT

- Strict protein restriction.
- Correction of fluids and electrolyte abnormalities.
- Lactulose and neomycin to clear the gut of bacteria and nitrogen products.
- Liver transplant may be lifesaving.
- See Table 8-3 for grading of hepatic encephalopathy.

Hepatorenal Syndrome (HRS)

DEFINITION

Acquired renal failure in association with liver failure; cause unknown.

CLINICAL FINDINGS

- Hypotension.
- Ascites:
  - Portal hypertension (high hydrostatic pressure)
  - Hypoalbuminemia (low oncotic pressure)
- Type 1 HRS: Rapid and progressive renal impairment, mostly due to SBP.
- Type 2 HRS: Moderate and stable reduction in glomerular filtration rate (GFR), commonly occurring in patients with preserved hepatic function.

DIAGNOSIS

- Azotemia, oliguria, hyponatremia, low urinary sodium.
- Sodium retention by kidneys from ↑ renin and angiotensin levels.
- Impaired liver clearance of aldosterone (all hormones).

Admit hepatitis if:
- Encephalopathic
- Excessive bleeding
- INR >3
- Intractable vomiting
- Immunosuppressed
- Due to alcohol
- Hypoglycemic
- Bilirubin >25

Reye syndrome: Acute hepatic encephalopathy associated with ASA use in children.

TABLE 8-3. Grading of Hepatic Encephalopathy

GRADE	LEVEL OF CONSCIOUSNESS	PERSONALITY AND INTELLECT	NEUROLOGIC SIGNS
0	Normal	Normal	None
1	Day/night sleep reversal Restlessness	Forgetfulness Mild confusion Agitation Irritability	Tremor Apraxia Incoordination Impaired handwriting
2	Lethargy Slowed responses	Disorientation to time Loss of inhibition Inappropriate behavior	Asterixis Dysarthria Ataxia, hypoactive reflexes
3	Somnolence Confusion	Disorientation to place Aggressive behavior	Asterixis Muscular rigidity Babinski signs Hyperactive reflexes
4	Coma	None	Decerebration

Hepatorenal syndrome has a bad prognosis. Mortality is almost 100%.

TREATMENT

- Low-salt diet
- Fluid restriction
- Diuretics (spironolactone and furosemide or hydrochlorothiazide)
- Paracentesis: Therapeutic in massive ascites with respiratory compromise; low risk of bleeding, infection, or bowel perforation
- Liver transplantation

Spontaneous Bacterial Peritonitis (SBP)

A 51-year-old man with a history of cirrhosis presents with confusion and mild abdominal pain. On exam, he is afebrile with a distended abdomen and mild asterixis. What procedure should be performed as part of his workup?

A diagnostic paracentesis should be performed to obtain fluid for cell counts and cultures. A high index of suspicion is necessary for diagnosis of SBP, as symptoms can be very mild.

ETIOLOGY

- Bacterial breach of intestinal barrier to peritoneum
- *Escherichia coli*, pneumococci (anaerobes rare)

CLINICAL FINDINGS

- SBP should be suspected in cirrhotics with fever, abdominal pain, worsening ascites, and encephalopathy.

- Mild tenderness or abdominal rigidity and guarding with rebound tenderness.
- Paracentesis:
    - Total white blood cell (WBC) count > 500 cells/mL
    - > 250 polymorphonuclear neutrophils/mL, very specific for SBP
    - Total protein > 1 g/dL
    - Glucose < 50 mg/dL
    - Cultures positive in > 90%

TREATMENT

Hospital admission for IV antibiotics (third-generation cephalosporin).

Hepatic Abscess

ETIOLOGY

- Ascending cholangitis:
    - Most common cause of hepatic abscess.
    - Frequent organisms include *E coli*, *Proteus vulgaris*, *Enterobacter aerogenes*, and anaerobes.
- Parasites (eg, *E histolytica*, *Echinococcus*): Travel history
- Idiopathic

GALLBLADDER

Cholangitis

DEFINITION

Obstruction of the biliary tract and biliary stasis → bacterial overgrowth and infection.

ETIOLOGY

- Common duct stone is the most common cause.
- Primary sclerosing cholangitis.

CLINICAL FINDINGS

- **Charcot's triad:** RUQ pain, jaundice, fever/chills
- **Reynolds' pentad:** Charcot's triad + shock and mental status change
- Labs: Elevated WBC, bilirubin (direct > indirect), and alkaline phosphatase ultrasound (95% sensitivity) reveals ductal dilatation and gallstones

TREATMENT

- ABCs.
- IV hydration.
- Correction of electrolytes.
- Antibiotics.
- Surgery consult.
- Endoscopic retrograde cholangiopancreatography (ERCP) may be effective in decompression.

Cholangitis is a surgical emergency with high mortality.

Gas in biliary tree is strong supportive evidence of cholangitis.

HIGH-YIELD FACTS

Gastrointestinal Emergencies

Murphy's sign: The arrest of inspiration while palpating the RUQ. This test is > 95% sensitive for acute cholecystitis, less sensitive in the elderly.

Sonographic Murphy's sign: The same symptom when the ultrasound probe is placed on the RUQ.

Gallstone composition:
- Cholesterol (70%): Radiolucent
- Pigment (20%): Radiodense
- Mixed (10%)

Cholelithiasis and Cholecystitis

A 45-year-old obese woman complains of fever, RUQ pain, and nausea that is worse when she eats. What is the imaging test of choice

The patient is presenting with symptoms of biliary tract disease. The fever raises the suspicion for acute cholecystitis. An RUQ ultrasound can help distinguish biliary colic from cholecystitis.

DEFINITIONS

- Cholelithiasis is a stone in the gallbladder.
- Choledocholithiasis is a stone in the common bile duct.
- Biliary colic: Transient gallstone obstruction of cystic duct causing intermittent RUQ pain lasting a few hours after a meal. No established infection.
- Acute cholecystitis is the obstruction of the cystic duct with pain lasting longer, fever, chills, nausea, and positive Murphy's sign.

DIAGNOSIS

- Labs: Alkaline phosphatase, bilirubin, LFTs, electrolytes, blood urea nitrogen (BUN), creatinine, amylase, lipase, CBC.
- Plain films may reveal radiopaque gallstones (10–15%).
- Ultrasound to look for presence of gallstones, thickened gallbladder wall, positive sonographic Murphy's sign, gallbladder distention, fluid collection. Presence of gallstones, thickened gallbladder wall, and pericholecystic fluid has a positive predictive value of > 90% (Figure 8-4).
- **Hepato-iminodiacetic acid (HIDA) scan:** For this test, technetium-99m-labeled iminodiacetic acid is injected IV and is taken up by hepatocytes. In normals, the gallbladder is outlined within 1 hour. Useful if diagnostic uncertainty exists.

TREATMENT

- Uncomplicated biliary colic may go home if pain controlled.
- Acute cholecystitis should be treated with antibiotics and be admitted to the surgical service.

PANCREAS

Acute Pancreatitis

A 50-year-old man alcoholic presents with midepigastric pain radiating to the back. He is leaning forward on his stretcher and vomiting. What is his diagnosis?

The patient is presenting with symptoms of pancreatitis. The diagnosis is confirmed by an elevated lipase. Treatment is mainly supportive with IV fluids, pain control, and antiemetics.

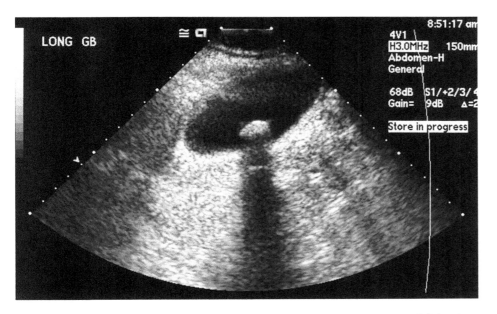

FIGURE 8-4. Sonogram demonstrating classic "headlight" appearance of cholelithiasis.

DEFINITION

Inflammation and self-destruction of the pancreas by its digestive enzymes.

RISK FACTORS

> A 66-year-old woman with hypertension and seizures for which she is on furosemide and valproic acid presents with abdominal pain, back pain, and fever. Her nonfasting glucose is noted to be 300. There is a large number of drugs that cause pancreatitis. Diuretics and anticonvulsants are common agents that can → pancreatitis.

- Gallstones and alcohol account for 85% of all cases.
- Pancreatic tumor (obstructing common duct).
- Hyperlipidemia.
- Hypercalcemia.
- Trauma.
- Iatrogenic (ERCP).
- Ischemia.
- Drugs (thiazide diuretics, steroids).
- Familial.
- Viral (coxsackievirus, mumps).

CLINICAL FINDINGS

- Abrupt onset of deep epigastric pain with radiation to the back.
- Positional preference—leaning forward.
- Nausea, vomiting, anorexia, fever, tachycardia, and abdominal distention with diminished bowel sounds.
- Jaundice with obstructive etiology.

Hypercalcemia can cause pancreatitis, and pancreatitis can cause hypocalcemia.

A sentinel loop is distention and/or air-fluid levels near a site of abdominal distention. In pancreatitis, it is secondary to pancreatitis-associated ileus.

DIAGNOSIS

- Leukocytosis, elevated amylase and lipase (lipase more specific).
- AXR: Sentinel loop, colon cutoff (distended colon to midtransverse colon with no air distally).
- Ultrasound: Good for pseudocyst, abscess, and gallstones.
- CT preferred diagnostic test (Figure 8-5).

PROGNOSIS

Ranson's criteria (see Table 8-4): Mortality rates correlate with the number of criteria present. Presence of < 3 criteria equals a < 5% mortality rate, while the presence of ≥ 6 criteria approaches a 100% mortality rate:

- At presentation:
  - Age > 55 years
  - WBC > 16,000/μL
  - Glucose > 200 mg/dL
  - Lactic dehydrogenase > 350 units/L
  - > 250 IU/L
- During initial 48 hours:
  - Hematocrit ↓ > 10 points
  - BUN ↑ > 5 mg/dL
  - Serum Ca^{2+} < 8 mg/dL
  - Arterial PO_2 < 60 mmHg
  - Base deficit > 4 mEq/L
  - Fluid sequestration > 6 L

TREATMENT

- Fluid resuscitation
- Electrolyte correction

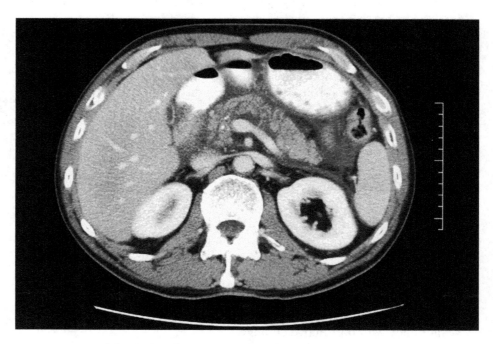

FIGURE 8-5. Abdominal CT demonstrating stranding in the peripancreatic region, consistent with acute pancreatitis.

TABLE 8-4. Mortality Rate Based on Number of Ranson's Criteria

NUMBER OF CRITERIA	MORTALITY RATE
0–2	< 5%
3–4	15–20%
5–6	30–40%
> 6	Almost 100%

- Prevention of vomiting with antiemetics
- Analgesia
- NPO (pancreatic rest)
- NG suction as needed

Pancreatic Pseudocyst

DEFINITION

- Encapsulated fluid collection with high enzyme content in a pseudocyst protruding from the pancreatic parenchyma.
- Most common complication of pancreatitis (2–10%).

CLINICAL FINDINGS

- Symptoms of pancreatitis.
- CT and ultrasonography (US) both have a sensitivity of 90%.

TREATMENT

- Surgical creation of fistula between cyst and stomach allowing for continuous decompression is most effective. Cyst eventually resolves without further intervention.
- Drain in 6 weeks when walls mature to reduce secondary infection, hemorrhage, or rupture.

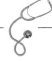

Suspect a pancreatic pseudocyst when patients with pancreatitis fail to resolve.

LARGE INTESTINE

Large Bowel Obstruction

ETIOLOGIES

- Tumor (most common)
- Diverticular disease
- Volvulus (sigmoid and cecal)
- Fecal impaction (especially elderly and mentally retarded)
- Adhesions
- Strictures (mostly related to IBD and chronic colon ischemia)
- Hernia
- Pseudo-obstruction

HIGH-YIELD FACTS

Gastrointestinal Emergencies

CLINICAL FINDINGS

- Intermittent crampy abdominal pain, vomiting, abdominal distention.
- Absence of bowel movements or flatulence for several days.

DIAGNOSIS

- AXR may demonstrate stepladder appearance of air-fluid levels, thickening of bowel wall, or loss of colonic markings (haustra).
- CT scan of abdomen to look for a transition point (open vs. closed loop obstruction).
- Colonoscopy and water-soluble contrast enema if cause is not known and urgent surgical intervention is not required.

TREATMENT

- IV fluids, NG suction, and early surgical consult.
- May consider antibiotics if infection present.
- Sigmoidoscopy may be done to decompress bowel.

Appendicitis

Appendicitis is the most common surgical emergency.

DEFINITION

Inflammation of the appendix.

PATHOPHYSIOLOGY

- The inciting event is obstruction of the lumen of the appendix.
- This → an ↑ in intraluminal pressure with vascular compromise of the wall of the appendix.
- The environment is now ripe for bacterial invasion.

Appendicitis in late pregnancy presents with RUQ pain due to displacement of appendix by gravid uterus.

ETIOLOGY

- Fecalith (most common cause)
- Lymphoid hyperplasia
- Worms
- Granulomatous disease
- Inspissated barium
- Tumors
- Calculus
- Adhesions
- Dietary matter such as seeds

CLINICAL FINDINGS

- Usually begins as vague periumbilical pain, then migrates to the RLQ where it becomes more intense and localized (McBurney's point).
- Retrocecal appendicitis can present as right flank pain.
- Anorexia.
- Nausea, vomiting.
- Low-grade fever.
- RLQ pain with rebound tenderness and guarding.
- **Rovsing's sign:** Pain in RLQ when palpation pressure is exerted in left lower quadrant (LLQ).
- **Iliopsoas sign:** Pelvic pain upon flexion of the thigh while the patient is supine.
- **Obturator sign:** Pelvic pain on internal and external rotation of the thigh with the knee flexed.

Appendicitis: **Do not delay the diagnosis.** Mortality of perforation is about 3%, and usually occurs within 24–36 hours.

DIAGNOSIS

- Labs: Leukocytosis, hematuria, pyuria.
- Pregnancy test for women of childbearing age.
- If the diagnosis is clear-cut, no imaging studies are necessary.
- AXR is of little utility, rarely demonstrates fecalith (5% of time) or loss of psoas shadow.
- Ultrasonography may show noncompressible appendix (operator dependent).
- CT scan with contrast may demonstrate periappendiceal streaking. CT is 90–95% sensitive for appendicitis.

TREATMENT

- Prompt appendectomy
- NPO
- IV hydration
- Perioperative antibiotics

COMPLICATIONS

- Perforation
- Appendiceal abscess
- Prolonged ileus
- Small bowel obstruction
- Urinary retention
- Pneumonia

Conditions that mimic appendicitis—
CODE APPY
Crohn disease
Ovarian cyst
Diverticulitis
Ectopic pregnancy
Adenitis of the mesentery
Pelvic inflammatory disease
Pyelonephritis
Yersinia gastroenteritis

Volvulus

ETIOLOGIES

- Closed loop obstruction of the large bowel resulting from the bowel twisting on itself.
- Sigmoid (more common) occurs in the elderly and associated with chronic constipation.
- Cecal (less common) is the result of a congenital abnormality → inadequate fixation of the cecum. Most common in the 20s and 30s.

DIAGNOSIS

AXR:

- Sigmoid: Reveals a loop arising out of the left lower quadrant like bird beak creating a dilated loop that resembles a bent inner tube toward the right side.
- Cecal: The dilated loop points toward the right, but given the mobility of the cecum can appear anywhere, resembling a coffee bean.

TREATMENT

- IV fluids, NG suction, and early surgical consult.
- May consider antibiotics if infection present.
- Sigmoidoscopy may be done to decompress bowel.

Gastrointestinal Emergencies

Ogilvie Syndrome

DEFINITION

Colonic pseudo-obstruction due to marked cecal dilatation.

RISK FACTORS

Due to its small radius, the cecum is normally the site of highest pressure in the GI tract.

- Use/abuse of opiates, tricyclic antidepressants, anticholinergics.
- Prolonged bed rest.

DIAGNOSIS

AXR reveals cecal dilatation. A cecum diameter > 12 cm is a risk for perforation.

TREATMENT

- Decompression with enemas.
- If unsuccessful, colonoscopic decompression.

Diverticular Disease

A 70-year-old man presents with LLQ pain, diarrhea, and fever. On exam he has rebound tenderness in the LLQ and guaiac-positive stool. What are the next steps in management?

The patient presents with symptoms suggestive of diverticulitis. The workup would include a complete blood count (CBC), initiation of antibiotics, and a possible CT scan of the abdomen.

DEFINITIONS

Diverticulosis is the most common cause of painless lower GI bleeding in older patients.

- **Diverticula** are saclike herniations of colonic mucosa (most common at sigmoid) occurring at weak points in the bowel wall (insertions of arteries) with ↑ luminal pressures.
- **Diverticulosis** is the presence of diverticula can → massive painless lower GI bleeding.
- **Diverticulitis** (diverticula + inflammation) is the most common complication of diverticular disease. Fecal material lodges in diverticula, leading to inflammation and ischemia and mucosal erosion.

EPIDEMIOLOGY

Diverticulitis is a common cause of large bowel obstruction.

- Prevalent in 35–50% of general population.
- ↑ in the elderly and industrialized nations.

ETIOLOGIES

- Low-fiber diet
- Chronic constipation
- Family history

CLINICAL FINDINGS

- Diverticulosis:
  - Rectal bleeding
  - Anemia
  - Hematochezia

- Diverticulitis:
    - Constant severe LLQ pain with guarding
    - Abdominal distention
    - Fever
    - Diarrhea
    - Anorexia
    - Nausea
    - Vomiting

DIAGNOSIS

- AXR: Ileus, air-fluid levels, free air if perforation.
- CT: Study of choice.
- Colonoscopy and barium enema are relatively contraindicated in acute diverticulitis due to risk of perforation.

TREATMENT

- ABCs.
- Treat any hemodynamic compromise associated with massive GI bleeding.
- Diverticular disease: High-fiber diet and stool softeners to ↓ luminal pressure and prevent constipation.
- Diverticulitis: IV fluids, NPO, NG suction (for ileus), and broad-spectrum antibiotics. Admit with surgical consult if severe.
- Diverticulosis: Address the bleeding.

COMPLICATIONS

Abscesses, obstruction, fistula, stricture, and perforation.

Lower GI Bleed

DEFINITION

Bleeding distal to the ligament of Treitz (small intestine or colon).

ETIOLOGIES

- Diverticulosis (70%)
- Angiodysplasia
- Colon cancer/polyps
- Hemorrhoids
- Trauma
- IBD
- Ischemic colitis
- Inappropriate anticoagulation
- Irradiation injury
- Rectal disease

CLINICAL FINDINGS

- Hematochezia
- Abdominal pain
- Weakness
- Anorexia
- Melena
- Syncope
- Shortness of breath

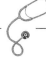

Barium enema and colonoscopy should be avoided in acute cases of diverticulitis due to risk of perforation.

Angiodysplasia is the most common cause of lower GI bleeding in younger patients. Diverticulosis is the most common cause in older patients.

Upper GI bleed is the most common cause of apparent lower GI bleed.

DIAGNOSIS

- NG lavage to rule out upper source (if blood is not seen and bile is aspirated, an upper source is unlikely).
- CBC (note acute blood loss will not be reflected in hematocrit).
- Colonoscopy to localize and possibly limit bleeding.
- If colonoscopy fails to reveal source, consider angiography or nuclear bleeding scan.

TREATMENT

- ABCs.
- Treat any hemodynamic compromise associated with massive GI bleeding similar to upper GI bleeding (stabilize first).
- Anoscopy and sigmoidoscopy for evidence of anorectal disease.
- Consider early GI/surgery consultation for large bleeds.
- Surgery if unstable or refractory to medical therapy.

Bright red blood that drips into the toilet or streaks stool suggests anorectal source.

RECTUM/ANUS

Anal Fissure

DEFINITION

Linear tear of the anal squamous epithelium.

ETIOLOGIES

- Most benign fissures occur in posterior or anterior line.
- Fissures in other location or multiple sites are associated with CD, infection, and malignancy.

CLINICAL FINDINGS

- Perianal pain during or after defecation with blood-streaked toilet paper (subsides between bowel movements).
- Diagnosis made by visual inspection.

TREATMENT

Sitz baths, stool softener, high-fiber diet, hygiene, and analgesics.

Anal fissures are the most common cause of anorectal pain (especially in children).

Hemorrhoids

DEFINITION

Dilated veins of the hemorrhoidal plexus (see Figure 8-6):

- Internal — arise above the dentate line and usually insensitive.
- External — below the dentate line, well innervated, painful!

CLINICAL FINDINGS

- External hemorrhoids present with painful thrombosis and tenderness to palpation.
- Painless bright red bleeding may occur if there is no thrombosis of veins.

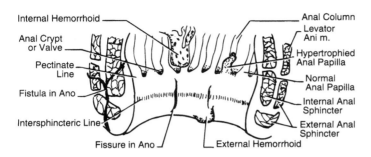

FIGURE 8-6. Anatomy of internal and external hemorrhoids.

(Reproduced, with permission, from DeGowin RL, Brown DD. *DeGowin's Diagnostic Examination*, 7th ed. New York: McGraw-Hill, 2000: 592.)

- Internal hemorrhoids are painless. Symptoms depend on the grade. Grade 1 internal hemorrhoids protrude into the anal canal. Grade 4 are irreducible and are permanently prolapsed, putting the tissue at risk for gangrene.

TREATMENT

If pain is severe, then excision of clot under local anesthesia followed by sitz baths and analgesics. Otherwise, manage expectantly with hydrocortisone cream, local anesthetic ointment, and sitz baths.

Perirectal Abscess

DEFINITION

An abscess in any of the potential spaces near the anus or rectum (perianal, ischiorectal, submucosal, supralevator, and intersphincteric); begins with infection of the anal gland as it drains into the anal canal.

CLINICAL FINDINGS

Extreme pain and mass on rectal exam.

TREATMENT

Evaluation, incision and drainage in the emergency department or operating room.

As with all abscesses, the treatment is drainage, and routine use of antibiotics is not warranted unless associated with cellulitis.

Perianal and Pilonidal Abscesses

ETIOLOGY

Ingrowing hair induces abscess formation.

CLINICAL FINDINGS

- Pain, swelling, redness, presence of fluctuant mass.
- Perianal is the most common anorectal abscess (40–50%).
- Pilonidal abscesses occur in the midline upper edge of the buttock.

TREATMENT

Incision and drainage followed by later surgical excision.

Gastrointestinal Emergencies

Renal and Genitourinary Emergencies

Classified as prerenal, intrinsic, or postrenal.

Prerenal ARF

DEFINITION

Decrease in renal perfusion and decrease in glomerular filtration rate (GFR) with normal tubular and glomerular function.

ETIOLOGY

- Hypovolemia (blood loss, vomiting, diarrhea, burns)
- Decreased cardiac output
- Sepsis
- Third spacing
- Hypoalbuminemia
- Drugs (nonsteroidal anti-inflammatory drugs [NSAIDs], angiotensin-converting enzyme [ACE] inhibitors, nitrates)
- Renal artery obstruction
- Nephrotic syndrome

DIAGNOSIS

- Urine sodium excretion is < 10 and fractional excretion of sodium (FeNa) is < 1%.

$$FeNa = \frac{(Urine\ Na) \times (Plasma\ creatinine) \times 100}{(Plasma\ Na) \times (Urine\ creatinine)}$$

- Blood urea nitrogen (BUN)-to-creatinine (Cr) ratio: > 20:1.

TREATMENT

- Volume replacement.
- Diuretics for congestive heart failure (CHF).
- Positive inotropics (eg, dobutamine) or afterload reduction (eg, ACE inhibitors) for pump failure.
- Mobilize third-space fluid.

Postrenal ARF

DEFINITION

Obstruction anywhere from renal parenchyma to urethra.

ETIOLOGY

- Nephrolithiasis
- Benign prostatic hyperplasia (BPH)
- Neurogenic bladder
- Bladder neck obstruction
- Urethral strictures, phimosis
- Substances causing renal tubular obstruction: acyclovir, methotrexate, uric acid, oxalate, sulfonamides, myeloma (Bence Jones) proteins
- Malignancy

Oliguria is the production of < 400 mL of urine in 24 hours.

Prerenal ARF is the most common cause of community acquired ARF (40–80% cases).

Most cases of prerenal failure will need FLUID, FLUID, and more FLUID.

Most common cause of postrenal failure is BPH.

TREATMENT

Depends on etiology, but may consist of the following:
- Foley catheter.
- Percutaneous nephrostomy tubes for obstructing renal stones.
- Urology consult if catheterization yields no urine.
- Aggressive hydration may be necessary if tubular obstruction is suspected.

Intrinsic ARF

A 7-year-old boy presents with oliguria and hematuria. His parents report that he had a sore throat 2 weeks prior to presentation. He is afebrile and has a blood pressure of 170/110 mm Hg. His BUN/Cr are elevated at 34/2.0 mg/dL. Urinalysis demonstrates RBC casts and proteinuria. What is the most likely diagnosis?

This child most likely has poststreptococcal glomerulonephritis (PSGN). An antistreptolysin (ASO) level if obtained will be elevated, as would be C3 complement levels. PSGN is a relatively uncommon complication of antecedent groups A streptococcus infection. It is seen 2 weeks after strep A pharyngitis infection, and 4 weeks after group A strep skin infection. Manifestation may be mild, in which case patients can be managed as outpatients, or may be severe in the form of significant hypertension, CHF, and uremia, in which case hospital admission is warranted.

An accurate history is imperative. Drugs, medical history, and family history are all important to help determine a cause of renal failure.

DEFINITION

Insult to the kidney parenchyma from disease states, drugs, or toxins.

ETIOLOGY

- Acute tubular necrosis:
  - Intravenous (IV) contrast
  - Acute renal ischemia secondary to surgery, trauma, shock, sepsis
  - Myoglobinuria from rhabdomyolysis
  - Drugs (aminoglycoside antibiotics, angiotensin-converting enzyme [ACE] inhibitors, nonsteroidal anti-inflammatory drugs [NSAIDs])
  - Third spacing in pancreatitis/peritonitis
- Glomerulonephritis (GN):
  - Antecedent streptococcal infection (group A, beta-hemolytic)
  - Systemic lupus erythematosus (SLE)
  - Wegener's granulomatosis
  - Polyarteritis nodosa
  - Goodpasture syndrome
  - Henoch-Schönlein purpura
  - Drugs (gold, penicillamine)
  - Immunoglobulin A nephropathy (Berger disease)
  - Idiopathic
- Acute interstitial nephritis
- Large-vessel and medium- and small-vessel disease

TREATMENT

Treat underlying cause.

- Discontinue any offending agents.
- Treat volume and metabolic abnormalities.
- ↑ urine output in oliguric patients with hydration and diuretics (mannitol, furosemide).
- ↑ renal perfusion with dopamine if needed.
- Consider dialysis for severe cases (if BUN >100 mg/dL or Cr >10 mg/dL).

Intractable volume overload and life-threatening hyperkalemia are the two most important indications for emergency dialysis.

CHRONIC RENAL FAILURE (CRF)/END-STAGE RENAL DISEASE (ESRD)

OVERVIEW

- Patients developing CRF are treated with diet and medications first and progress to use of intermittent dialysis and finally chronic dialysis.
- Uremia, electrolytes, anticoagulants, immunosuppression, vascular access, and cardiovascular stress with hemodialysis all contribute to potential problems.
- It leads to a state of general hyporesponsiveness.

An 81-year-old woman is brought in by ambulance. She was found lying on the floor of her apartment after sustaining a fall 3 days ago. Her creatine kinase is 12,500 U/L. Her BUN/Cr is 100/45 mg/dL. *Think: Rhabdomyolysis.*

COMPLICATIONS/SEQUELAE

- Arrhythmias: Due to electrolyte imbalances and drug toxicities:
  - Hyperkalemia is the most common when dialysis appointments are missed. Treatment: intravenous calcium (see Diagnostics chapter for more details).
  - Others include hypocalcemia, hypokalemia (during or immediately after dialysis), and hypermagnesemia.
- Hypertension: Due to increased intravascular volume—need dialysis but may temporize with IV nitroprusside, hydralazine, or labetalol.
- Hypotension: Due to ultrafiltration during dialysis—give IV fluid and pressors as necessary.
- **Neurological:**
  - Peripheral neuropathy: Manifested by impaired vibration sense and stocking-and-glove pain/anesthesia. It occurs in > 50% of ESRD patients.
  - Lethargy, seizures, coma, headache, and confusion all may occur.
  - Electrolytes, hypoglycemia, and concurrent illness (eg, sepsis) all may be contributing factors.
  - Must rule out intracranial bleed (especially if projectile vomiting or focal neurological exam) because of use of IV heparin during hemodialysis. Most common intracranial bleed here is subdural hematoma.
- **Hemodialysis disequilibrium:**
  - Syndrome that occurs toward the end of dialysis, usually after the first dialysis treatment.
  - Characterized by nausea, vomiting, hypertension, and a feeling of light-headedness. Can progress to seizures, coma, death.
  - Treatment consists of raising serum osmolality with mannitol and terminating dialysis.
- **Gastrointestinal (GI):**
  - Upper GI bleeds from anticoagulation, uremic gastritis, and peptic ulcer disease are more common than in the general population.

CRF patients have high mortality from many causes. Anything out of the ordinary in these patients should be investigated.

HIGH-YIELD FACTS

Renal and Genitourinary Emergencies

- Bowel obstruction may occur due to use of oral phosphate binders. Avoid Mg^{2+}-containing antacids and Fleet enemas (contain phosphate).
- **Vascular:**
  - External vascular access devices or internal shunts and grafts may become clotted or infected.
  - Strictures, aneurysms, vascular steal syndromes, or excessive bleeding may occur in the extremity with a graft.
  - Avoid blood draws, blood pressure measurements, or other procedures in an extremity with a graft.
- **Genitourinary:** Uremia (discussed below).

EMERGENT HEMODIALYSIS

Indications:

- Electrolyte abnormalities: Hyperkalemia is the most common and potentially the most dangerous, even at moderate levels.
- Volume overload and its various manifestations—the patient may be oliguric; also may have uncontrollable hypertension.
- Intractable acidosis; $HCO_3^- < 10$.
- Severe uremia.
- Dialysis may also be necessary to treat certain drug overdoses.

PERITONEAL DIALYSIS

Problems occur with the intraperitoneal catheter:

- Can become clogged or kinked, resulting in fluid overload and abdominal distention.
- Adhesions may form in the peritoneal space, decreasing fluid drainage.
- If aseptic technique is not followed, peritonitis may occur manifested by abdominal tenderness and GI symptoms.
- If systemic symptoms are present, IV antibiotics are necessary. Otherwise, antibiotic infusion into the peritoneum suffices as treatment.
- Lower rate of sepsis than hemodialysis.

Most common indication for initiating dialysis in ESRD is pulmonary edema.

HEMATURIA

ETIOLOGY

- Acute GN
- BPH
- Vascular:
  - Renal vessel thrombosis
  - Abdominal aortic aneurysm (AAA)
  - Arteriovenous malformation
- Urologic cancer:
  - Bladder cancer
  - Renal cell carcinoma
  - Rhabdomyosarcoma
- Urolithiasis/nephrolithiasis
- Pseudohematuria:
  - Vegetable dyes (eg, beets, rhubarb)
  - Phenolphthalein
  - Phenazopyridine

Urinary sediment:
- Granular casts → acute tubular necrosis
- WBC casts → pyelonephritis/ interstitial nephritis
- RBC casts → glomerulonephritis, malignant hypertension

- Porphyria
- Contamination from menstrual blood
- Sickle cell disease
- Trauma
- Infection:
  - *Schistosoma haematobium*
  - Sexually transmitted disease (STD)
  - Urinary tract infection (UTI)
- Inflammation

The most common causes of nontraumatic hematuria in order of frequency are:
- Nephrolithiasis
- Carcinoma of GU tract
- Urethritis
- UTI
- BPH
- Glomerulonephritis

CLINICAL FINDINGS

- Start with a urinalysis and go from there.
- Timing of hematuria:
  - At initiation of the stream suggests a urethral source.
  - At the end of the stream suggests prostate or bladder neck problems.
  - Continuous hematuria has a renal, bladder, or ureteral source.
- "Brown" or "Coca-Cola" urine has a renal source: hematuria, GN, and myoglobinuria.

PROTEINURIA

DEFINITION

> 150 mg/24 hours in adult patients, or > 140 mg/m^2 in children.

CLINICAL FINDINGS

- Tubular source (impaired reabsorption) has > 2 g/day excretion (eg, diabetic or hypertensive nephropathy).
- Glomerular source (diffusion across glomerular membrane) may have up to 10 g/day excretion (eg, nephrosis).
- These criteria apply if proteinuria is isolated. A nephritic picture will have proteinuria but other urinalysis findings as well (eg, casts).
- Nephrotic-range proteinuria: Excretion of > 3.5 g of protein/24 hours.

NEPHROLITHIASIS

EPIDEMIOLOGY

- Peak incidence in midlife (~70% occur between ages 20–50 years)
- Twice as common in men

PATHOPHYSIOLOGY

- Most originate in kidney and pass in to collecting system.
- ~90% of stones are radiopaque.
- Stone composition:
  - Calcium oxalate: 75%, radiopaque.
  - Struvite: 15%, radiopaque—magnesium ammonium phosphate stones, also called **infectious stones.** They are in the shape of staghorn calculi; also called **coffin lid crystals.** They occur exclusively in UTI patients.
  - Urate: 10%, radiolucent.
  - Cystine: 1%, radiopaque—due to inborn error of metabolism.

- Stones partially obstruct at five different places where the most pain occurs:
  - Renal calyx
  - Ureteropelvic junction
  - Pelvic brim
  - Ureterovesicular junction (tightest space)—most common location for impacted stone
  - Vesicular orifice
- Stone passage:
  - Rarely fully obstruct the ureter due to their shapes.
  - < 5-mm stones—most pass freely.
  - 5- to 8-mm stones—15% will pass freely.
  - > 8-mm stones—only 5% will pass freely.

RISK FACTORS

- Medications (hydrochlorothiazide, acetazolamide, allopurinol, antacids, excess vitamins, laxative abuse)
- Male gender
- Dehydration
- Hot climate
- Family history
- Inflammatory bowel disease—Crohn
- Gout
- Hyperparathyroidism
- Immobilization
- Sarcoidosis
- Malignancy
- Recurrent UTI

DIFFERENTIAL DIAGNOSIS

- Abdominal aortic aneurysm (AAA)
- Testicular/ovarian torsion
- Ectopic pregnancy
- Salpingitis
- Pyelonephritis
- Renal infarction
- Appendicitis
- Drug-seeking behavior
- Musculoskeletal strain
- Incarcerated hernia
- Papillary necrosis (due to NSAID abuse, infection, sickle cell disease, diabetes)
- Carcinoma
- Renal tuberculosis

CLINICAL FINDINGS

- Pain: Acute, severe.
- Flank, abdominal, or back pain, with radiation to groin.
- Patients are very restless and cannot sit (opposite of patients with peritonitis, who tend to lie perfectly still).
- Waxes and wanes.
  - Cause of colicky pain: Hyperperistalsis of smooth muscle of calyx, pelvis, and ureter.
  - Cause of dull pain: Acute obstruction and renal capsular tension.

- Possibly nausea, vomiting, ileus, hematuria (micro- or macroscopic), low-grade fever, urinary urgency/frequency.

DIAGNOSIS

- Urinalysis: Dipstick test, microscopic analysis and culture.
- More than 10% of patients with kidney stones will have no hematuria on urine dip.
- Although intravenous pyelogram (IVP) has historically been the gold standard, in most emergency departments (EDs), noncontrast abdominal CT (Figure 9-1) is the first-line test.
- Ultrasonography is another good imaging option (Table 9-1).
- KUB (kidney, ureter, and bladder) may be able to detect a stone, but it is not helpful to determine pyelonephritis or hydronephrosis. It may be a good screening tool to look for other abdominal pathology.
- Testing is recommended in first-time presentations and in the elderly (rule out AAA, other causes).

TREATMENT

- Analgesia with NSAIDs and opiates as needed.
- Hydration.
- Nifedipine or tamsulosin may increase likelihood of stone passage.
- Admit for:
  - Urinary extravasation
  - Obstructing stone
  - Infected stone
  - Intractable pain (most common indication)
  - Patient with single kidney
- Nephrostomy tubes may be necessary to relieve severe hydronephrosis.
- Extracorporeal shockwave lithotripsy, cystoscopy, and ureteroscopy may be necessary to mobilize obstructing stones.
- Discharged patients should be instructed to strain their urine to screen for passage of the stone and to return if fever, vomiting, or severe exacerbation of pain should occur.

A 34-year-old man presents with left flank pain radiating to his left testicle. The pain does not change with movement or position and is colicky in nature. Urine dip is positive for blood. *Think: Renal colic.*

It is unusual to see first-time presentation of kidney stone in the elderly. Even when the story seems classic, investigate symptoms in the elderly carefully. A commonly missed diagnosis is AAA.

HIGH-YIELD FACTS

Renal and Genitourinary Emergencies

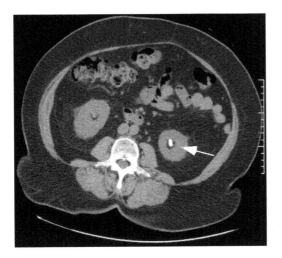

FIGURE 9-1. Noncontrast abdominal CT demonstrating nephrolithiasis (arrow) in the right kidney, which shows up as radiopaque (white).

TABLE 9-1. Imaging Modalities for Urolithiasis

	IVP	CT	US
Positive findings	▪ Delay in appearance of nephrogram ▪ Distention of renal pelvis ▪ Distortion of calyx ▪ Hydronephrosis ▪ Extravasation of dye	▪ Presence of suspicious calculi ▪ Dilation of collecting system ▪ Hydronephrosis ▪ Ureteral caliber changes ▪ Stranding of perinephral fat	▪ Hydronephrosis ▪ Detection of stones in ureter (> 5 mm) ▪ Provides anatomic information only
Sensitivity (%)	64–90	95–97	84–97% for hydronephrosis
Specificity (%)	94–100	96–98	~100% for hydronephrosis
Advantages	Provides information on kidney function in addition to anatomy as well as degree of obstruction	▪ Fast, easy ▪ No contrast dye ▪ Recognizes other pathology also (AAA, malignancy, renal abscess)	▪ Provides an option for patients who cannot undergo CT or IVP ▪ Especially useful for pregnant women and children (to avoid excess radiation exposure) and also obese patients ▪ Excellent for detecting hydronephrosis
Disadvantages	▪ Involves use of contrast dye, which can be nephrotoxic ▪ Time consuming and complex	▪ Does not give functional information ▪ More radiation than IVP or US ▪ Does not define degree of obstruction ▪ Underestimates the size of stone by around 12%	▪ Limited ability to detect smaller stones ▪ Does not give functional information (< 5 mm diameter)

NEPHROTIC SYNDROME

A 10-year-old boy with nephrotic syndrome presents with flank pain, and hematuria. There is no history of trauma. Vital signs are normal, and he is afebrile. Laboratory analysis reveals worsening renal function. What is the next step in the management of this patient?

This patient has renal vein thrombosis as a consequence of his nephrotic syndrome. Patients with nephrotic syndrome can develop a hypercoagulable state due to nephrotic loss of antithrombin III, increasing the risk of thrombosis. The next step would be to perform renal vein US to look for the thrombosis. Due to the risk for thrombosis, deep vein punctures should be avoided in children with nephrotic syndrome.

It is important to note that children with nephrotic syndrome are relatively immunocompromised, so if this child had fever or signs of peritonitis, prompt workup including paracentesis would have been indicated.

DEFINITION

- Protein-losing nephropathy with protein loss > 3.5 g/day.
- In primary nephrotic syndrome the diseases are limited to kidney, while secondary nephritic syndrome results from systemic diseases such as PSGN.

ETIOLOGIES

- Most common cause in adults: Membranous nephropathy
- Most common cause in children: Minimal change disease
- Idiopathic

CLINICAL FINDINGS

- Classic features are edema, hypoalbuminemia, proteinuria, and hyperlipidemia.
- The edema is often insidious (slow onset) and may begin with preorbital edema.
- Other features may include hypertension, hematuria, or oliguria.
- Acute renal failure is rare.

DIAGNOSIS

- Urinalysis shows oval fat bodies (tubular epithelial casts with cholesterol), proteinuria (3–4+ on urine dipstick), high specific gravity, and sometimes microscopic hematuria.
- Serum studies demonstrate hypoalbuminemia, hypercholesterolemia. Usually, BUN, creatinine, and hematocrit are normal.
- Chest x-ray may demonstrate bilateral pleural effusions or pulmonary edema.

TREATMENT

- Fluid resuscitation for hypovolemia (despite the edema).
- Corticosteroids.
- Diuretics such as furosemide for respiratory distress or ascites. If diuretics alone do not suffice, then consider salt or fluid restriction in that order.
- Other immunosuppressive agents possible for refractory cases.
- Diuretics if respiratory distress or ascites.

NephrOtic syndrome: Associated with prOteinuria

NephrItic syndrome: Associated with hematuria and Inflammation

Clinical features of nephrotic syndrome —
LEAP
Hyper**L**ipidemia
Edema
Hypo**A**lbuminemia
Proteinuria

TESTICULAR TORSION

A 19-year-old man presents with severe pain to the right testicle, which occurred suddenly while he was playing baseball. Physical exam reveals a tender, swollen, firm testicle with a transverse lie. There is no cremasteric reflex on that side. What diagnosis should you immediately suspect?

The presentation is highly suspicious for testicular torsion. Indeed, testicular ultrasound revealed hypoechoic areas within the right testicle suggesting necrosis. There was no vascular flow signal within the testis on Doppler. The patient subsequently underwent inguinal orchiectomy. Pathology showed testicular parenchymal edema with ischemia and hemorrhage consistent with a clinical picture of torsion. *(continued)*

Testicular torsion, or rotation of the testes with twisting of the spermatic cord, is a common surgical emergency. Incidence follows a bimodal peak, highest around puberty, with a smaller peak in infancy. Differential diagnoses include scrotal edema, epididymitis, hernia, tumor, varicocele, hydrocele and trauma. This condition warrants strong clinical suspicion, early diagnosis and expeditious surgical management.

DEFINITION

Twisting of a testicle on its root—"bell clapper deformity."

EPIDEMIOLOGY

Most common in infants under age 1 and in young adults (peripubertal period).

CLINICAL FINDINGS

- Usually occurs during strenuous activity (eg, athletic event), but sometimes occurs during sleep.
- Pain may be in the lower abdomen, inguinal canal, or testicle. No change in pain with position. Pain may be sudden or severe and constant or intermittent.
- Twisting is usually in a horizontal direction.
- Physical exam alone is not sufficient to exclude the diagnosis.
- No cremasteric reflex.

DIAGNOSIS

Doppler US to look for flow to testicle: No flow, asymmetric testicle and diffusely hypoechoic is highly suggestive of torsion (Figure 9-2).

TREATMENT

- Immediate urology consult.
- Attempt manual correction of the torsion—untwist from medial to lateral (ie, patient's right testicle gets rotated counterclockwise and the left clockwise).
- If Doppler US is equivocal and manual detorsion does not work, immediate exploratory surgery is necessary to prevent death of the testicle.
- Time is testicle! (The longer the delay to definitive treatment, the lower the chance of salvaging the testicle.)

Manual detorsion is like "opening a book." Imagine a book standing on its spine and the front and back covers are the right and left testes, respectively. "Open" the front cover to untwist the right and likewise for the left.

TORSION OF APPENDIX TESTIS OR APPENDIX EPIDIDYMIS

DEFINITION

Both the testis and epididymis have a small appendix that can become twisted.

CLINICAL FINDINGS

- "Blue dot" sign: Palpation of a tender nodule on transillumination of the testes
- Localized pain

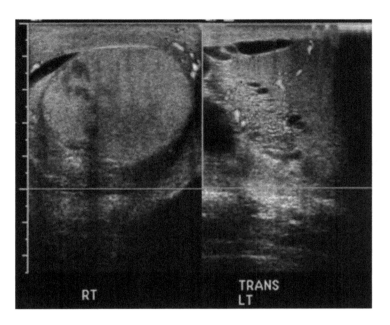

FIGURE 9-2. Doppler ultrasound of bilateral testes shows swollen right testis with hypoechoic areas within and reduced arterial signal suggesting testicular torsion with necrosis *(left panel)*. This is compared to the left testis, which has normal flow *(right panel)*.

Also see Color Insert.

TREATMENT

- Get a US/Doppler to look for blood flow to testes (need to rule out testicular torsion).
- If normal, then appendix testis can be allowed to degenerate/calcify.
- Analgesia as needed.
- Scrotal support, ice.

ORCHITIS

DEFINITION

Inflammation of the testicles.

ETIOLOGIES

- Mumps
- Syphilis

CLINICAL FINDINGS

- Presents with history of bilateral testicular pain
- Usually will remit after a few days
- Fever, nausea, vomiting, myalgias

TREATMENT

- Treat symptomatically (pain management).
- Disease-specific treatment (eg, antibiotics for syphilis).
- Local scrotal care.

HYDROCELE

DEFINITION

Fluid accumulation in a persistent tunica vaginalis due to obstruction, which impedes lymphatic drainage of the testicles (see Figure 9-3).

ETIOLOGY

- Trauma
- Neoplasia
- Congenital
- Infection: Elephantiasis
- CHF

CLINICAL FINDINGS

- May cause much discomfort and pain when distended.
- Other scrotal masses must be ruled out (eg, torsion).
- Transilluminates on physical exam.

TREATMENT

- Surgical follow-up for drainage.
- Reassurance is usually necessary.

VARICOCELE

DEFINITION

Varicose vein in scrotal sac.

ETIOLOGY

- Caused by venous congestion in the spermatic cord due to incomplete drainage for pampiniform plexus.

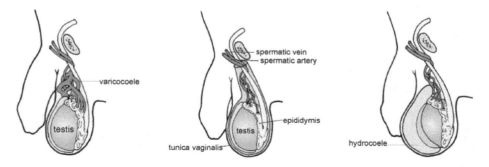

FIGURE 9-3. Varicocele vs. normal vs. hydrocele.

- Left-sided varicocele is due to left renal obstruction.
- Right-sided varicocele is due to inferior vena cava obstruction/compression.

CLINICAL FINDINGS

- Palpating "a bag of worms" in the testis.
- Accentuated by Valsalva maneuver and supine position.
- Usually asymptomatic, but persistence has been implicated in sterility.

TREATMENT

May be surgically excised to improve spermatogenesis (elective procedure).

EPIDIDYMITIS

A 27-year-old man presents with lower left abdominal pain, bilateral testicular pain (left > right), and fever for 2 weeks. He denies any history of STDs. On exam, the abdomen is soft, and palpation of the testes is normal except for isolated tenderness of the epididymis. Cremasteric reflex is normal. Urinalysis reveals pyuria. Testicular ultrasound reveals an enlarged, hypoechoic epididymis, with increased vascularity to the left testicle. How would you treat this patient?

This patient has epididymitis. Sexually active patients should always be checked or empirically treated for gonorrhea and *Chlamydia*. Treatment consists of a 2-week course of antibiotics for STD-related disease and 4 weeks for more complicated urinary tract pathologies. Untreated, it can lead to orchitis, testicular abscess, and rarely sepsis. Long-term sequelae can include infertility secondary to peritubular fibrosis.

DEFINITION

Inflammation of the epididymis.

ETIOLOGY

- Bacterial infection: Most common organisms are *Escherichia coli, Chlamydia trachomatis*, and *Neisseria gonorrheae*.
- Congenital abnormalities with reflux.
- STDs with urethral stricture.
- Amiodarone (due to lymphocytic infiltration and epididymal fibrosis).

CLINICAL FINDINGS

- Gradual onset of lower abdominal or testicular pain (vs. typical sudden onset of pain in torsion).
- Pyuria (50–95%).
- Fever (75%).
- Dysuria, urethral discharge (10–30%).
- Positive Prehn's sign: Transient pain relief on elevating scrotal contents while recumbent (10%).

TREATMENT

- Antibiotics for infection (note longer duration of 10–14 days for uncomplicated cases)
- Bed rest
- Scrotal elevation (scrotal support when ambulating)
- Cold compress
- NSAIDs
- Stool softener

FOURNIER'S GANGRENE

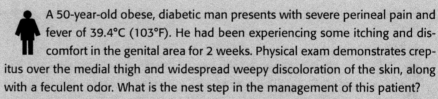

A 50-year-old obese, diabetic man presents with severe perineal pain and fever of 39.4°C (103°F). He had been experiencing some itching and discomfort in the genital area for 2 weeks. Physical exam demonstrates crepitus over the medial thigh and widespread weepy discoloration of the skin, along with a feculent odor. What is the nest step in the management of this patient?

This patient has Fournier's gangrene, which is a urological emergency. He requires fluid resuscitation, broad-spectrum parenteral antibiotics, and surgical debridement.

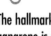

The hallmark of Fournier's gangrene is pain of genital area out of proportion to physical exam early in the course. In late stages, the patient may actually report less pain, as necrosis sets in.

DEFINITION

Rapidly progressive gangrene of groin.

ETIOLOGY

- Usually polymicrobial origin from skin, rectum, or urethra.
- Subcutaneous spread becomes virulent and causes end-artery thrombosis and extensive necrosis in scrotal, medial thigh, and lower abdominal areas.

EPIDEMIOLOGY

Especially prevalent in diabetic and other immunocompromised patients.

TREATMENT

- Broad-spectrum IV antibiotics
- Aggressive fluid resuscitation with normal saline
- Surgical debridement
- Hyperbaric oxygen therapy shown to be of benefit
- Tetanus prophylaxis if soft-tissue injury is present

A 41-year-old man presents stating he heard his penis "crack" while having intercourse. Vital signs are normal. Physical exam reveals an edematous, purplish penis. What is the next step in the management of this patient?

This patient has a penile fracture. He requires analgesia and urologic consultation for surgical repair.

CLINICAL FINDINGS

- "Snapping sound" during sexual intercourse due to tearing of the tunica albuginea.
- Penis is tender, swollen, and discolored, "eggplant" deformity.
- Urethra is usually spared.

TREATMENT

- Urologic consultation
- Surgery necessary to evacuate hematoma and to repair the tunica

BALANOPOSTHITIS

DEFINITION

Inflammation of the glans penis and foreskin:

- Balanitis = inflammation of glans
- Posthitis = inflammation of foreskin

ETIOLOGY

- Allergy to latex condoms
- Diabetes mellitus
- Infection—most commonly with *Candida albicans*
- Drugs—sulfonamides, tetracyclines, phenobarbital
- Trauma

Often seen in diabetics and in children who have not learned to clean themselves properly.

CLINICAL FINDINGS

Areas (glans and prepuce) are purulent, excoriated, malodorous, and tender.

TREATMENT

- Preventative therapy with adequate cleaning and drying.
- Topical therapy useful.
- Consider circumcision, especially if recurrent.
- Look for phimosis/paraphimosis.

HIGH-YIELD FACTS

Renal and Genitourinary
Emergencies

PEYRONIE DISEASE

PEYRONIE DISEASE

DEFINITION

Gradual or sudden dorsal curvature of the penis with erections.

ETIOLOGY

- Due to thickened plaque on tunica—may be associated with Dupuytren contractures in the hand.
- May be painful and preclude sexual intercourse.

TREATMENT

Spares urethra and not emergent; reassurance and referral.

PHIMOSIS

DEFINITION

Inability to retract foreskin over glans (proximally).

ETIOLOGY

May be from infection, poor hygiene, old injury with scarring, congenital abnormalities.

CLINICAL FINDINGS

May cause urinary retention secondary to pain or obstruction of urethra.

TREATMENT

- Patient will need circumcision or dorsal slit to foreskin or preputial plasty.
- Topical steroids might avert circumcision or balloon dilatation.

Do not force retraction of foreskin. May lead to paraphimosis.

PARAPHIMOSIS

DEFINITION

Inability to reduce proximal edematous foreskin over glans (distally).

PATHOPHYSIOLOGY

Edema of the glans leads to venous engorgement, decreased arterial flow, and eventual gangrene.

TREATMENT

Attempt manual reduction or emergent circumcision.

- Manual reduction: Wrap glans with elastic banding for several minutes. Alternatively, several small punctures to edematous area can be made with a 27G needle to express fluid. Local anesthetic block prior to making the punctures is advisable.
- Dorsal slit: See Procedures chapter.

Paraphimosis is a true urologic emergency!

Replace the foreskin when you insert Foley catheters in uncircumcised patients to prevent paraphimosis.

DEFINITION

Painful pathologic erection dorsally.

ETIOLOGY

- Sickle cell disease: Sickling in corpus cavernosum
- Drugs (eg, prostaglandin E, papaverine, phentolamine, sildenafil, phenothiazines, trazodone)
- Leukemic infiltrate
- Idiopathic
- Spinal cord injury
- Immunosuppressive disorders

CLINICAL FINDINGS

Corpus cavernosum with stagnant blood—spongiosum and glans are usually soft.

TREATMENT

- Intramuscular (IM) terbutaline (smooth muscle relaxer)
- Aspiration of blood from cavernosum plus irrigation
- Hydration and hyperbaric oxygen for sickle cell disease
- Urologic consult

COMPLICATIONS

Urinary retention, infection, and impotence and penile fibrosis.

BENIGN PROSTATIC HYPERPLASIA (BPH)

DEFINITION

The prostate undergoes two growth spurts during life, the second of which begins at around 40 years. This second spurt focuses around the urethra and later in life may cause urinary obstruction.

CLINICAL FINDINGS

- Decreased urinary stream
- Hesitancy
- Dribbling
- Incomplete emptying of bladder
- Nocturia
- Overflow incontinence
- Chronic urinary retention
- Obstruction
- Enlarged prostate on rectal exam

ETIOLOGY

Infection, drugs (eg, alpha agonists), and alcohol may exacerbate symptoms to the point where patients are seen in the ED.

Many over-the-counter cold medications contain pseudoephedrine, which can cause complete prostatic obstruction.

DIAGNOSIS

- Urinalysis to look for infection.
- BUN/Cr to look for postrenal failure.
- Prostate-specific antigen (PSA) to monitor for prostate cancer (not done in the ED).
- Foley to check postvoiding residual volume.
- Sonogram to measure prostate size and look for hydronephrosis.
- Urodynamic studies to determine effect of BPH on urinary flow (outpatient).
- Other outpatient studies such as cystoscopy and IVP are helpful for planning surgical procedures.

TREATMENT

- Avoid things that exacerbate symptoms (eg, caffeine).
- Leuprolide or finasteride to ↓ testosterone levels (factor in growth), which results in ↓ of prostate size.
- Alpha blockers to ↓ internal sphincter tone (doxazosin, terazosin, tamsulosin, prazosin).
- Transurethral resection of the prostate (TURP) for definitive treatment.

PROSTATITIS

DEFINITION

Inflammation of the prostate.

ETIOLOGY

UTI and STD pathogens (mainly gram-negative organism).

CLINICAL FINDINGS

- May present with chills, back pain, perineal pain.
- Recurrent UTIs despite treatment.
- Rectal exam will reveal a firm, warm, swollen, tender, boggy prostate.
- If exudate is expressed via the urethra, send it for culture.
- Dysuria, ↑ frequency and urgency.

TREATMENT

- Requires 1 month of total antibiotic therapy because of typically poor penetration into the prostate.
- Acute prostatitis is susceptible to antibiotic treatment with usual UTI antibiotics since inflammation renders the prostate more penetrable.
- Chronically infected prostate without acute inflammation is a relatively "protected" area. Choose your antibiotics wisely—fluoroquinolones have good penetration.
- Do not perform urethral catheterization if patient has painful urinary retention. Perform suprapubic needle aspiration/catheterization.

Do not massage the prostate on rectal exam if prostatitis is suspected due to ↑ risk of bacteremia.

HIGH-YIELD FACTS

Renal and Genitourinary Emergencies

A 25-year-old man presents with right-sided groin pain that occurred after he attempted to lift a refrigerator. On physical exam, there is a bulge in the inguinal canal. Bowel sounds can be heard over the canal. What is the cause of his acute scrotal mass?

He has an inguinal hernia. An inguinal hernia is the most common cause of a scrotal mass. Listen for bowel sounds over the mass. Transilluminate to rule out hydrocele. When you're convinced, try to reduce. If it reduces, patient can be managed as an outpatient with referral for elective repair. If it cannot be reduced, then it is incarcerated and requires emergent surgical consultation.

EPIDEMIOLOGY

- **Adults:**
  - Male > female by 9-to-1 ratio (indirect inguinal hernia most common for both sexes)
  - Lifetime incidence: 5–25% of males, 2% of females.
  - Bimodal peaks before 1 year of age and then again after age 40.
  - Groin hernias (femoral and inguinal) = 75% of abdominal wall hernias.
  - Inguinal hernias account for 70–95% groin hernias; two-thirds of these indirect.
  - Bilateral in 20% of cases.
  - Ninety percent of cases in children and young adults have **indirect inguinal hernias.** As age of patient ↑, so does incidence of acquired (direct) hernias. See Table 9-2.
- **Pediatrics:**
  - Incidence: 3–5% of full-term infants and up to 30% of preterm infants.
  - More common in boys, premature infants, and on the right.

TABLE 9-2. Types of Inguinal Hernias

Type	Description	Relationship to Inferior Epigastric Vessels	Covered by Internal Spermatic Fascia?	Usual Onset
Indirect	Protrudes through the inguinal ring and is ultimately the result of the failure of the processus vaginalis not obliterating in infancy; hernia sac passes outside of Hesselbach's triangle	Lateral	Yes	Congenital
Direct	Acquired deficiency in transversus abdominis muscle—enters through a weak point in the fascia of the abdominal wall; hernia sac passes through Hesselbach's triangle	Medial	No	Adult

- Bilateral in 5–30% of cases.
- An incarcerated inguinal hernia is the most common cause of intestinal obstruction from the first week to the fifth month of life.

RISK FACTORS

- ↑ intra-abdominal pressure:
- Obesity
- Pregnancy
- Ascites
- ↓ muscle tone and deterioration of connective tissue:
- Aging
- Systemic disease
- Malnutrition
- Smoking

CLINICAL FINDINGS

- Presents as a palpable mass in the inguinal canal or as a scrotal mass.
- The mass is usually reducible (either spontaneously or manually). If not, it is incarcerated. Incarceration can lead to strangulation then necrosis.
- Emergent situations occur when signs and symptoms of intestinal obstruction or severe pain or inability to reduce the mass lead to the diagnosis of incarcerated hernia. It is present as tense blue mass in scrotum.
- There might be bowel sounds in the scrotal sac.

TREATMENT

- Firmer manual reduction may be attempted in the ED, but if irreducible, surgical intervention is necessary.
- Reducible hernias should be referred for eventual repair to avoid incarceration.
- For irreducible/strangulated hernia, give fluid resuscitation, broad-spectrum parenteral antibiotics along with emergent surgical intervention.

URETHRAL STRICTURE

DEFINITION

Fibrotic narrowing of urethral lumen.

ETIOLOGY

- Often due to STDs (urethral inflammation → fibrosis)
- Urethral instrumentation

CLINICAL FINDINGS

- Urinary retention, difficulty voiding
- Difficulty placing Foley or coudé catheter

TREATMENT

- Catheterization or expansion of urethra with filiform rods
- Retrograde urethrography to delineate the location and extent of stricture
- Suprapubic cystotomy

DEFINITION

Inability to void completely.

ETIOLOGY

- BPH
- Drugs (anticholinergics, antihistamines, antispasmodics, alpha-adrenergic agonists, antipsychotics, tricyclic antidepressants)
- Mechanical: Stenosis of urethral meatus, bladder neck contracture, urethral stricture
- Cancer (bladder and prostate)
- Neurogenic bladder (consider patient may have spinal cord issue)
- Infrequent ejaculation
- Urethral tumor or foreign body
- Infection: Prostatitis (caused by *E coli/Proteus mirabilis*)
- Pelvic masses and prolapse of pelvic organs: Most common cause of urinary retention in women
- Congenital posterior urethral valves: Most common cause of acute urinary retention in children

> **Urethral stricture:**
> Differential includes voluntary tightening, bladder neck contraction, and BPH.

CLINICAL FINDINGS

- Inability to void for > 7 hours/straining to void
- Hesitancy
- ↓ urinary stream
- Interruption of urinary stream
- Lower abdominal pain
- Distended bladder
- Nocturia
- Nocturnal incontinence

DIAGNOSIS

- Urinalysis to look for infection
- BUN/Cr to evaluate renal function

TREATMENT

- Catheterization is both diagnostic and therapeutic. Patients can be discharged after observation for a few hours with outpatient urology referral.
- Antibiotics for concurrent UTI.
- Belladona and opium suppositories to avoid constant urge to void.

COMPLICATIONS

- Patients with chronic urinary retention can develop postobstructive diuresis when Foley relieves retention.
- Postobstructive diuresis is characterized by massive urine output, which can → hypotension due to hypovolemia and electrolyte imbalances.
- Urethritis, cystitis, prostatitis, sepsis.

Consider nosocomial UTI infections with *Pseudomonas* and methicillin-resistant *Staphylococcus aureus* in institutionalized or recently hospitalized patients.

URINARY TRACT INFECTION (UTI)

DEFINITION

Infection anywhere from kidney parenchyma (pyelonephritis) to urethral orifice (urethritis).

ETIOLOGY

- UTIs in men often due to anatomical defect and related instrumentation.
- Usual culprits are gram-negative aerobes (eg, *E coli*) but spectrum varies: *Staphylococcus saprophyticus*, *Proteus* (alkaline urine), *Klebsiella*, *Enterobacter*.

EPIDEMIOLOGY

- Women: 10–20% lifetime incidence
- Men: 1–10% lifetime incidence
- Institutionalized patients: 50% incidence
- Children: 5–14%

CLINICAL FINDINGS

- Presentation varies with sites of involvement.
- Pyuria.
- Bacteriuria.
- Dipstick may be positive for leukocyte esterase and nitrites.
- Microscopic or gross hematuria.
- Urine culture and sensitivity.
- White blood cells (WBC) in urinary sediment (> 5 to 10 WBC/hpf).

DIAGNOSIS

- Urine dip, urinalysis, urine Gram stain, and culture.
- Imaging studies (IVP, ultrasound, CT scan, or retrograde urogram) may be indicated for:
  - Children under 5 years (rule out pyelonephritis).
  - All male children (rule out anatomic defect).
  - Recurrent UTIs in women.
  - Fever for more than 3 days with treatment.
  - Recurrent pyelonephritis.
  - In severely ill patients, must rule out things such as perinephric abscess and pyoureter.

TREATMENT

- Trimethoprim-sulfamethoxazole, fluoroquinolones, and aminopenicillins have all been used and are effective; may need urine culture to streamline treatment.
- Three days for simple UTI (nonpregnant reproductive-age female), 7 days for others.
- Patients with chronic Foley catheters can have asymptomatic bacteruria and need not be treated; if symptomatic, change catheter and treat (probably need admission for IV antibiotics; also beware of fungal infection in these patients if unresponsive to therapy).
- Stable pyelonephritis (no signs and symptoms of sepsis) may be treated as an outpatient with close follow-up.

- In pregnant patients, all bacteriuria must be treated, and all pyelonephritis must be admitted for IV antibiotics due to higher risk of miscarriage with UTI.

Gonorrhea

Second most frequently reported STD.

ETIOLOGY

Neisseria gonorrhoeae: Gram-negative diplococcus involves columnar or transitional epithelium.

SIGNS AND SYMPTOMS (NONULCERATIVE DISEASE)

- Purulent discharge.
- Dysuria, epididymitis, inguinal lymphadenitis, proctitis (in homosexuals).
- Oral or pharyngeal lesions may be present if acquired through oral sex.
- Systemic infection may present as fever, rash, or monoarticular arthritis (usually the knee).
- Urethritis, cervicitis, pelvic inflammatory disease (PID), infertility in women.
- Urethritis, epididymitis/orchitis and prostatitis in men.

TREATMENT (CDC GUIDELINES)

- Recommended regimens for all adult and adolescent patients, regardless of travel history or sexual behavior:
    - Ceftriaxone 125 mg IM in a single dose or
    - Cefixime 400 mg orally in a single dose or 400 mg by suspension (200 mg/5 mL)
    - **Plus** treatment for chlamydia if chlamydial infection is not ruled out.
- Alternative regimens:
    - Spectinomycin (currently not available in the United States) 2 g in a single IM dose or
    - Single-dose cephalosporin regimens

Chlamydia

A medical student couple, each 24 years old, presents with genitourinary symptoms. The woman complains of dyspareunia, dysuria, and a yellow mucopurulent discharge. Physical exam reveals a friable erythematous cervix, and bilateral adnexal tenderness. The man presents with painful urination and some testicular pain, and states his symptoms seem to "come and go." Physical exam reveals a mild, sticky, milky mucus-like discharge from penis and irritation around the opening of his penis. What infection do they have?   *(continued)*

Due to a high rate (~60%) of concurrent chlamydia infection, treatment for chlamydia should always be included with that for gonorrhea.

Chlamydia is the most common organism causing STD infection.

ETIOLOGY

Specific serotypes of *Chlamydia trachomatis* infects columnar/pseudostratified columnar epithelial surfaces.

SIGNS AND SYMPTOMS

- Dyspareunia.
- Pelvic pain.
- Yellow mucopurulent discharge.
- Friable, erythematous cervix.
- Tender epididymis if causing epididymitis.
- Peritonitis.
- Urethritis.
- Seventy-five percent of females and 50% of males are asymptomatic.

TREATMENT

- **First-line:**
  - Azithromycin 1 g PO once or
  - Doxycycline 100 mg PO bid × 7 days
- **Alternatives:**
  - Ofloxacin 300 mg PO bid × 7 days or
  - Erythromycin base 500 mg PO qid × 7 days or
  - Erythromycin ethylsuccinate 800 mg PO × 7 days or
  - Levofloxacin 500 mg PO × 7 days

Lymphogranuloma Venereum (LGV)

ETIOLOGY

Specific serotypes of *C trachomatis* (different from the ones that cause chlamydia).

SIGNS AND SYMPTOMS

- Initial small painless papule that quickly disappears.
- Inguinal lymphadenopathy appears 2–6 weeks later, which may suppurate through the skin—these remain painless (bubo formation).
- Extensive scarring and strictures may result.
- Painful mucopurulent/bloody proctitis with anal intercourse.

TREATMENT

- Recommended regimen: Doxycycline 100 mg PO bid × 21 days.
- Alternative regimen: 500 mg PO erythromycin 4×/day × 21 days.

Due to a high rate (~60%) of concurrent gonorrhea infection, treatment for gonorrhea should always be included with that for chlamydia.

HIGH-YIELD FACTS

Renal and Genitourinary Emergencies

- Buboes might require aspiration through intact skin or incision and drainage to prevent the formation of inguinal/femoral ulcerations.
- Persons who have had sexual contact with a patient who has LGV within the 60 days before onset of the patient's symptoms should be examined, tested for urethral or cervical chlamydial infection, and treated with a standard chlamydia regimen. Optimum contact interval is unknown; some specialists use longer contact intervals.

Chancroid

ETIOLOGY

- *Haemophilus ducreyi,* gram-negative bacillus.
- Also a cofactor for HIV transmission.

SIGNS AND SYMPTOMS

Painful inguinal adenopathy.

- Tender, shallow ulcers with irregular reddish borders: "kissing lesions"
- Inguinal mass/abscess from coalesced nodes (bubo)

TREATMENT

- Azithromycin 1 g PO once *or*
- Ceftriaxone 250 mg IM once *or*
- Erythromycin 500 mg PO tid × 7 days *or*
- Ciprofloxacin 500 mg PO bid × 3 days.
- If required, aspiration of buboes to relieve pain (not to be excised).
- Patient should be tested for HIV at the time of treatment and, if negative, 3 months later.
- Sex partners of patients who have chancroid should be examined and treated, regardless of whether symptoms of the disease are present, if they had sexual contact with the patient during the 10 days preceding the patient's onset of symptoms.

Syphilis

ETIOLOGY

Treponema pallidum.

SIGNS AND SYMPTOMS

- **Primary stage:** Painless ulcer (chancre) with indurative borders, which is highly ineffective; ulcers heal spontaneously 3–6 weeks after primary infection.
- **Secondary stage:**
  - Occurs 3–6 weeks after primary chancre heals.
  - Fever, sore throat, rash (trunk with spread to palms and soles), malaise, warts (condylomata lata), aseptic meningitis, lymphadenopathy; also spontaneously resolves.
- **Tertiary stage:**
- May occur after many years of latency.
- Various manifestations in multiple systems:
  - **Argyll Robertson pupil** (small pupil that reacts to accommodation but not light).

PainFUL ulcers:
- Chancroid
- Herpes

PainLESS ulcers:
- LGV
- Syphilis

Urethral discharge:
- Gonococcus
- *Chlamydia*
- *Trichomonas*

HIGH-YIELD FACTS

Renal and Genitourinary Emergencies

269

The **Jarisch-Herxheimer reaction** is an acute febrile reaction that occurs ~24 hours after treatment for early syphilis. It presents with headache and severe myalgias. It can cause early labor and fetal distress in pregnancy.
Syphilis buzzwords:
- Stage 1: Painless chancre
- Stage 2: Condyloma lata
- Stage 3: Gummas, Argyll Robertson pupil, tabes dorsalis

There are several preparations of penicillin G, including benzathine, aqueous procaine, and aqueous crystalline. The mixed forms are not appropriate therapy for syphilis.

- **Tabes dorsalis** (posterior column disease presenting with loss of position, deep pain and temperature sensation, ataxia, ↓ or absent deep tendon reflexes, wide-based gait, urinary retention or incontinence, impotence, sharp leg pain, meningitis, dementia).
- **Gummas** (granulomatous, necrotic lesions on the skin and submucosa involving the palate, nasal septum, or other organ).
- **Thoracic aortic aneurysm/dissection** (due to spirochetes in aortic vasa vasorum).

TREATMENT

- **For primary and secondary:**
  - Benzathine penicillin G 2.4 million units IM once for *early* latent syphilis (Bicillin LA). Repeat the dose three times at 1-week intervals for *late* latent syphilis.
  - Dose for children is 500,000 U/kg IM up to adult dose.
  - If penicillin-allergic, consider desensitization or doxycycline or tetracycline PO × 2 weeks.
- **For neurosyphilis:**
  - Aqueous penicillin G 2.4 million units every 4 hours × 10–14 days *or*
  - Ceftriaxone 1 g IV/IM daily × 14 days.
- **For sex partners:**
  - Persons who were exposed within the 90 days preceding the diagnosis of primary, secondary, or early latent syphilis in a sex partner might be infected even if seronegative; therefore, such persons should be treated presumptively.
  - Persons who were exposed > 90 days before the diagnosis of primary, secondary, or early latent syphilis in a sex partner should be treated presumptively if serologic test results are not available immediately and the opportunity for follow-up is uncertain.

Human Papillomavirus (HPV)

ETIOLOGY

Human papillomavirus.

SIGNS AND SYMPTOMS

- Genital and anal warts causing discomfort but not pain
- Condylomata acuminata when warts coalesce

TREATMENT

HPV Vaccine
- Quadrivalent HPV vaccine protects against four HPV types (6, 11, 16, 18), which are responsible for 70% of cervical cancers and 90% of genital warts.
- Recommended for girls and women ages 9–26, before the onset of sexual activity.
- The vaccine is effective for at least 5 years.

Self-Treatments (Applied by Patient)
- Podofilox 0.5% solution or gel:
  - Applied to visible genital warts bid × 3 days, followed by 4 days of no therapy; cycle can be repeated up to four times.
  - Total wart area treated should not exceed 10 cm².
  - Total volume of podofilox should be limited to 0.5 mL/day.

- Imiquimod 5% cream:
  - Applied once daily at bedtime, three times a week for up to 16 weeks.
  - Treatment area should be washed with soap and water 6–10 hours after the application.

Physician Treatments

- Cryotherapy with liquid nitrogen or cryoprobe. Applications repeated every 1–2 weeks until eradicated.
- Podophyllin resin 10–25% in a compound tincture of benzoin. Treatment can be repeated weekly if needed. A small amount should be applied to each wart and allowed to air dry. Avoid in pregnant patients because of teratogenic effects.
- Trichloroacetic acid (TCA) or bichloroacetic acid (BCA) 80–90%: Small amount should be applied only to warts and allowed to dry, at which time a white "frosting" develops. If an excess amount of acid is applied, the treated area should be powdered with talc, sodium bicarbonate (ie, baking soda), or liquid soap preparations to remove unreacted acid. This treatment can be repeated weeky as needed.
- Surgical removal either by tangential scissor excision, tangential shave excision, curettage, or electrosurgery.

The safety of podofilox and imiquimod during pregnancy has not been established.

Trichomoniasis

A 31-year-old sexually active female presents with vaginal burning, itching, and discharge. Abdominal tenderness is noted. She admits to having sexual intercourse with a few different men about a week ago. The vaginal discharge is a yellowish gray, frothy, and malodorous. The pH of vaginal secretion is 5.0–6.5. Whiff test is positive. What is the diagnosis, and how would you treat it?

This is the classic description for trichomoniasis. However, the whiff test and vaginal pH are rudimentary techniques. A wet mount, where the trichomonad organisms can be identified under a microscope, is only about 60% sensitive. A DNA test is most accurate, and is available as a point-of-care test. Treatment for nonpregnant patients is with metronidazole. Remember to warn patients that this medication cannot be taken with alcohol; the combination can cause a disulfuram reaction, which consists of severe nausea, vomiting and malaise. All sex partners should be treated with a one time does of 2 g of metronidazole. The patient should avoid intercourse until therapy is completed and all partners are asymptomatic.

Most common nonviral STD in the world.

ETIOLOGY

Trichomonas vaginalis.

SIGNS AND SYMPTOMS

- Copious, foamy, yellow-green, malodorous discharge with pH > 4.5.
- Punctate red spots on cervix or vaginal wall ("strawberry cervix").
- Labial irritation or swelling.
- Dyspareunia.
- Dysuria.
- Men may be asymptomatic.

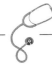

Trichomoniasis: Flagellated organisms are seen swimming under the wet mount.

"Whiff test": Two drops of KOH mixed with the discharge and heated onto a slide produces a fishy smell. This is characteristic of both *Trichomonas* and bacterial vaginosis.

TREATMENT

- Single-dose metronidazole (2 g) or 500 mg bid × 1 week. Abstain from alcohol while on the drug, to avoid disulfuram reaction.
- Clotrimazole for first-trimester pregnancy.

Herpes

EPIDEMIOLOGY

More than 50 million people in the United States are infected.

ETIOLOGY

Herpes simplex virus (HSV). Most caused by HSV-2. Infections caused by HSV-1 tend to have lower recurrence rates.

SIGNS AND SYMPTOMS

- Painful pustular or ulcerative lesions.
- Initial infection more severe than recurrences.
- May have systemic effects (fever, headache, myalgias), left axis deviation, aseptic meningitis.
- Also a causative agent in encephalitis and esophagitis.
- Adenopathy develops during second and third weeks of illness and is bilateral, mildly tender, and nonfluctuant.

TREATMENT

- Oral antiviral therapy helps to control acute symptoms and is also useful for chronic suppressive therapy. However, they do not eradicate the virus and do not ↓ the risk, frequency, or severity of recurrences.
    - Acyclovir 400 mg PO tid × 7–10 days *or*
    - Acyclovir 200 mg PO 5×/day × 7–10 days *or*
    - Famciclovir 250 mg PO tid × 7–10 days *or*
    - Valacyclovir 1 g PO bid × 7–10 days
- Duration of oral treatment may be extended if healing is incomplete at 10 days.
- Topical antiviral therapy is not recommended.
- Sex partners of patients who have genital herpes can benefit from evaluation and counseling. Symptomatic sex partners should be evaluated and treated in the same manner as patients who have genital lesions. Asymptomatic sex partners of patients who have genital herpes should be questioned concerning histories of genital lesions and offered type-specific serologic testing for HSV infection.

SEXUAL ASSAULT

EPIDEMIOLOGY

- An estimated 6% of crimes are rapes.
- Approximately one in eight women have been raped, with only 25% of cases reported.
- Two to 4% of rapes are committed against males.

CLINICAL FINDINGS

- The interviewer must determine from the patient the identity and number of persons involved, details on what happened (what kind of assault), areas of pain, how long ago it happened, what happened after the incident, last menstrual period, oral contraceptive use, last consensual intercourse, and allergies.
- Other signs of physical abuse:
  - Facial and extremity injuries are more common than actual injuries to the genitalia.
  - When males are sodomized, they may have thorax and abdomen abrasions because of the position they are in; also anal fissures and lacerations may be seen.
  - ↓ sphincter tone or severe hemorrhoids may indicate chronic sodomy.
- When examining a rape victim, most EDs use a standardized kit provided by the police:
  - All physical injuries (all lacerations and bruises) are documented.
  - A pelvic exam is done, and all mucosal surfaces (oral, vaginal, and anal) are sampled.
  - Testing for STDs is done.
  - Skin and fingernail scrapings are collected.
  - Semen can be sampled if found with the use of a Wood's lamp (fluoresces, but this is not specific for semen).

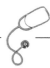

The most important aspect of dealing with sexual assault victims is to ensure their psychological well-being. This very traumatic experience could potentially be made worse by the victim's being surrounded and "interrogated" by hospital and police personnel. Every effort should be made to make the patient as comfortable as possible.

TREATMENT

- Addressing all physical injuries (admission if necessary).
- Tetanus prophylaxis.
- STD and pregnancy testing (offer prophylaxis).
- Hepatitis B prophylaxis.
- Human immunodeficiency virus counseling (offer prophylaxis).
- Most physicians will empirically treat for gonorrhea and chlamydia.
- Medical and psychiatric follow-up should be arranged within 2 weeks.
- Ensure that patient has a safe place to go; arrange for social worker to see patient if needed.

HIGH-YIELD FACTS

Renal and Genitourinary
Emergencies

Hematologic and Oncologic Emergencies

Primary and Secondary Hemostasis

- Primary hemostasis is the initial superficial clotting performed by **platelets.** Defects (eg, thrombocytopenia) typically result in oozing from IV sites and bleeding from mucous membranes, nose, and gastrointestinal (GI) tract. Also manifest and petechiae and ecchymoses.
- Secondary hemostasis is a function of the coagulation cascade and clotting factors. Defects in this process (eg, hemophilia) result in large, deep bleeds such as hemarthrosis (bleeding into a joint).

Coagulation Cascade

See Figure 10-1.

Heparin

- ↑ activated partial thromboplastin time (aPTT).
- Affects intrinsic pathway.
- ↓ fibrinogen levels.
- Primarily affects factors **VIII,** IX, X, XI, XII.
- Low-molecular-weight heparins have 10 times activity against factor Xa.
- Safe in pregnancy.
- Adverse effects include bleeding, thrombocytopenia, and osteoporosis.

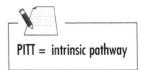

PITT = intrinsic pathway

Heparin goes with **Intrinsic** pathway because **H** comes right before **I.**

PeT = PT measures extrinsic pathway.

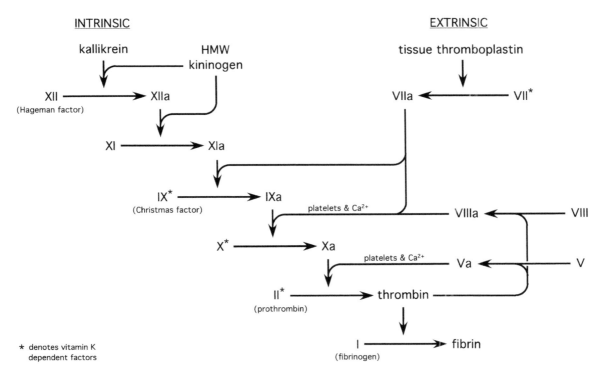

FIGURE 10-1. Coagulation cascade.

Leafy green vegetables
have high vitamin K
content and can make the
International Normalized
Ratio (INR) become
subtherapeutic for patients
on warfarin.

Warfarin

- ↑ prothrombin time (PT).
- Affects extrinsic pathway.
- ↓ vitamin K.
- Primarily affects II, V, **VII.**
- Teratogenic.
- Has an initial *pro*coagulant effect, taking 48–72 hours to become anti-coagulant. Concurrent bridging with heparin during this time is needed, and oral warfarin dose is titrated slowly.

aPTT

- Tests extrinsic and common pathways.
- Isolated elevation of aPTT (with normal PT) seen in:
  - Heparin therapy
  - Deficiencies of factors VIII (hemophilia A), factor IX (hemophilia B), factor XI, and factor XII (asymptomatic)

PT

- Tests intrinsic and common pathways.
- Isolated elevation of PT (with normal PTT) seen in:
  - Vitamin K deficiency
  - Warfarin therapy
  - Liver disease (↓ factor production)
  - Congenital (rare)

Thrombin Time

- Measures the time it takes to convert fibrinogen into a fibrin clot.
- Elevated in:
  - Diffuse intravascular coagulation (DIC—consumes fibrinogen)
  - Liver disease (↓ production of fibrinogen)
  - Heparin therapy (inhibits fibrinogen formation)
  - Hypofibrinogenemia (low fibrinogen to start)

Bleeding Time

- Measures time from start of skin incision to formation of clot (normal = 3–8 minutes).
- Independent of coagulation cascade.
- Elevated in:
  - Thrombocytopenia
  - Qualitative platelet disorders
  - von Willebrand disease (VWD)

HEMOPHILIA A

PATHOPHYSIOLOGY

Sex-linked recessive disease causing a deficiency of factor VIII.

SIGNS AND SYMPTOMS

- Severity of disease varies depending on amount of factor VIII activity.
- Deep tissue bleeding, hemarthrosis (secondary hemostasis problems).

DIAGNOSIS

- Prolonged aPTT, normal bleeding time.
- Clinical picture, family history, and the factor VIII coagulant activity level.

TREATMENT

- Recombinant factor VIII
- Cryoprecipitate

Unlike in VWD, bleeding time in hemophilia A is unaffected because no abnormality with platelets is present.

HEMOPHILIA B (CHRISTMAS DISEASE)

PATHOPHYSIOLOGY

X-linked recessive disease that causes a deficiency of factor IX.

SIGNS AND SYMPTOMS

Identical to hemophilia A.

DIAGNOSIS

Factor IX assay.

TREATMENT

- Fresh frozen plasma (FFP)
- Recombinant factor IX

VON WILLEBRAND DISEASE (vWD)

DEFINITION

- Type I: Partial quantitative deficiency of von Willebrand factor (vWF) (most common)
- Type II: Qualitative defect of vWF
- Type III: Almost total absence of vWF

vWD is the most common inherited bleeding disorder.

PATHOPHYSIOLOGY

- vWF is a glycoprotein that is synthesized, stored, and secreted by vascular endothelial cells.
- It functions to (1) allow platelets to adhere to the damaged endothelium and (2) carry factor VIII in the plasma.

ETIOLOGY

Usually autosomal dominant inheritance.

EPIDEMIOLOGY

- One in 100 live births have some defect in vWF.
- Only 1 in 10,000 manifests a clinically significant bleeding disorder.

SIGNS AND SYMPTOMS

Primary hemostasis problems: Epistaxis, GI bleeding, easy bruising, menorrhagia, prolonged bleeding after dental extraction.

DIAGNOSIS

- Prolonged bleeding time (platelets don't adhere well).
- Prolonged aPTT (factor VIII is ↓).
- Normal PT.
- Normal platelet count.
- Definitive diagnosis is made with abnormal assay of vWF, vWF:antigen, or factor VIII:C (usually not in the emergency department [ED]).

TREATMENT

- Type I: Desmopressin
- Types II and III:
  - Factor VIII concentrates with large amounts of vWF:
    - Synthetic-treated product, no risk of infection
    - Provides VWF most efficiently, with the least amount of volume
  - Cryoprecipitate and FFP: Will also work, but carry risk of infection and provide low concentration of VWF for given volume, resulting in volume overload for severe cases.

ANTIPHOSPHOLIPID ANTIBODY SYNDROME

- Defined as presence of lupus anticoagulant or anticardiolipin antibodies in addition to thrombosis and/or pregnancy complications.
- Most commonly manifests as recurrent fetal losses in women of childbearing age.
- Antiphospholipid antibody impairs in vivo anticoagulant pathways.
- Diagnosis is by lupus anticoagulant and anticardiolipin antibody detection. Tests to detect presence: dilute Russell's viper venom time (dRVVT), kaolin clotting time, dilute phospholipid time.
- Asymptomatic patients need no treatment. Patients with thrombosis need long-term anticoagulation. Pregnant patients can be treated with heparin.

THROMBOCYTOPENIA

DEFINITION

Platelet count < 140,000/mm³.

Platelets < 50,000/mm³: Bleeding with trauma. Platelets < 20,000/mm³: Spontaneous bleeding can occur. Platelets < 10,000/mm³: High risk for potentially life-threatening bleeding.

280

ETIOLOGY

↑ destruction
- Antibody-coated platelets removed by macrophages:
  - Idiopathic thrombocytopenic purpura (ITP)
  - Human immunodeficiency virus (HIV)-associated thrombocytopenia
  - Transfusion reactions
  - Some drug-induced thrombocytopenias
- Thrombin-induced platelet damage: DIC (seen with obstetrical complications, metastatic malignancy, septicemia, and traumatic brain injury)
- Removal by acute vascular abnormalities:
  - Thrombotic thrombocytopenic purpura (TTP)
  - Hemolytic uremic syndrome (HUS)
- Adult respiratory distress syndrome–induced thrombocytopenia

↓ Production
- ↓ megakaryocytes in marrow:
  - Leukemia
  - Aplastic anemia
- Normal megakaryocytes:
  - Alcohol-induced reactions
  - Megaloblastic anemias
  - Some myelodysplastic syndromes
  - Medications (eg, antibiotics)

Sequestration in Spleen
- Cirrhosis with congestive splenomegaly
- Myelofibrosis with myeloid metaplasia

Causes of thrombocytopenia— PLATELETS
Platelet disorders: TTP, HUS, ITP, DIC
Leukemia
Anemia
Trauma
Enlarged spleen
Liver disease
EtOH
Toxins (benzene, heparins, aspirin, chemotherapy agents, etc)
Sepsis

RISK FACTORS

- Drugs (chemotherapeutic agents, ethanol, thiazides, antibiotics)
- Prior thrombocytopenic episodes
- Underlying immunologic disorder
- Massive blood transfusions
- Significant EtOH consumption
- Term pregnancy

SIGNS AND SYMPTOMS

Primary hemostasis signs:

- Petechiae
- Purpura
- Heme-positive stool
- Recurrent epistaxis, gingival bleeding, or menorrhagia
- Hepatosplenomegaly (jaundice, spider angiomas, and palmar erythema may be present if condition is due to EtOH abuse)

DIAGNOSIS

- Complete blood count (CBC) with platelet morphology and manual platelet count
- PT/PTT
- Bleeding time
- Liver function tests (LFTs)

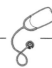

TREATMENT

- Treatment depends on cause.
- Typically, no need to give platelets unless < 10,000/µL or active bleed.
- Platelets are contraindicated in TTP.

CHEMICALLY INDUCED PLATELET DYSFUNCTION

Antiplatelet Therapy

- Platelets are significant components of the thrombotic response to damaged coronary and cerebral artery plaques.
- Prompt antiplatelet therapy can halt progression and significantly reduce morbidity/mortality from acute myocardial infarction and cerebrovascular accident.
- **Aspirin (ASA):** *Irreversibly* acetylates platelet cyclooxygenase: As platelets have no biosynthetic machinery, it is *inactivated for the life span of the platelet* (8–10 days).
- **Ticlopidine (Ticlid):**
  - Irreversibly inhibits conversion of platelet surface receptor to its high-affinity binding state
  - Prevents fibrinogen receptor expression
  - Lasts for life span of platelet
- **Clopidogrel (Plavix):**
  - Ticlopidine analog, similar mechanism
  - Rapid onset of action, can be used acutely
  - Intravenous (IV) administration possible

TREATMENT

With all of these drugs, if significant bleeding occurs, platelets should be given because although the patient may have a normal count, the platelets are dysfunctional.

IDIOPATHIC THROMBOCYTOPENIC PURPURA (ITP)

A 42-year-old woman with no past medical history presents due to petechiae that have erupted over her arms and legs in the past 2 days. She also reports gingival bleeding. Physical exam reveals petechiae within the oral cavity as well. Labs demonstrate a platelet count of 7,000/mm³, normal PT/aPTT, and a prolonged bleeding time. What is the diagnosis and treatment for this patient?

She has ITP and would benefit from initiation of glucocorticoids. Although the thrombocytopenia will likely return after steroids are stopped, she is unlikely to have a life-threatening bleed.

DEFINITION

An autoimmune-mediated destructin of platelets.

- Adult ITP usually results from antibody development against a structural antigen present on the platelet surface.
- Childhood ITP is thought to be triggered by a virus, which produces an antibody that cross-reacts with an antigen on the platelet surface.

DIAGNOSIS

- Peripheral blood smear should be unremarkable with the exception of ↓ platelets.
- Bone marrow is normal with the exception of possibly ↑ megakaryocytes.

TREATMENT

- **Adults:**
  - Initial treatment is prednisone 1 mg/kg/day. Platelet levels usually rise over the coming weeks, during which time the steroid dosage is tapered.
  - Most patients will have a recurrence of thrombocytopenia after steroids discontinued.
  - Splenectomy is traditional second-line treatment, providing complete remission in most patients with ITP.
  - However, given the benign course of ITP and risks of splenectomy, many patients have more conservative management.
- **Patients with ITP and life-threatening bleeding:**
  - High-dose steroids.
  - Suppress mononuclear phagocyte clearance of platelets by administering IV immunoglobulin (IVIG) at 1 g/kg for 1 day.
  - Platelet transfusion for life-threatening bleeding.
- **Children:**
  - Seventy to 80% of children have complete remission without therapy.
  - Those with more severe symptoms or lack of spontaneous remission can be treated with steroids, IVIG.

THROMBOTIC THROMBOCYTOPENIC PURPURA (TTP)

A 52-year-old man presents to the ED "not feeling well." His wife has noticed he is a bit confused and "not acting right." He has bruising over his left arm that was just noticed today. His past medical history is significant for a hospitalization 1 month ago for a myocardial infarction. His medications include losartan and clopidogrel. His vital signs reveal a temperature of 37.9°C (100.2°F), pulse of 120 bpm, and BP of 88/40 mm Hg. Labs demonstrate a platelet count of 15,000/mm³, hemoglobin of 7.1 g/dL, normal PT/aPTT, elevated bilirubin, and a BUN/Cr of 28/1.6 mg/dL. What is the diagnosis and appropriate treatment?

His symptoms are suggestive of TTP. He has thrombocytopenia, hemolytic anemia, mild renal insufficiency, and altered mental status. If obtained, a peripheral smear would also show schistocytes. Untreated, the mortality for TTP is around 80%. He should be admitted for treatment with plasma exchange.

TTP diagnostic pentad:
- Fever
- Altered mental status
- Renal dysfunction
- Microangiopathic hemolytic anemia
- Thrombocytopenia

You do *not* need all present for diagnosis!

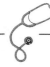

Do not transfuse platelets in patients with TTP — this could kill them.

TTP is a disease with high mortality when not diagnosed and treated early. Also, it is a disease that recurs, with each subsequent episode being slightly worse. Patients eventually die of multiple thrombi lodged in the brain, kidneys, and other organs.

DEFINITION

Life-threatening disorder due to uncleaved, giant von Willebrand proteins clogging up microvasculature causing sheering of RBCs and consumption of platelets.

EPIDEMIOLOGY

- Female > male
- Age 10–45 years

RISK FACTORS

- Most commonly idiopathic cause
- Pregnancy
- Drugs: Quinine, cyclosporine, mitomycin C, ticlopidine, clopidogrel, H_2 blockers, oral contraceptives, penicillin
- Autoimmune disorders (eg, systemic lupus erythematosus)
- Infection (including *Escherichia coli* O157:H7, *Shigella dysenteriae*, and HIV)
- Allogeneic bone marrow transplantation

SIGNS AND SYMPTOMS

- Fever
- Waxing and waning mental status (correlates with lodging and dislodging of thrombus in cerebral vessels)
- Pallor
- Petechiae
- Colicky pain of various body parts (again due to thrombus in vessels)

DIAGNOSIS

- TTP should be assumed if thrombocytopenia and microangiopathic hemolytic anemia without other known source (DIC, lupus, etc).
- Peripheral blood smear: Schistocytes and helmet cells.
- CBC: Anemia, thrombocytopenia, elevated reticulocyte count.
- Blood urea nitrogen/creatinine (BUN/Cr): Azotemia.
- Urinalysis: Hematuria, red cell casts, and proteinuria.
- LFTs: Elevated lactic dehydrogenase, elevated bilirubin (unconjugated > conjugated), low haptoglobin.

TREATMENT

- **Do not transfuse platelets—can worsen disease process.**
- Plasma exchange is mainstay of treatment (given daily, until platelet count rises to normal).
- May give FFP if plasmapheresis not available.
- Transfuse packed RBCs if anemia is symptomatic (tachycardia, orthostatic hypotension, hypoxia).
- Consider corticosteroids, vincristine, antiplatelet agents, and splenectomy for refractory cases.
- Monitor for and treat acute bleeds (remember to look for intracranial bleed as well).
- Admit patients to the intensive care unit.

A 6-year-old boy presents with abdominal pain, oliguria, diarrhea, and fever. Several kids from his school came down with the same thing after his birthday party at a local hamburger chain. His vital signs are stable. He appears pale. Labs demonstrate a hemoglobin of 8.3 g/dL, creatinine of 2.2 mg/dL, and a platelet count of 20,000/mm³. What is the diagnosis and appropriate treatment for this child?

He has HUS, likely from undercooked and contaminated ground beef. He should be admitted to a facility with hemodialysis capabilities.

HUS diagnostic triad:
- Renal failure
- Microangiopathic hemolytic anemia
- Thrombocytopenia

DEFINITION

A similar syndrome to TTP, with the primary manifestation being renal failure.

ETIOLOGY

Unknown.

EPIDEMIOLOGY

- Most common in childhood
- Adult form also seen

RISK FACTORS

- Infection with *E coli* O157:H7 or *Shigella dysenteriae*
- Ingestion of undercooked meats and unpasteurized products

SIGNS AND SYMPTOMS

- GI symptoms (nausea, vomiting, abdominal pain).
- Oliguria.
- Pallor.
- GI bleeding.
- Seizures can result as a complication of renal failure, due to hypertension, hyponatremia, fluid overload, and electrolyte imbalances.

DIAGNOSIS

Same as TTP. Can test stool for *E coli* O157:H7 infection, but not likely to come back in ED.

Platelet transfusion is not contraindicated for HUS as it is for TTP.

TREATMENT

- Dialysis and supportive care.
- Plasmapheresis is sometimes used in adults.

PROGNOSIS

- The time for highest mortality is during the course of the disease, when central nervous system (CNS) complications can result.
- Most children recover without sequelae after the acute illness.
- Some children will have progressive renal dysfunction and hypertension and should be monitored for a period of at least 5 years.
- Adults do not recover so well and usually have residual renal failure.

> A 27-year-old woman who is 39 weeks pregnant is the victim of a high-speed motor vehicle crash. She presents with vaginal bleeding and uterine irritability. A few hours later, she goes into shock and begins bleeding profusely from her multiple lacerations. She is unstable, with tachycardia and hypotension. Labs show prolonged PT/aPTT, platelets of 30,000/mm³, and elevated fibrin split products. What should her treatment include?
>
> She has DIC secondary to abruptio placentae. Aggressive supportive care (airway, IV fluid) need to be given. She should receive FFP to improve PT/PTT, platelet transfusion, and OB consult for emergency caesarean section. Unlike TTP, platelet transfusion is safe in DIC.

DEFINITION

DIC is a coagulopathy that happens when both the fibrinolytic and coagulation cascades are activated.

RISK FACTORS

- Infection: Usually from gram-negative organisms (endotoxin causes generation of tissue factor activity on the plasma membrane of monocytes and macrophages); probably the most common cause.
- Trauma: Crush injuries, brain trauma, burns.
- Obstetrical complications:
  - Abruptio placentae
  - Saline-induced therapeutic termination
  - Retained products of conception
  - Amniotic fluid embolism
- Malignancy:
  - Mucin-secreting adenocarcinomas of pancreas and prostate
  - Acute promyelocytic leukemia
- Shock from any cause.
- Snake bites.
- Heatstroke.
- Severe transfusion reaction.
- Drugs.
- Foreign bodies such as peritoneovenous shunts.

PATHOGENESIS

- Results from generation of tissue factor in the blood or the introduction of tissue factor–rich substances into the circulation.
- Tissue factor is the most fibrinogenic substance known, and it initiates coagulation.
- Coagulative activity is difficult to regulate once it is begun in this fashion, and soon the factors of coagulation have been exhausted, resulting in coagulopathy.

SIGNS AND SYMPTOMS

- Sites of recent surgery or phlebotomy bleed profusely and cannot be controlled with local measures.

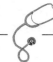

PT/aPTT are normal in ITP, TTP, and HUS. They are abnormally elevated in DIC.

- Ecchymoses form at sites of parenteral injections.
- Serious GI bleeding may ensue at sites of erosion of the gastric mucosa.

DIAGNOSIS

- Presence of fibrin split products
- Thrombocytopenia
- Markedly prolonged PT/PTT
- Low fibrinogen concentration
- Elevated plasma D-dimers (cross-linked fibrin degradation by-products)
- Schistocytes on peripheral smear

TREATMENT

- Treat underlying cause.
- If a transient process, give cryoprecipitate (has fibrinogen) and platelets for temporary support.
- For DIC-associated bleeding with raised PT and aPTT, use FFP.

HEPARIN-INDUCED THROMBOCYTOPENIA (HIT)

DEFINITION AND CLINICAL MANIFESTATIONS

- Type I HIT is a transient, harmless, and mild drop in platelets, usually 1 or 2 days after initiation of heparin. Patient may be kept on heparin and platelets will return to normal.
- Type II HIT (true HIT) is an immune-mediated process against the heparin-platelet complex. It is manifested by arterial and venous **thrombosis** as well as thrombocytopenia. It is life threatening. It typically presents 4–10 days after heparin exposure *or* after several hours if patient has had prior heparin exposure.

DIAGNOSIS

- Clinical suspicion.
- More common with unfractionated heparin (around 2%) but can occur with low-molecular-weight heparin (LMWH, <1%).
- Heparin-induced platelet aggregation assay (HIT assay)—specific but insensitive.
- Serotonin release assay.

TREATMENT

- Immediate removal of any heparin exposure (including LMWH), including flushes and locks.
- Anticoagulation is the mainstay of treatment, as most complications are caused by thrombosis. Lepirudin and argatroban are direct thrombin inhibitors used in this setting. Warfarin **should not** be used initially as it can precipitate worsening thrombosis.
- Platelet transfusions relatively contraindicated, but can be given for severe bleeding.

Several entities must be considered in the differential. The outcomes and treatments are very different.

- **Gestational thrombocytopenia:** Mild and asymptomatic, usually with platelet count > 70,000 μL, typically occurring in the third trimester. There are no sequelae, and it resolves after delivery.
- **Preeclampsia** (discussed in greater detail in the Obstetric Emergencies chapter): Hypertension, proteinuria, and edema typically developing in the third trimester. Eclampsia is the above with the addition of seizures. Typically, platelets are ↓ in these patients more than usual gestational thrombocytopenia. Delivery of the child is the mainstay of treatment.
- **HELLP syndrome** (hemolytic anemia, elevated liver enzymes, low platelets): Has the same features as preeclampsia with the addition of hemolysis and elevated liver function tests (LFTs) (thrombocytopenia can be seen in both). This is life threatening, and delivery is indicated. Diagnose by platelet count, lactic dehydrogenase (LDH) (high indicates hemolysis), LFTs, and peripheral blood smear (schistocytes indicate microangiopathic hemolysis).

HEREDITARY HEMOLYTIC ANEMIAS

Sickle Cell Anemia (SCA)

Features of SCA—
SICKLE
Splenomegaly/Sludging
Infection
Cholelithiasis
Kidney—hematuria
Liver congestion/Leg ulcers
Eye changes

A 1-year-old child recently adopted from Liberia is brought in to the ED by parents with increasing lethargy over the past 3 days. The parents also note that he is more pale than usual. Past medical history is unknown, and he is taking no medications. Splenomegaly is noted on exam. His temperature is 37.8°C (100.0°F), pulse 180 bpm, blood pressure 85/50 mm Hg, and respiratory rate 26 bpm. Laboratory studies reveal a hemoglobin of 7.4 g/dL. What is the cause of his symptoms?

This child has an acute splenic sequestration crisis secondary to sickle cell anemia. This is a relatively common presentation of sickle cell anemia in children < 4 years of age (infarction → fibrosis and destruction of spleen in older children and adults). The initial treatment is supportive, including packed RBC transfusions. About half will have a recurrence, so splenectomy should be considered.

DEFINITION

- Genetic disease characterized by the presence of hemoglobin S in RBCs.
- Hemoglobin S is formed by substitution of valine for glutamine in the sixth position of the β-hemoglobin chain.
- During periods of high oxygen consumption, this abnormal hemoglobin distorts and causes cell to sickle.
- Sickle cell trait: Heterozygous for sickle gene.
- Sickle cell disease: Homozygous for sickle gene.

EPIDEMIOLOGY

- In the United States, primarily affects African-Americans.
- ↑ incidence in populations from Africa, the Mediterranean, Middle East, and India.

PATHOPHYSIOLOGY

- Deoxygenated hemoglobin S undergoes a conformational change with low O_2 tension.
- When enough hemoglobin S molecules change conformation, the hemoglobin molecules crystallize, forming a semisolid gel in the interior of the RBC.
- This causes the RBC to adopt a sickle shape (Figure 10-2).
- The distorted RBCs are inflexible and plug small capillaries, → occlusion and ischemia/infarction.
- The sickled cells also have an ↑ propensity to adhere to the capillary endothelium.
- The distortion also results in a weakening of the RBC membrane, and the cells have a ↓ life span in the circulation, causing the chronic hemolytic anemia.
- Early in the sickling process, the RBCs can resume their normal shape if O_2 tension is restored; later, the sickling becomes irreversible.
- Low RBC H_2O content can also trigger sickling.
- Early in life, the spleen removes most of the sickled cells from the circulation, causing splenomegaly. Eventually, the toll of continuous sequestration damages the spleen to the point of infarction. The spleen fibroses and shrivels to a fraction of its normal size, often termed *autosplenectomy*.
- Absence of splenic function renders these patients more susceptible to infections, particularly by encapsulated organisms (*Haemophilius influenzae*, pneumococci, meningococci, *Klebsiella*).

DIAGNOSIS

- All newborns at risk in the United States are screened for the disease.
- Peripheral smear: Howell-Jolly bodies (cytoplasmic remnants of nuclear chromatin that are normally removed by the spleen), sickled cells.
- Blood tests show anemia, ↑ reticulocyte count, and ↑ indirect bilirubin.
- Hemoglobin electrophoresis will show hemoglobin S.
- Anemia (mean hemoglobin ~8 g/dL).
- Reticulocytes ~3–15%.

Patients with SCA are prone to infection with encapsulated organisms. *Salmonella* osteomyelitis is most common among patients with SCA.

Life span of erythrocytes in patients with SCA is 17 days vs. 120 days for normal adults.

A 24-year-old man with known sickle cell disease presents with pain in his lower back and knees. He is afebrile, has an O_2 saturation of 100%, and normal labs. *Think: Vaso-occlusive crisis of sickle cell disease.*

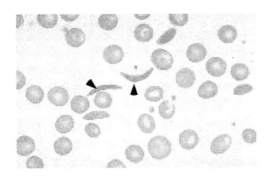

FIGURE 10-2. **Peripheral smear demonstrating sickled RBCs (arrows).**

Treat sickle cell vaso-occlusive pain crisis aggressively with analgesics, generally opioids.

- **Typical vaso-occlusive crisis:**
  - Symptoms include arthralgias and pain.
  - Caused by vascular sludging and thrombosis. Uncomplicated crisis is treated with hydration and aggressive use of analgesics.
  - May be precipitated by infection.
  - Reticulocytes elevated.
  - Most sickle cell emergencies are due to vaso-occlusive crisis infarcting a particular organ.
  - Transfusion generally not recommended in acute setting (may ↑ viscosity and worsen symptoms).
- **Acute chest syndrome:**
  - Fever, chest pain, cough, shortness of breath, and pulmonary infiltrates on chest radiograph.
  - Thought to be due to infection and occlusion of pulmonary microvasculature.
  - Major cause of mortality in patients > 5 years old.
  - Oxygenation should be monitored. Antibiotics and hydration are treatment. Exchange transfusion if severe. Always give supplemental oxygen as well.
- **Aplastic crisis:**
  - Life-threatening complication characterized by severe pancytopenia.
  - Low reticulocyte count.
  - Due to medullary sickling, common complication of infection with parvovirus B19.
- **CNS crisis:**
  - The only type of vaso-occlusive crisis that is painless (no pain receptors).
  - Cerebral vascular occlusion is more common in children, and cerebral hemorrhage is more common in adults.
  - Evaluation should include computed tomographic (CT) scanning.
  - Lumbar puncture should be performed if CT is negative and headache is present to exclude diagnosis of subarachnoid hemorrhage.
- **Priapism:** Sickling in corpus cavernosum of penis causing protracted painful erection. This can → impotence. Draining of corpora cavernosa can be done. Also, subcutaneous terbutaline can be used.
- **Acute hepatic sequestration crisis:** Sequestration and sickling of RBCs in liver → high bilirubin and severe anemia. Aggressive transfusion is treatment as well as exchange transfusion if severe.
- **Acute splenic sequestration:**
  - Second most common cause of death in children with SCA (by adulthood, autosplenectomy will have disposed of this source of morbidity/mortality).
  - Sickled cells block outflow from the spleen, causing pooling of blood and platelets in the spleen. In major sequestration crisis, the hemoglobin drops three points from baseline or to a level < 6 g/dL.
- **Renal papillary necrosis:**
  - Characterized by flank pain and hematuria.
  - Occurs because of the very high osmolalities in renal medulla needed to pull the water from the collecting ducts, causing the RBCs to sickle.

Thalassemias

ETIOLOGY

- Defective globin chain synthesis.
- Patients with β-thalassemia have ↓ production of β-globin chain. Likewise, patients with α-thalassemia have defective production of α chains and accumulate excessive β-globin chains.

CLINICAL FEATURES

- Severity of anemia dependent on extent of disease
- Hepatosplenomegaly
- Bone marrow expansion causing osteopenia

DIAGNOSIS

- Microcytosis, hypochromasia on peripheral smear.
- CBC may or may not reveal anemia.
- Hemoglobin electrophoresis.

TREATMENT

- Thalassemia carrier and traits are asymptomatic and need no treatment.
- Patients with hemoglobin H (one functional α-globin chain) and β-thalassemia major may or may not require intermittent transfusions.
- In all such cases presenting to the ED with manifestations of severe anemia or hemolysis, a thorough search for precipitating events like infection or oxidative stress should be undertaken.

Glucose-6-Phosphate Dehydrogenase (G6PD) Deficiency

- G6PD maintains glutathione in reduced state to prevent oxidative damage to RBCs.
- Males are affected more commonly as the gene for G6PD is carried on X chromosome.
- Severity is proportional to magnitude of enzyme deficiency.
- Majority of patients stay asymptomatic unless exposed to infections or oxidative stress.
- Diagnosis is by quantitative assay.
- Treatment is primarily preventive and symptomatic management.

BLOOD PRODUCTS

Packed RBCs

- Treatment of choice for hemorrhagic shock.
- Type O negative blood is the universal donor and should be used for life-threatening bleeding until type-specific blood is available.
- Aproximately 250 mL per unit; generally start with 2 units or 15 mL/kg in children.
- Risk of infectious disease transmission.

6 units of platelets ("6-pack") will raise platelet count about 25,000–50,000/mm³.

Platelets

- Bleeding from thrombocytopenia or inadequate platelet function (platelet inhibitors).
- Avoid in TTP and relatively contraindicated in HIT.
- ABO matching is preferred.
- Risk of infectious disease transmission.

Fresh Frozen Plasma (FFP)

- Contains all coagulation factors; dosing at 10–15 mL/kg.
- Used primarily to reverse elevated INR (warfarin effect), replace multiple clotting factors (DIC).
- ABO compatibility is required.
- Risk of infectious disease transmission.

Prothrombin Complex Concentrate (PCC)

- Contains vitamin K–dependent clotting factors.
- More expensive than FFP.
- Faster reversal of INR than FFP, but clinical outcomes similar and PCC more expensive.
- Does not require ABO compatibility.

Cryoprecipitate

- Contains large amounts of factor VIII and vWF.
- ABO compatibility is not required.
- Risk of infectious disease transmission.

Clotting Factor Concentrates

- Factors VII, VIII, IX.
- Very expensive.
- Do not require ABO compatibility.
- Almost no risk of infectious disease transmission.

TRANSFUSION REACTIONS

ABO Incompatibility

- Most common transfusion reaction.
- Almost invariably due to **human error.**
- Patients are immunized against A/B antigen (Ag) without prior exposure because endogenous bacteria produce glycoproteins with structures similar to the A/B Ag.
- Which antibody (Ab) form is actually determined by the patient's own A/B status.

Non-ABO Incompatibility

- Uncommon, occurring mostly in multitransfused patients.
- One to 1.5% risk of red cell alloimmunization per unit transfused.
- Fifteen to 20% incidence in multitransfused patients.
- Most commonly Ab to Rh and Kell (K) Ag, less frequently Duffy (Fy) and Kidd (Jk) Ag.
- Rh-negative mothers who give birth to Rh-positive children have a 15–20% chance of developing anti-Rh Ab due to fetal-maternal hemorrhage.
- Anti-Rh_0 immune globulin is routinely given to Rh-negative mothers prenatally and perinatally to prevent Rh immunization.

Patients developing shortness of breath around the time of transfusion of blood products may have transfusion-related acute lung injury (TRALI); treatment is primarily supportive.

COMMON ED PRESENTATIONS OF CANCER COMPLICATIONS

Malignant Pericardial Effusions

- Seen with cancers of lung and breast, Hodgkin's and non-Hodgkin's lymphoma, leukemia, malignant melanoma, and postradiation pericarditis.
- Large effusions can → cardiac tamponade.

Syndrome of Inappropriate Antidiuretic Hormone Hypersecretion (SIADH)

- Most commonly associated with small cell carcinoma.
- Other cancers that can cause SIADH are brain, thymus, pancreas, duodenum, prostate, and lymphosarcoma.
- See Diagnostics chapter for description.

Adrenal Crisis

- Seen with malignant melanoma and cancers of breast, lung, and retroperitoneal organs.
- See Endocrine Emergencies chapter for description.

Neutropenic Fever

- Defined as fever and absolute granulocyte count < 500/mm^3.
- Patients are at great risk of developing overwhelming sepsis; 70% mortality if antibiotics delayed.
- Treated with hydration, broad-spectrum antibiotics, and reverse isolation. Start antibiotics immediately; do not wait for a source.
- Blood, urine, and sputum cultures as well as chest x-ray for diagnosis. Lumbar puncture only if change in mental status.

HIGH-YIELD FACTS

Hematologic and Oncologic Emergencies

A 53-year-old woman with 50-pack-year history of smoking presents with facial and upper extremity edema and distended neck veins. She states the symptoms are worse in the morning. She is afebrile and her vital signs are stable; her lungs reveal mild crackles bilaterally to auscultation. Her chest x-ray reveals bilateral pleural effusions. What should be done now?

Her symptoms suggest SVC syndrome. She should have the head of the bed elevated, receive steroids, and undergo a chest CT. She also needs to be monitored closely for any signs of airway obstruction.

DEFINITION

Acute or subacute obstruction of the SVC due to compression, infiltration, or thrombosis.

EPIDEMIOLOGY

- Usually from a malignant tumor (80%). Almost exclusively (95%) lung cancer and lymphoma.
- Presenting symptom of undiagnosed malignancy in 60% of cases.
- Nonmalignant causes are increasing because of use of invasive vascular devices (catheters, pacemaker wires). Thrombosis (most common), goiter, and aortic aneurysm are examples.

PHYSIOLOGY

- Blood flow: Internal jugular and subclavian veins → brachiocephalic (innominate) veins → SVC ← azygous vein ← bronchial veins.
- Blockade above the azygous vein manifests less severely, as chest wall collaterals allow bypass of the obstruction and because unobstructed drainage of the bronchial veins avoids many of the pulmonary problems.
- Due to lack of gravitational assistance with drainage, many symptoms are more severe in the recumbent position and in the morning after sleep.
- Slow-growing tumors allow more time for collateral development, and thus a less severe picture, than rapidly growing ones.

SIGNS AND SYMPTOMS

- Dyspnea (most common), facial swelling, head fullness.
- Distended neck or chest wall veins (67%), isolated upper extremity edema, particularly periorbital and facial (56%), pulmonary manifestations (40%) including tachypnea, cyanosis, crackles, rales.
- Less commonly, sequelae of ↑ intracranial pressure (ICP): Papilledema, cerebral edema, altered mental status, visual disturbances, headache, seizures, coma, cerebral hemorrhage, death.

DIAGNOSIS

- Chest x-ray: Mediastinal widening and pleural effusion most common. Mass apparent in only 10% of cases.

- Contrast-enhanced chest CT usually diagnostic—defines level of blockage and usually underlying mass/etiology.
- If mass detected, biopsy for definitive diagnosis.

TREATMENT

- Stridor with central airway obstruction or laryngeal edema and ↑ ICP are emergencies and require endovascular stenting +/– radiation.
- For most cases, treatment consists of elevating head of bed, steroids to ↓ any inflammatory component, and diuretics until tissue diagnosis is obtained.
- Removal of catheter if thrombotic etiology.
- Definitive treatment depends on etiology of obstruction (usually chemotherapy +/– radiation).

SPINAL CORD COMPRESSION

DEFINITION

Malignancy metastasizing to and destroying vertebral bodies and extending in the epidural space, causing thecal sac or cord impingement.

ETIOLOGY

- Most common malignancies: Prostate, breast, lung.
- Other causes: Renal cell cancer, lymphoma, myeloma, melanoma, vertebral subluxation, epidural hematomas, and intramedullary metastasis.

SIGNS AND SYMPTOMS

- Back pain is most common symptom (90%). Usually, it is localized to level of compression but later stages may have radicular quality.
- Weakness is often present (75%), usually in lower extremities.
- Loss of sensation is also common (60%). Saddle anesthesia is classic for cauda equina syndrome.
- Loss of bladder and bowel function (incontinence or retention) is a late finding.

DIAGNOSIS

- Diagnostic study of choice is magnetic resonance imaging (MRI). Imaging of entire thecal sac is important for prognostic reasons as well as to guide treatment decisions (surgery vs. radiation).
- Myelography can also be used. Positive myelogram shows dye obstruction at level of lesion.
- Plain films of spine have 10–15% false-negative rate and should not be relied upon for screening. Back pain and corresponding bone lesion on plain film in a cancer patient predicts 80% chance of cord compression.

TREATMENT

- Rapid treatment is essential as duration of symptoms is inversely proportional to chances of recovery. Pretreatment neurologic status is most important prognostic factor (ie, the best chance of walking out is for those who walk in).

The location of spinal cord compression mirrors the number vertebrae: 68% thoracic, 19% lumbosacral, and 15% cervical.

New back pain in a patient with a history of malignancy should be considered spinal cord compression until proven otherwise.

- Ideally, treatment is initiated at first sign of compression and before any signs or symptoms of neurologic compromise.
- High-dose steroids to control inflammation/edema.
- Oncology consult.
- Radiation for patients with multiple areas of compression, poor prognosis, or radiosensitive tumor (small cell lung cancer, myeloma).
- Surgery is superior for patients with single area of compression, radioresistant tumors (renal cell, melanoma, prostate cancer) or have mechanical cause such as a posterior protuberant bone from a pathologic fracture.

TUMOR LYSIS SYNDROME

DEFINITION

Acute life-threatening condition arising from massive release of lysed tumor cell cytosol and nucleic acids. Complications include renal failure and life-threatening electrolyte disturbances.

ETIOLOGY

- Usually occurs 1–5 days after instituting antineoplastic therapy (chemotherapy or radiation). Can occur spontaneously before treatment initiated.
- Likelihood of syndrome ↑ with tumor bulk (tumor >10 cm or WBCs > 50,000) and sensitivity to antineoplastic therapy.
- Generally low risk with solid tumors.
- Most common with hematologic malignancies: Acute leukemias, lymphomas (particularly Burkitt's).

DIAGNOSIS

Two or more serum abnormalities from the following:

- Hyperuricemia: Due to DNA breakdown and urate nephropathy.
- Hyperkalemia: Due to release of cytosol.
- Hyperphosphatemia: Due to protein breakdown and nephropathy due to precipitation of calcium phosphate crystals.
- Hypocalcemia: Due to hyperphosphatemia driving renal excretion of Ca^{2+}.

SIGNS AND SYMPTOMS

- Mostly due to electrolyte disturbances.
- Nausea, vomiting, diarrhea, anorexia, lethargy.
- Neuromuscular symptoms: Muscle cramps, tetany, convulsions.
- Cardiac: Dysrhythmias, heart failure, sudden death, syncope.
- CNS: Confusion, seizures.
- Renal: Uremia (due to protein breakdown), renal failure (due to urate and Ca^{2+} crystal deposition).

TREATMENT

- Aggressive hydration.
- Loop diuretics to wash out crystals if no oliguria or hypovolemia.
- Rasburicase/allopurinol to ↓ uric acid.
- Close monitoring and correction of electrolytes.
- Corrected hyperphosphatemia before replacing Ca^{2+} to prevent calcium-phosphate precipitation unless patient is severely symptomatic (tetany, cardiac dysrhythmia).
- May require nephrology consultation and dialysis.

Gynecologic Emergencies

Ovarian Cysts

TYPES

- Follicular cysts:
  - First 2 weeks of menstrual cycle (most common).
  - Pathologic when > 2.5 cm of diameter.
  - Pain secondary to stretching of capsule/rupture of cyst.
  - Usually regress spontaneously in 1–3 months.
  - Rarely associated with hemorrhage.
- Corpus luteum cysts:
  - Last 2 weeks of menstrual cycle (less common).
  - Pathologic when > 3 cm of diameter.
  - Bleeding into cyst cavity may cause stretching or rupture of capsule.
  - Usually regress at end of menstrual cycle.
  - Associated with significant degree of hemorrhage.
- Polycystic ovaries (PCO):
  - Endocrine disorder: Hyperandrogenism and anovulation.
  - Menses occur infrequently but are heavy and painful.
  - Ovarian cysts possibly secondary to chronic anovulation.
  - Long-term management is with oral contraceptives.

SIGNS AND SYMPTOMS

Cysts are usually asymptomatic unless complicated by rupture, torsion, or hemorrhage.

DIAGNOSIS

Ultrasound is useful for visualizing cysts and signs of rupture (free fluid in pelvis).

TREATMENT

- Supportive, pain medications.
- Complications are treated surgically.

Ovarian Torsion

DEFINITION

Twisting of the ovary on its stalk.

EPIDEMIOLOGY

Most common in the mid-20s (years old).

PATHOPHYSIOLOGY

- Venous drainage is occluded, but arterial supply remains patent due to double supply from ovarian and uterine arteries.
- Ovarian edema, hemorrhage, necrosis, and infarction may occur rapidly.

SIGNS AND SYMPTOMS

- Sudden onset of severe unilateral pelvic pain.
- More commonly associated with the presence of enlarged ovary (tumor, cyst, abscess, or hyperstimulated with fertility drugs).

PCO classic triad:
- Obesity
- Hirsutism
- Oligomenorrhea

HIGH-YIELD FACTS

Gynecologic Emergencies

- Patients often give history of similar pain that resolved spontaneously (twisting/untwisting).
- Unilateral adnexal tenderness on pelvic exam.

DIAGNOSIS

Doppler ultrasound reveals ↓ or absent flow to ovary and can demonstrate location of an adnexal mass. See Figure 11-1.

Adnexal torsion is a gynecologic emergency.

TREATMENT

- Laparotomy/laparoscopy usually successful early on.
- Advanced cases may require oophorectomy.

Ovarian Tumors

- Malignant tumors are less common than benign ones but have the highest mortality of all gynecologic malignancies.
- They usually present late in course with abdominal distention (secondary to massive ascites).

The most common ovarian tumor is a benign cystic teratoma (dermoid cyst).

VAGINAL DISORDERS

Bacterial Vaginosis

A 21-year-old sexually active woman who is 10 weeks pregnant presents with a 3-day history of a homogenous grayish-white malodorous discharge. pH of vaginal secretions is 5.5, and combining the secretions with 10% KOH yields a fishy odor. What organisms are most likely to cause this and how would you treat it? *(continued)*

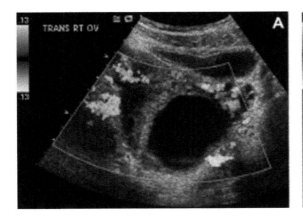
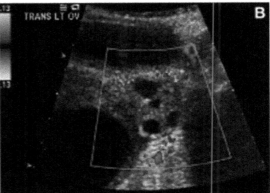

FIGURE 11-1. Sonogram of ovaries.

Panel A is an ultrasound Doppler depicting hypoechoic enlarged right ovary with a large cystic area and lack of vascular signal on Doppler, consistent with torsion. **Panel B** shows normal left-side ovary with normal vasculature. (Reproduced, with permission, from Stead L, Kaufman M, Stead SM, Bhagra A, Dajani N. *First Aid for Radiology.* New York: McGraw-Hill, 2008: Figure 5-11.)

The KOH test described is the "whiff" test, which is nonspecific, but yields a fishy odor if amines are present. This patient has bacterial vaginosis, which is caused by *Gardnerella vaginalis* most commonly. Other causative organisms may include *Bacteroides* non-*fragilis*, *Mobiluncus*, *Peptostreptococcus*, and *Mycoplasma hominis*. It is especially important in pregnancy to treat bacterial vaginosis, as untreated it can cause preterm labor. Treatment for first-trimester pregnancy consists of clindamycin 2% vaginal gel bid × 7 days or clindamycin 300 mg PO or 100 g intravaginally × 3 days.

If this patient were not pregnant, treatment would consist of metronidazole 500 mg PO bid × 7 days or metro vaginal gel 0.75% qd × 5 days. Treatment of sexual partners is not necessary unless balanitis is present. A woman's response to therapy and the likelihood of relapse or recurrence are not affected by treatment of sex partner.

Lactobacilli are abundant in yogurt. A Yoplait® (yogurt) a day keeps vaginitis away.

Bacterial vaginosis in pregnancy can cause preterm labor, so it should always be treated, even if the patient is asymptomatic.

DEFINITION

Most common vulvovaginitis.

ETIOLOGY

- Marked ↓ in numbers of lactobacilli are protective.
- Infection with organisms such as *Peptostreptococcus* species, *Bacteroides* species, and *Gardnerella vaginalis*.

SIGNS AND SYMPTOMS

Fishy-smelling itchy discharge.

DIAGNOSIS

- Via wet mount of vaginal smear.
- **Diagnostic criteria for bacterial vaginosis—AMSEL criteria:**
  - White, noninflammatory vaginal discharge (relative absence of white blood cells [WBCs])
  - Clue cells (epithelial cells coated by bacteria) on microscope (Figure 11-2)
  - pH > 4.5
  - "Whiff test" (fishy odor to discharge after adding KOH)

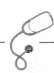

Warn patients against having *any* alcohol while on metronidazole (not even a teaspoonful of alcohol-containing mouthwash). It can cause a disulfiram-like reaction when coingested with alcohol, resulting in severe retching.

TREATMENT

- **First-line:**
  - Metronidazole 500 mg PO bid × 7 days
  - Metronidazole 0.75% gel intravaginally bid × 5 days
  - Clindamycin cream 2% 5 g intravaginally hs × 7 days
- **Alternatives:**
  - Single 2-g PO metronidazole (causes extreme nausea)
  - Clindamycin 300 mg PO bid × 7 days
  - Clindamycin ovules 100 g intravaginally hs × 3 days

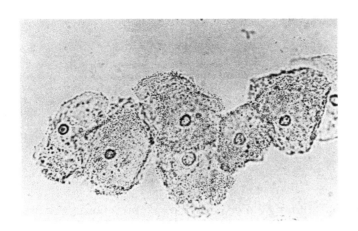

FIGURE 11-2. Clue cells in bacterial vaginosis.

(Reproduced, with permission, from Knoop K, Stack LB, Storrow AB. *Atlas of Emergency Medicine*. New York, NY: McGraw-Hill, 1997: 488.)

Candidiasis

A 47-year-old woman presents with vaginal and vulvar pruritus and dysuria. Physical exam reveals a white, curdy discharge and beefy red labia. Wet prep demonstrates pseudohyphae. pH is 4.0–5.0. Whiff test is negative. Patient is afebrile, and other vitals are stable. Urine is positive for glucose. What is patient's most likely diagnosis and how would you treat it?

This patient has candidiasis, most commonly caused by the fungus *Candida albicans*. Oral treatment consists of a single dose of fluconazole 150 mg or itraconzaole 200 mg by mouth. Several vaginal preparations can also be used, for 3–7 days' duration. The duration of treatment must be doubled during pregnancy. Treat male partners only if balanitis is present. If a woman has 4+ episodes per year, then she should be treated with a prophylactic regimen for 6 months.

DEFINITION

Most common fungal infection.

ETIOLOGY

Candida albicans.

RISK FACTORS

- Diabetes mellitus
- Stress
- Human immunodeficiency virus (HIV)
- Post antibiotic therapy
- Pregnancy
- Oral contraceptive therapy

SIGNS AND SYMPTOMS

- White "cottage cheese" discharge (pH < 4.5)
- Beefy red swollen labia
- Raised white adherent vaginal plaques
- Pruritus
- Dyspareunia, dysuria

DIAGNOSIS

Presence of pseudohyphae on 10% KOH prep (Figure 11-3).

TREATMENT

- Multiple antifungal preparations (oral and intravaginal) are available.
- Fluconazole 150 mg single dose—the only FDA-approved oral agent.

Contact Vulvovaginitis

DEFINITION

Vulvovaginitis caused by exposure to chemical irritant or allergen (douches, soaps, tampons, underwear, topical antibiotics).

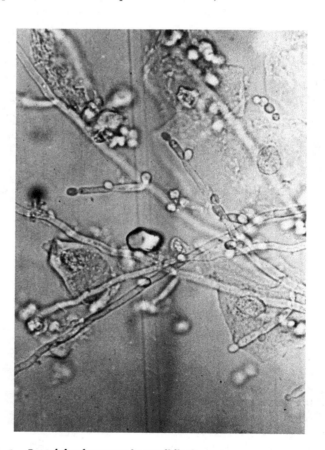

FIGURE 11-3. Pseudohyphae seen in candidiasis.

(Reproduced, with permission, from Pearlman MD, Tintinalli JE, eds. *Emergency Care of the Woman.* New York: McGraw-Hill, 1998: 544.)

SIGNS AND SYMPTOMS

- Erythema and edema of labia
- Clear watery discharge

TREATMENT

- Removal of offending substance
- Sitz baths for mild cases
- Topical steroids for severe cases

Atrophic Vaginitis

DEFINITION

↓ estrogen stimulation of vagina → mucosal atrophy.

ETIOLOGY

- Pregnancy and lactation
- Postmenopause

SIGNS AND SYMPTOMS

- Red, dry-appearing labial mucosa.
- Atrophic vagina is predisposed to ulceration and superinfection.
- Dyspareunia, vulvar discomfort.

TREATMENT

- Topical vaginal estrogen cream.
- Hormone replacement therapy for postmenopausal women.

Endometriosis

DEFINITION

Presence of endometrial glands/stroma outside the uterus that may affect ovaries, fallopian tubes, bladder, rectum, or appendix.

PATHOPHYSIOLOGY

Most commonly accepted hypothesis is "retrograde menstruation":

- During menses, uterus contracts against partially closed cervix.
- Menstrual flow passes retrograde into fallopian tubes and pelvic cavity.
- Ectopic endometrial tissue then responds to cyclic hormonal influence.

SIGNS AND SYMPTOMS

- Pain most often occurs just before and during menses—unilateral or bilateral and often recurrent.
- Classic triad of endometriosis: Dysmenorrhea, dyspareunia, dyschezia.

DIAGNOSIS

Suspected clinically, confirmed by direct visualization (laparoscopy).

Every woman who presents with abdominal/pelvic pain or vaginal bleeding should have a documented β-hCG test. All women are pregnant until proven otherwise.

TREATMENT

- Analgesia for acute episodes (nonsteroidal anti-inflammatory drugs [NSAIDs] or opiates)
- Hormonal therapy (suppress normal menstrual cycle) for long-term control
- Surgery for cases refractory to medical management

Dysfunctional Uterine Bleeding

TYPES AND CAUSES

- Ovulatory: Regular menstrual periods with intermenstrual bleeding: Causes include oral contraceptives, persistent corpus luteum, and uterine fibroids.
- Anovulatory: Chronic estrogen stimulation without cyclic progesterone:
  - Hyperstimulated endometrium thickens and sheds irregularly.
  - Most common during menarche and menopause.
  - ↑ risk of endometrial hyperplasia/adenocarcinoma.
- Miscellaneous: Carcinoma, polyps, condylomata, lacerations (trauma), retained foreign bodies, endometriosis, blood dyscrasias, anticoagulant use.

TREATMENT

- Treatment in the hemodynamically stable, nonpregnant patient is primarily supportive.
- Oral contraceptive pills (several regimens) will stop the bleeding and may be useful to "jump start" a regular cycle, although still anovulatory.
- Refer for gynecologic follow-up.

> Bleeding in postmenopausal women (over 6 months after cessation of menopause) may represent early signs of cervical or endometrial neoplasia and should be referred for urgent gynecologic follow-up.

> Warn patients that heavy withdrawal bleeding may follow cessation of oral contraceptive therapy.

CERVIX

Anatomy

- The cervix is the lowest portion of the uterus, composed primarily of collagen with 10% smooth muscle.
- Cervical dysplasia may occur secondary to infection, inflammation, or neoplasia.
- Abnormalities noted on speculum exam should be referred for gynecologic follow-up.

Cervicitis

DEFINITION

Inflammation of the cervix, most often due to infection.

ETIOLOGY

- *Neisseria gonorrhoeae*
- *Chlamydia trachomatis*
- *Trichomonas vaginalis*

RISK FACTORS

Unsafe sexual practices.

SIGNS AND SYMPTOMS

- Yellow mucopurulent discharge
- Dysuria
- Friable cervix

DIAGNOSIS

- Culture of discharge
- Wet mount to look for WBCs or motile trichomonads

TREATMENT

See Renal and Genitourinary Emergencies chapter for specific treatment regimens for gonorrhea, chlamydia, and trichomoniasis.

Due to the high rate of concurrent chlamydia and gonorrhea infection, treatment for both is given when either is suspected.

BARTHOLIN'S GLAND ABSCESS

PATHOPHYSIOLOGY

- Bartholin's (vestibular) gland lies at 5 and 7 o'clock positions of vestibule.
- Secretions normally provide lubrication during intercourse.
- Obstruction of gland → cyst formation, which may develop into abscess on secondary infection.

ETIOLOGY

Most common pathogens:

- Polymicrobial
- *Neisseria gonorrhoeae*
- *Chlamydia trachomatis*
- *Staphylococcus aureus*
- *Streptococcus faecalis*
- *Escherichia coli*
- Anaerobes
- Normal vaginal flora

TREATMENT

- Incision and drainage (usually under conscious sedation).
- Once the abscess cavity is drained, a balloon catheter is left in the cavity for continuous drainage while healing (6 weeks). The patient may engage in all activities including intercourse while it is in place.
- Antibiotics.
- Definitive surgical excision may be indicated for recurrent abscesses.
- Sitz bath.

There is a high rate of recurrence of Bartholin's abscess secondary to fistulous tract formation.

A 19-year-old sexually active woman presents with left lower crampy pelvic pain for 1 week. Physical exam reveals temperature of 38.3°C (101.0°F), cervical motion tenderness, and a mucopurulent vaginal discharge. Laboratory results reveal erythrocyte sedimentation rate (ESR) 65 and white blood cell count (WBC) 16. What is the diagnosis?

This patient has pelvic inflammatory disease (PID). The Centers for Disease Control and Prevention (CDC) diagnostic criteria for PID include:

- Lower abdominal pain
- Tenderness to pelvic exam
- Cervical motion and adnexal tenderness
- *Plus one or more of the following:*
  - Fever > 101 degrees
  - Abnormal vaginal/cervical discharge
  - Lab evidence of gonococci or *C trachomatis*
  - Elevated ESR or C-reactive protein

DEFINITION

PID is a leading cause of female infertility.

Spectrum of inflammatory disorders of the female upper genital tract, including any combination of endometritis, salpingitis, tubo-ovarian abscess, and pelvic peritonitis.

PATHOPHYSIOLOGY

Bacterial infection involving female upper reproductive tract cases are presumed to originate with a sexually transmitted disease of the lower genital tract, resulting in inflammation and scarring.

RISK FACTORS

The most accurate way to diagnose PID is via laparoscopy.

- Young age
- Previous PID
- Multiple sexual partners
- Intrauterine device use (risk is only in the first month after insertion)
- Douching
- Instrumentation of cervix
- Smoking

ETIOLOGY

- The most common pathogens are *N gonorrhoeae* and *C trachomatis*.
- Anaerobes, gram-negatives, and *Mycoplasma* are less common.

CLINICAL PRESENTATION

PID is a risk factor for infertility, chronic pelvic pain, and ectopic pregnancy.

- Can be subtle
- Adnexal/uterine tenderness
- Cervical motion tenderness
- Fever may be present
- Abnormal bleeding

DIAGNOSIS

- **Most common:**
  - Abnormal cervical or vaginal mucopurulent discharge.
  - Presence of WBC on saline microscopy of vaginal secretions (wet mount).
  - Laboratory documentation of cervical infection with *N gonorrhoeae* or *C trachomatis.*
- **Most specific criteria:**
  - Endometrial biopsy with histopathologic evidence of endometritis.
  - Transvaginal sonography or magnetic resonance imaging (MRI) techniques showing thickened, fluid-filled tubes with or without free pelvic fluid or tubo-ovarian complex.
  - Laparoscopic abnormalities consistent with PID.
- **Nonspecific:** Elevated ESR or C-reactive protein.

PID is uncommon in pregnancy due to the plug formed by the fusion of the chorion and decidua, providing an additional natural barrier to infection.

CDC GUIDELINES FOR INPATIENT ADMISSION

- Uncertain diagnosis
- Suspected tubo-ovarian abscess (TOA)
- Fever > 39.0°C (102.2°F)
- Failure of outpatient therapy
- Pregnancy
- First episode in a nulligravida
- Inability to tolerate PO intake
- Inability to follow up in 48 hours
- Immunosuppressed patient
- Other considerations for admission:
  - Pediatric patient
  - Presence of infected foreign body

TREATMENT

- **Inpatient therapy (parenteral):**
  - Cefotetan 2 g IV every 12 hours *or*
  - Cefoxitin 2 g IV every 6 hours *plus*
  - Doxycycline 100 mg orally or IV every 12 hours
- **Outpatient therapy:**
  - Ceftriaxone 250 mg IM in a single dose *plus*
  - Doxycycline 100 mg orally twice a day for 14 days *with or without*
  - Metronidazole 500 mg orally twice a day for 14 days

COMPLICATIONS

- TOA
- Fitz-Hugh–Curtis syndrome
- Septic abortion
- Intrauterine growth retardation
- Premature rupture of membranes
- Preterm delivery

The most common organism in TOA is *Bacteroides*.

TUBO-OVARIAN ABSCESS (TOA)

- Common and potentially fatal complication of PID.
- Intravenous antibiotics curative in 60–80% of cases.
- Surgical drainage or salpingectomy/oophorectomy in resistant cases.
- Ruptured TOA presents with shock and 15% mortality rate.

FITZ-HUGH–CURTIS SYNDROME

- "Perihepatitis" secondary to ascending gonorrhea/chlamydia infection (infection tracks up fallopian tubes into paracolic gutters).
- Mild elevations of liver function tests with symptoms of diaphragmatic irritation.
- "Violin string" adhesions are classic anatomic findings.
- Treatment with IV antibiotics (as for PID) is usually curative.

Obstetric Emergencies

Human Chorionic Gonadotropin (hCG)

- Presence of beta subunit of hCG is used as criteria for positive pregnancy test.
- Produced by trophoblastic tissue ~8–9 days after ovulation; may be detectable in the urine 1–2 days after implantation.
- Maintains corpus luteum (which maintains progesterone production).
- After 6–8 weeks, progesterone production shifts to placenta.

Human Placental Lactogen (hPL)

- Produced by placenta, ↑ throughout pregnancy.
- Antagonizes insulin → ↑ glucose levels.

Prolactin

- Rises in response to increasing maternal estrogen.
- Stimulates milk production.

Progesterone

- Produced by the ovaries (up to 8 weeks) and placenta (after 8 weeks).
- Prevents uterine contractions.

Estrogens

- Produced by both fetus and placenta.
- Limited role in monitoring course of pregnancy and fetal well-being.

Cortisol

- Both maternal and fetal adrenal production.
- Responsible for differentiation of type II alveoli → surfactant production.
- Antagonizes insulin → increased glucose levels.

Cardiovascular

- Plasma volume ↑ to ~150% of pregestational levels.
- ↑ in red blood cell (RBC) mass less than plasma volume → hemoglobin/hematocrit will drop slightly ("anemia of pregnancy").
- Heart rate and stroke volume both rise → ↑ cardiac output.
- Systolic blood pressure (BP)/diastolic BP/mean arterial pressure all decrease until 20 weeks, then rise again.
- Gravid uterus obstructs venous return from lower extremities.
- ↑ blood flow to kidneys (waste) and skin (heat).

Patients in second and third trimester of pregnancy may experience a significant drop in BP when lying down. This "supine hypotensive syndrome" is relieved by turning onto the left side, taking weight of the uterus off the vena cava.

313

Respiratory

- Functional residual capacity decreases due to effects of gravid uterus.
- ↑ tidal volume and minute ventilation.
- Hyperventilation leads to chronic respiratory alkalosis.

Renal

- Progesterone causes smooth muscle dilatation (ureters, bladder).
- Renal bicarbonate excretion compensates for respiratory alkalosis.
- Both renal plasma flow and glomerular filtration rate increase.
- Renin levels are elevated → ↑ angiotensin levels.

Metabolic

- By 10th week, ↑ insulin levels and anabolic activity.
- Insulin resistance and human placental lactogen (hPL)/cortisol activity → elevated glucose levels.

Endocrine

- Estrogen stimulates thyroxine-binding globulin → ↑ triiodothyronine (T_3)/thyroxine (T_4) levels.
- Both adrenocorticotropic hormone and cortisol levels ↑ after 3 months.

PRENATAL CARE

Routine Tests

- Blood tests (blood counts, type and screen, Rh factor, glucose screen)
- Syphilis, rubella, hepatitis B, human immunodeficiency virus (HIV)
- Serum alpha-fetoprotein (between 16 and 20 weeks)
- Ultrasonography (around 16–20 weeks)
- Cervical cultures for gonorrhea, chlamydia, group B strep, and cytology

With sudden weight gain in the third trimester, consider preeclampsia.

Monitoring

- Weight gain (26–28 pounds is average).
- Urinalysis (glucose, protein).
- BP.
- Fundal height:
  - Barely palpable at ~12 weeks.
  - Top of uterus is halfway between pubic symphysis and umbilicus at 16 weeks.
  - Top of uterus at umbilicus ~20–22 weeks.
  - Centimeters above pubic symphysis approximates age of fetus after ~20 weeks.
- Fetal assessment: Attitude, lie, presentation, position.
- Nonstress test (NST): Assess for fetal heart rate accelerations in response to movement.
- Amniotic fluid index (AFI): Assess for oligohydramnios (AFI < 5 cm).

Asymptomatic bacteriuria in the pregnant woman is treated with antibiotics (eg, nitrofurantoin).

- Reactive NST and adequate AFI with normal fetal movement constitutes a normal biophysical profile.

Ectopic Pregnancy (EP)

A 30-year-old woman presents to the emergency department (ED) with a 3-day history of abdominal pain and spotting. Her last menstrual period was 4.5 weeks prior. Pelvic examination revealed a closed os and was otherwise unremarkable. She is afebrile, with a pulse of 110 bpm. The human chorionic gonadotropin (β-hCG) value is 1,283 mIU/mL. What is the next step in the management of this patient?

Ectopic pregnancy needs to be ruled out in this patient. An EP is a potentially life-threatening emergency. This diagnosis should be considered in any pregnant patient who presents within the first trimester with abdominal pain or vaginal bleeding. Transvaginal ultrasongraphy (US) is an excellent diagnostic tool and, if patient is not unstable, should be the next step in this case. The threshold for detecting an intrauterine pregnancy (IUP) on transvaginal US is a value of ~1,000 mIU/mL, or 4–6 weeks' gestation. The presence of an echogenic adnexal mass, an empty uterus, and free fluid in the pelvis are suggestive of an EP. If cardiac activity is identified outside the uterus, then the diagnosis of EP is confirmed. Treatment consists of hemodynamic stabilization, $Rh_O(D)$ immune globulin for Rh-negative women, and treatment of the ectopic mass either surgically (preferred) or medically with methotrexate. Methotrexate is not a universally available option. It is generally reserved for the hemodynamically stable patient with an ectopic size < 3.5–4.0 cm and no sonographic evidence of rupture. Success rate is approximately 85%.

EPIDEMIOLOGY

- Leading cause of pregnancy-related death in the first trimester.
- Third leading cause of all maternal mortality.
- ~6 % mortality rate.

PATHOPHYSIOLOGY

- Zygote implants outside uterus (95% in fallopian tubes).
- Aborts when vascular supply to abnormal placenta disrupted, but may rupture as well.

RISK FACTORS

Risk: **APPRAISE IT!**
- **A**ge
- **P**revious EP
- **P**elvic inflammatory disease (PID)
- **R**ace
- **A**IDS and other sexually transmitted diseases (STDs)
- **I**ntrauterine device (IUD)
- **S**moking

- Elective abortion
- Infertility treatment
- Tubal surgery or scarring

SIGNS AND SYMPTOMS

- Classic triad:
    - Abdominal pain
    - Vaginal bleeding
    - Amenorrhea
- Spectrum anywhere from asymptomatic up to hemorrhagic shock.

DIAGNOSIS

- β-hCG:
    - Sensitivity of pregnancy tests: Urine positive > 20 mIU/mL.
    - Serum normal pregnancy: β-hCG ↑ by at least 66% for the first 6–7 weeks from day 9. If it does not, suspect ectopic pregnancy.
- **Progesterone in the presence of classic triad:**
    - < 5 ng/mL highly suggestive of EP.
    - > 25 ng/mL highly suggestive of IUP.
- **Ultrasound:**
    - Used to establish presence or absence of IUP (Figure 12-1).
    - Imaging findings associated with EP (Figure 12-2):
        - Presence of an echogenic adnexal mass
        - Empty uterus
        - Free fluid in the pelvis
        - Cardiac activity outside the uterus confirms diagnosis
- Can usually visualize IUP (gestational sac) by transvaginal sonogram at β-hCG > 1,000 (approximately 5 weeks) and by transabdominal sonogram at 5,000 (discriminatory threshold).
- Incidence of coexisting EP/IUP (heterotopic) is 1/4,000, but ↑ to 1/100 in women on fertility drugs.

TREATMENT

- Medical management: Methotrexate for termination.
- Surgery for hemodynamic instability or if medical management not feasible.
- Rh-immune globulin for Rh-negative women.

β-hCG level doubles approximately every 2–3 days in normal early pregnancy.

Transvaginal IUP sono findings:
- Gestational sac: ~1,000
- Yolk sac: ~2,500
- Heart tones: ~10,500–17,000

HIGH-YIELD FACTS

Obstetric Emergencies

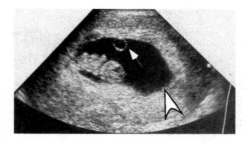

FIGURE 12-1. Intrauterine pregnancy.

Arrowhead shows gestational sac; small arrow shows yolk sac.

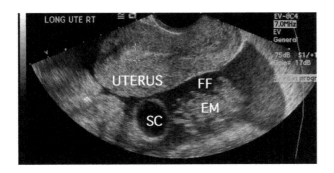

FIGURE 12-2. Transvaginal sonogram demonstrating an ectopic pregnancy.

Note the large amount of free fluid (FF) in the pelvis. No intrauterine pregnancy was seen. A large complex echogenic mass (EM) was seen in the left adnexa, consistent with an ectopic pregnancy. A simple cyst (SC) is also seen in the right adnexa. The area within the uterus represents a small fibroid.

Hyperemesis Gravidarum

DEFINITION

- Syndrome of intractable nausea and vomiting in a pregnant woman.
- Usually occurs early in pregnancy and resolves by end of first trimester.

TREATMENT

- Fluid and electrolyte abnormalities are common and should be replaced as indicated.
- Metoclopramide and ondansetron are both class B in pregnancy.

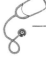

Eating small frequent meals and things such as toast and crackers may help ease the nausea and vomiting and keep some food down.

Rhesus (Rh) Isoimmunization

DEFINITION

Immunologic disorder that affects Rh-negative mothers of Rh-positive fetuses.

PATHOPHYSIOLOGY

- Occurs with maternal exposure to fetal Rh-positive blood cells in the setting of transplacental hemorrhage (typically occurs during delivery, may also occur with abortions and trauma).
- Initial exposure leads to primary sensitization with production of immunoglobulin M antibodies.
- In subsequent pregnancies, maternal immunoglobulin G antibody crosses placenta and attacks Rh-positive fetal RBCs.

Rh immunoprophylaxis should be considered for all pregnant patients who sustain any abdominal trauma regardless of the amount of vaginal bleeding.

PREVENTION

- Prevention of Rh isoimmunization is by administering Rh_o immune globulin (RhoGAM) to mothers during time of potential antigen exposure (amniocentesis, threatened abortion, trauma, delivery, etc).
- RhoGAM is also administered prophylactically to all Rh-negative mothers ~28 weeks' gestation.

The Kleihauer-Betke test allows quantification of the amount of maternal–fetal blood mixing.

First-trimester vaginal bleeding occurs in approximately 25% of all pregnancies, one half of which will eventually result in miscarriage.

Threatened Abortion

DEFINITION

Abdominal pain or vaginal bleeding in first 20 weeks' gestation.

SIGNS AND SYMPTOMS

- Closed cervix
- No passage of fetal tissue by history or exam

DIAGNOSIS

β-hCG and ultrasound to confirm IUP and rule out EP.

TREATMENT

- Bed rest for 24 hours.
- Avoid intercourse, tampons, and douching until bleeding stops.
- Arrange outpatient follow-up for repeat β-hCG/sonogram in 24–48 hours.
- Rh isoimmunization prophylaxis as needed.

Inevitable Abortion

DEFINITION

Vaginal bleeding with open cervical os but no passage of fetal products.

TREATMENT

- Dilation and curettage (D&C, evacuation of pregnancy).
- Rh isoimmunization as needed.

Incomplete Abortion

DEFINITION

Incomplete passage of fetal products, usually between 6 and 14 weeks of gestation.

SIGNS AND SYMPTOMS

- Open cervical os
- Pain and bleeding

TREATMENT

- D&C
- Rh isoimmunization prophylaxis as needed

Complete Abortion

DEFINITION

Complete passage of fetal products and placenta before 20 weeks of gestation.

- Closed cervical os.
- Uterus contracts.
- Pregnancy-induced changes begin to resolve.

TREATMENT

- Supportive management with outpatient follow-up for ultrasound-confirmed complete abortion.
- D&C if unsure all products have been passed.
- Rh isoimmunization prophylaxis as needed.

Septic Abortion

DEFINITION

Uterine infection during any stage of an abortion.

CAUSES

Bowel and genital flora are most often implicated.

SIGNS AND SYMPTOMS

- Fever
- Bleeding
- Cramping pain
- Purulent discharge from cervix
- Boggy, tender, enlarged uterus

TREATMENT

- Prompt evacuation
- Broad-spectrum antibiotics
- Rh isoimmunization prophylaxis as needed

Embryonic Demise (Missed Abortion)

DEFINITION

Embryo larger than 5 mm without cardiac activity.

SIGNS AND SYMPTOMS

May progress to spontaneous abortion with expulsion of products.

TREATMENT

- D&C
- Rh isoimmunization prophylaxis as needed
- Complications may occur secondary to infection or coagulopathy

HIGH-YIELD FACTS

Obstetric Emergencies

Abruptio Placentae

DEFINITION

Premature separation of normally implanted placenta from uterine wall (usually third trimester).

RISK FACTORS

- Previous abruptio placentae
- Abdominal trauma
- Hypertension
- Cocaine use
- Smoking
- Multiparity
- Advanced maternal age

Hypertension is the most common risk factor for abruptio placentae.

SIGNS AND SYMPTOMS

- Vaginal bleeding with dark clots.
- Abdominal pain.
- Uterine pain/irritability.
- Uterus may be soft or very hard.

DIAGNOSIS

- Ultrasound is not reliable in the diagnosis of abruptio placentae.
- Fetal heart monitoring for signs of fetal distress.

TREATMENT

- Emergent obstetrical consultation for maternal/fetal monitoring and possible delivery.
- Rh isoimmunization prophylaxis as needed.

COMPLICATIONS

- Fetal distress
- Diffuse intravascular coagulation
- Amniotic fluid embolism
- Maternal/fetal death

Placenta Previa

DEFINITION

Implantation of placenta overlying internal cervical os.

RISK FACTORS

- Previous placenta previa
- Prior C-section
- Multiple gestations
- Multiple induced abortions
- Advanced maternal age

HIGH-YIELD FACTS

Obstetric Emergencies

SIGNS AND SYMPTOMS

- Painless vaginal bleeding
- Soft, nontender uterus

DIAGNOSIS

Ultrasonography will confirm placental location.

TREATMENT

- Pelvic/cervical exam is *not* performed in the emergency department (ED), as this can precipitate massive bleeding. It is done in the operating room (OR) where emergency C-section can be performed if massive bleeding does occur.
- Emergent obstetrical consultation for maternal/fetal monitoring and possible delivery.
- Rh isoimmunization prophylaxis as needed.

Do not perform bimanual pelvic exam on patient with late pregnancy vaginal bleeding until placenta previa is ruled out.

PREGNANCY-INDUCED HYPERTENSION

Defined as BP > 140/90 mm Hg, increase in systolic BP > 20 mm Hg, or ↑ in diastolic BP > 10 mm Hg.

Preeclampsia and Eclampsia

A 42-year-old woman arrives at the ED seizing. The patient's friend states that she delivered a baby boy 8 days ago at an outside hospital. Her friend also states she has no history of seizures or overdose. Her BP is 192/125 mm Hg. Her urine dipstick shows 1+ protein. What is the drug of choice for this patient's seizures?

Given that the patient is 8 days postpartum with no prior seizure history, this patient must be presumed to have eclampsia. Twenty-five percent of seizures associated with eclampsia occur up to 10 days postpartum. Immediate treatment with IV magnesium would be appropriate to terminate the seizure. Other resuscitative measures such as correcting hypoxia and hypoglycemia must occur concurrently.

Seizures in eclampsia:
- 25% are before labor
- 50% are during labor
- 25% are up to 10 days postpartum

DEFINITIONS

- Preeclampsia is a syndrome of hypertension, proteinuria, and generalized edema that occurs in weeks 20–24 of pregnancy.
- Eclampsia is preeclampsia plus seizures.

RISK FACTORS

- Primigravida
- Very young or advanced maternal age
- History of hypertension or kidney disease
- Diabetes mellitus

Morbidity and Mortality Associated with Eclampsia

Mother:
- Intracranial hemorrhage
- Acute renal failure
- HELLP syndrome
- Hepatic encephalopathy
- Pulmonary edema

Fetus:
- Intrauterine growth restriction
- Placental abruption
- Oligohydramnios

HELLP syndrome complicates ~10% of preeclampsia: **H**emolysis, **E**levated **L**iver enzymes, **L**ow **P**latelets

Rapid BP reduction in preeclamsia/eclampsia may decrease uterine blood flow and → fetal distress.

Magnesium for eclampsia:
- Terminates seizure
- Prevents recurrence of seizures
- ↓ risk of placental absorption
- Associated with fewer NICU admissions
- Drug of choice—better than phenytoin or placebo

Signs of magnesium toxicity:
- Hyporeflexia or loss of deep tendon reflexes
- Respiratory depression
- Bradydysrhythmias

- Hydatidiform mole
- Multiple gestations
- Family history of pregnancy-induced hypertension
- Obesity

ETIOLOGY

The cause is unknown but might be due to ↓ in uteroplacental blood flow.

SIGNS AND SYMPTOMS

- Weight gain > 5 lbs/week
- Headache, visual disturbances
- Peripheral edema
- Pulmonary edema
- Oliguria
- Abdominal pain

DIAGNOSIS

- **Diagnostic triad:**
  - Hypertension as defined above
  - Proteinuria > 300 mg/24 hours (corresponds to 1+ protein on urine dipstick)
  - Generalized edema (recently, edema has been eliminated as a diagnostic criterion, as many pregnant women have edema as part of their pregnancy without ever developing preeclampsia).
- **Laboratory findings:**
  - Elevated uric acid, serum creatinine, liver function tests, and bilirubin
  - Thrombocytopenia

TREATMENT

- Absolute bed rest.
- Left lateral decubitus position to ↑ blood flow to uterus.
- Hydralazine for BP control (labetalol for refractory cases).
- Magnesium sulfate for seizure and secondary BP control (phenytoin or diazepam for refractory cases). Watch for signs of magnesium toxicity.
- Maintain urine output at 30 mm Hg, as many of the drugs used are cleared through the kidney.
- Definitive treatment is delivery of the fetus.

HYDATIDIFORM MOLE

A 17-year-old girl who is 11 weeks pregnant by dates presents with severe vomiting. Her BP is 190/120 mm Hg. Her fundal height is at the umbilicus. Sonogram reveals echogenic material in the uterus, but no gestational sac or fetal heartbeat is present. What diagnosis are you suspicious for?

This patient's fundal height at the umbilicus would suggest 20 weeks of gestation but she is only 11 weeks. Also, the lack of gestational sac or fetal heartbeat is not consistent with an 11-week pregnancy either (should be seen earlier, around 6 weeks). This patient is also hypertensive, suggesting preeclampsia. Together, these features suggest a diagnosis of hydatiform mole, which is treated by D&C.

DEFINITION

- "Molar pregnancy" secondary to overproduction of chorionic villi
- Partial mole: Triploid (two sets paternal, one maternal), presence of fetal parts, higher tendency to progress to choriocarcinoma
- Complete mole: Diploid (two sets maternal), absence of fetal parts

RISK FACTORS

- Previous history of molar pregnancy.
- Very young or advanced maternal age.

SIGNS AND SYMPTOMS

- Severe nausea and vomiting
- Uterus larger than expected for dates
- Passage of grapelike clusters of vesicles through vagina
- Intermittent vaginal bleeding during early pregnancy
- Preeclampsia before 20 weeks' gestation

DIAGNOSIS

- Anemia
- β-hCG higher than expected
- Ultrasonography:
  - Complete mole: Complex, echogenic intrauterine mass containing many small cystic spaces "snowstorm appearance." Fetal tissues and amnionic sac are absent (Figure 12-3).
  - Partial mole: Thickened, hydropic placenta with a concomitant fetus.

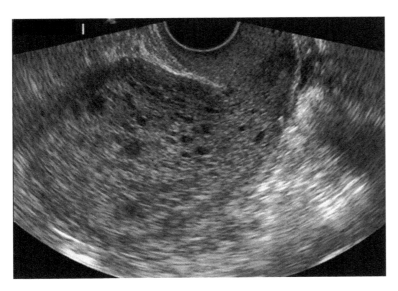

FIGURE 12-3. Sonogram of a complete hydatidiform mole.

The classic "snowstorm" appearance is created by the multiple placental vesicles, which completely fill this uterine cavity. (Reproduced, with permission, from Schorge JO, Schaffer JL, Halvorson LM, Hoffman BL, Bradshaw DKD, Cunnigham FG. *Williams Gynecology*; http://accessmedicine.com. Copyright © McGraw-Hill Companies, Inc.)

TREATMENT

- D&C
- Follow-up to monitor for choriocarcinoma

NORMAL LABOR AND DELIVERY

- Progressive cervical effacement and/or dilatation in the presence of uterine contractions occurring < 5 minutes apart and lasting 30–60 seconds at a time (Table 12-1).
- "False" labor—during last 4–8 weeks of pregnancy, contractions (Braxton Hicks) occur in the absence of cervical dilatation or effacement.

First Stage

- Starts with onset of labor, ends with complete dilatation (10 cm) of cervix.
- "Latent" phase—effacement with minimal dilatation.
- "Active" phase—accelerated rate of cervical dilatation.

Second Stage

- Starts with complete cervical dilatation, ends with delivery of baby.
- Six cardinal movements of labor: Descent, flexion, internal rotation, extension, external rotation, expulsion.

Third Stage

- Starts with delivery of baby, ends with delivery of placenta.
- Assess external genitalia for signs of perineal/rectal tears.

Fourth Stage

- Starts with delivery of placenta, ends with stabilization of mother.
- Monitor for hemodynamic instability and postpartum hemorrhage.

TABLE 12-1. Duration of the Stages of Labor

	PRIMIPAROUS	MULTIPAROUS
First stage	6–18 hours	2–10 hours
Cervical dilatation (active phase)	1.0 cm/h	1.2 cm/h
Second stage	0.5–3.0 hours	5–20 minutes
Third stage	0–30 minutes	0–30 minutes
Fourth stage	~1 hour	~1 hour

Premature Rupture of Membranes (PROM)

DEFINITION

Rupture of fetal membranes before labor begins.

SIGNS AND SYMPTOMS

Leakage of amniotic fluid prior to onset of labor at any stage of gestation.

DIAGNOSIS

- Pooling of amniotic fluid in vaginal fornix.
- Nitrazine paper test: Turns blue in presence of amniotic fluid (false positive seen with use of lubricant).
- Ferning pattern on microscopic paper (false negative seen with blood) (Figure 12-4).

TREATMENT

- If fetus > 37 weeks, delivery within 24 hours.
- If fetus < 37 weeks, timing of delivery is weighed against risks of fetal immaturity.

Preterm Labor

DEFINITION

Defined as labor occurring after 20 weeks' and before 37 weeks' gestation.

Patients with PROM are at risk for chorioamnionitis.

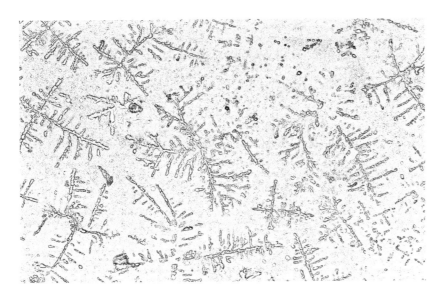

FIGURE 12-4. "Ferning" pattern of amniotic fluid when exposed to air.

Can be useful for diagnosing PROM. Photo contributed by Robert Buckley, MD. (Reproduced, with permission, from Knoop KJ, Stack LB, Storrow AB, Thurman RJ. *The Atlas of Emergency Medicine*, 3rd ed. New York: McGraw-Hill, 2010: 848.)

HIGH-YIELD FACTS

Obstetric Emergencies

DIAGNOSIS

Diagnosed by regular uterine contractions in the presence of cervical dilatation/effacement.

RISK FACTORS

- PROM
- Abruptio placentae
- Multiple gestation
- Drug use
- Polyhydramnios
- Incompetent cervix
- Infection (including STDs)

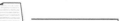
TREATMENT

- Hydration and bed rest (successful in ~20% cases).
- Glucocorticoids (betamethasone) to accelerate fetal lung maturity.
- Tocolysis with magnesium sulfate, beta blockers (terbutaline, ritodrine), and prostaglandin synthetase inhibitors (indomethacin).
- Contraindications to tocolysis:
  - Severe preeclampsia
  - Severe bleeding from placenta previa or abruptio placentae
  - Chorioamnionitis

Strategies for Assessing Potential Fetal Distress

1. Assess for short-term (beat-to-beat) and long-term variability of fetal heart rate (normal).
2. Assess for response of fetal heart rate to uterine contractions:
   - Accelerations are a normal response to uterine contractions.
   - Early decelerations are usually related to head compression (normal).
   - Variable decelerations may be related to intermittent cord compression.
   - Late decelerations are often related to uteroplacental insufficiency.
3. Fetal tachycardia may be a sign of maternal fever or intrauterine infections.
4. Presence of "heavy" meconium in amniotic fluid ↑ risk of aspiration.

POSTPARTUM COMPLICATIONS

Postpartum Hemorrhage

DEFINITION

- Classified as early (within 24 hours of delivery) or late (up to 1–2 weeks postpartum)
- > 500 mL blood loss (vaginal delivery) or 1,000 mL (cesarean delivery)

CAUSES OF EARLY POSTPARTUM HEMORRHAGE

- **Uterine atony:** Most common cause (overdistended uterus, prolonged labor, oxytocin use).
- **Genital tract trauma:** Vaginal or rectal lacerations.

- **Abnormal placental attachment:** Placenta accreta, results in bleeding at time of placental delivery.
- **Retained products of conception:** Acts as a wedge preventing uterine contractions, → ↑ bleeding.
- **Uterine inversion:** Uterus turns inside out, → vasodilatation and ↑ bleeding.

CAUSES OF LATE POSTPARTUM HEMORRHAGE

- Endometritis
- Retained products of conception

SIGNS AND SYMPTOMS

- Vaginal bleeding
- Soft, atonic uterus

TREATMENT

- Repair any lacerations.
- Manually remove placenta if it does not pass.
- Bimanual massage and/or intravenous oxytocin to stimulate uterine contractions.
- Methylergonovine for refractory cases.

Endometritis

DEFINITION

Infection of the endometrium.

CAUSES

Majority of infections are caused by normal vaginal/cervical flora (enterococci, streptococci, anaerobes).

SIGNS AND SYMPTOMS

- Fever
- Tender, swollen uterus
- Foul-smelling lochia

DIFFERENTIAL DIAGNOSIS

In patients who do not respond to antibiotic therapy, consider:

- Pelvic abscess (requires surgical drainage) *or*
- Pelvic thrombophlebitis (requires anticoagulation)

TREATMENT

- Broad-spectrum antibiotics
- Hospitalization

HIGH-YIELD FACTS

Obstetric Emergencies

Musculoskeletal Emergencies

DEFINITIONS

- Sprain:
  - A partial or complete rupture of the fibers of a ligament.
  - First degree: Joint is stable; integrity of the ligament is maintained with a few fibers torn.
  - Second degree: Joint stability is maintained but ligamentous function is ↓.
  - Third degree: Joint instability with complete tearing of ligament.
- Strain:
  - A partial or complete rupture of the fibers of the muscle-tendon junction.
  - First degree: Mild.
  - Second degree: Moderate, associated with a weakened muscle.
  - Third degree: Complete tear of the muscle-tendon junction with severe pain and inability to contract the involved muscle.

ETIOLOGY

Trauma: Indirect or direct, causing the ligaments of any joint to stretch beyond their elastic limit.

SIGNS AND SYMPTOMS

- Pain and swelling over area involved.
- Patient may have experienced a snap or pop at time of injury.

TREATMENT

- **For first- and most second-degree sprains:**
  - Rest, ice, compression, and elevation ("RICE" therapy) for 24–36 hours.
  - Weight bearing as tolerated in the case of lower extremity sprain.
  - Early ambulation associated with ↓ healing time.
  - Air cast or wrap can be used for support.
  - Crutches only if unable to ambulate.
  - Orthopedic follow-up is generally not necessary.
  - Analgesia (eg, ibuprofen—to be taken with food to ↓ gastric irritation).
- **For third-degree sprains:**
  - Splint that prevents range of motion (ROM) of joint.
  - Crutches: Provide non-weight-bearing status in lower extremity injuries.
  - RICE and pain medications.
  - Orthopedic follow-up for appropriate treatment, which may include operative repair in the young.

RICE therapy:
Rest (although return to activity as soon as pain allows)
Ice
Compression (splint)
Elevation

Herpetic Whitlow

DEFINITION

Painful infection of the terminal phalanx.

ETIOLOGY

- Initiated by viral inoculation.
- Sixty percent of cases are herpes simplex virus type 1 (HSV-1); 40% are HSV-2.
- Incubation period is 2–20 days.

SIGNS AND SYMPTOMS

- Prodrome of fever and malaise.
- Initial pain and burning or tingling of the infected digit, followed by erythema, edema, and the development of 1- to 3-mm grouped vesicles on an erythematous base over the next 7–10 days.
- Complete resolution occurs over subsequent 5–7 days.
- Recurrences observed in 20–50% of cases are usually milder and shorter in duration.

DIAGNOSIS

- Primarily clinical diagnosis
- Laboratory tests (not usually required):
  - Tzanck test.
  - Viral culture of aspirated vesicle (requires 24–48 hours).
  - Serum antibody titers.

TREATMENT

- Self-limited disease.
- Symptomatic relief.
- Acyclovir may be beneficial and may prevent recurrrence.
- Use antibiotic in bacterial superinfection.
- Incision is contraindicated.

Felon

DEFINITION

Infection of the pulp space of any of the distal phalanges (Figure 13-1).

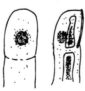

FIGURE 13-1. Felon (infection of pulp space).

(Reproduced, with permission, from DeGowin RL, Brown DD. *DeGowin's Diagnostic Examination*, 7th ed. New York: McGraw-Hill, 2000: 703.)

ETIOLOGY

Caused by minor trauma to the dermis over the finger pad.

COMPLICATIONS

Results in ↑ pressure within the septal compartments and may → cellulitis, flexor tendon sheath infection, or osteomyelitis if not effectively treated.

TREATMENT

- Using a digital block, perform incision and drainage with longitudinal incision over the area of greatest induration but not over the flexor crease of the distal interphalangeal (DIP).
- A drain may be placed and the wound checked in 2 days.
- Seven- to 10-day course of antibiotics: Usually first-generation cephalosporin or anti-*Staphylococcus* penicillin.

Paronychia

DEFINITION

Infection of the lateral nail fold (Figure 13-2).

ETIOLOGY

Caused by minor trauma such as nail biting or manicure.

TREATMENT

- Without fluctuance, this may be treated with a 7-day course of antibiotics, warm soaks, and retraction of the skin edges from the nail margin.
- For more extensive infections, an 18-gauge needle or scalpel can be used to gently lift and unroll (not cut) the skin at the base of the nail and at the lateral nail. This is relatively painless and will allow drainage of purulent material. A digital block and incision are rarely needed.
- Pus below the nailbed may require partial or total removal of the nail.
- Advise patient to do warm soaks and return for wound check in 2 days.
- Antibiotics may not be necessary unless area is cellulitic.

Flexor Tenosynovitis

DEFINITION

- This is a surgical emergency requiring prompt identification.
- Infection of the flexor tendon and sheath is caused by penetrating trauma and dirty wounds (ie, dog bite).

FIGURE 13-2. Paronychia.

(Reproduced, with permission, from DeGowin RL, Brown DD. *DeGowin's Diagnostic Examination*, 7th ed. New York: McGraw-Hill, 2000: 703.)

■ Infection spreads along the tendon sheath, allowing involvement of other digits and even the entire hand, causing significant disability.

ETIOLOGY

■ Polymicrobial.
■ *Staphylococcus* most common.
■ *Neisseria gonorrhoeae* with history of sexually transmitted disease.

SIGNS AND SYMPTOMS

Kanavel criteria:

■ Digit is flexed at rest.
■ Passive extension produces pain.
■ Symmetrical swelling of finger.
■ Tenderness over flexor tendon sheath.

TREATMENT

■ Immobilize and elevate hand.
■ Immediate consultation with hand surgeon.
■ Intravenous (IV) antibiotics.

Cellulitis

A 17-year-old high school wrestler returns to the emergency department (ED) with worsening cellulitis over his left thigh. Two days ago he was seen in the ED and started on a 10-day course of cephalexin which he states he has been taking as prescribed. He is well in appearance and not febrile. There is no evidence of abscess, but there is a small amount of purulent drainage and the area of erythema and warmth has ↑ in size since you saw him 2 days ago. Why is he not responding to the antibiotic and what is the next step in his management?

The most likely explanation for his lack of response to the current therapy is that he has an infection with methicillin-resistant *Staphylococcus aureus* (MRSA). Further history reveals that other members of his wrestling team have also had skin infections recently. He should be transitioned to an antibiotic with coverage against MRSA, such as clindamycin or trimethoprim-sulfamethoxazole (TMP-SMX). If he required admission, IV vancomycin would be a good choice.

DEFINITION

A local erythematous inflammatory reaction of the subcutaneous tissue following a cutaneous breach, which → infection.

ETIOLOGY

■ *Streptococcus pyogenes* (most common)
■ *Staphylococcus*
■ *Haemophilus influenzae* in unimmunized individuals
■ Enterobacteriaceae in diabetics
■ Methicillin-resistant *S aureus* (MRSA)

Kanavel criteria for tenosynovitis—STEP
Symmetrical swelling of finger
Tenderness over flexor tendon sheath
Extension (passive) of digit is painful
Posture of digit at rest is flexed

SIGNS AND SYMPTOMS

- Localized tenderness and swelling
- Warmth
- Erythema
- If immunocompromised, may see fever and leukocytosis

TREATMENT

- For uncomplicated cellulitis in healthy individuals, cephalexin or dicloxacillin 500 mg qid × 10 days or azithromycin 500 mg × 1, then 250 mg qd × 4 days.
- IV antibiotics for head and face involvement and the immunocompromised: Cefazolin 1 g IV qid and nafcillin or oxacillin 2 g IV q4h. Ceftriaxone or imipenem for severe cases.
- MRSA infections:
  - TMP-SMX or clindamycin for outpatient therapy
  - Vancomycin if IV needed
- Antibiotic resistance patterns vary based on region and change frequently. Always consult an up-to-date source for current antibiotic recommendations.

Gas Gangrene

ETIOLOGY

A life- and limb-threatening soft-tissue infection caused by one of the spore-forming *Clostridium* spp., resulting in myonecrosis, gas production, and sepsis.

- *Clostridium perfringens* (80–90%).
- *Clostridium septicum.*
- These are spore-forming gram-positive anaerobic bacilli found in soil, gastrointestinal tract, and female genitourinary tract.

PATHOPHYSIOLOGY

- Dirty wounds with jagged edges become infected with the ubiquitous organism that produces exotoxins.
- These cause systemic toxicity and cellular destruction.
- Bacteremia is rare.

SIGNS AND SYMPTOMS

- Three-day incubation period.
- Patient complains of **pain out of proportion** to physical findings.
- Limb feels heavy.
- Skin becomes discolored (brown).
- Crepitance.
- Fever.
- Tachycardia.
- Diabetics are particularly susceptible due to immunocompromise (impaired white blood cell [WBC] chemotaxis), peripheral neuropathy (delaying detection of small wounds), and impaired peripheral perfusion.

Features of gas gangrene —
CLOSTRIDiuM P
Clostridium spp./**C**repitance of skin
Leukocytosis
COagulopathy
Spore-forming gram-positive anaerobic bacilli, found in soil
Thrombocytopenia/ **T**achycardia
Radiograph shows gas in soft tissue
Irritability
Discoloration of skin
Myoglobinemia
Painful

DIAGNOSIS

- Metabolic acidosis
- Leukocytosis
- Myoglobinuria, myoglobinemia
- Coagulopathy
- Elevated creatine phosphokinase (CPK)
- Gas in soft-tissue planes on radiograph

TREATMENT

- Fluid resuscitation, may require transfusion.
- Monitor intake and output.
- Antibiotics: Penicillin G or clindamycin; metronidazole or chloramphenicol if penicillin allergic.
- Surgical debridement is definitive treatment.
- Hyperbaric O_2 may be helpful.

Septic Arthritis

DEFINITION

Infection of joint space.

The most common organism to cause septic arthritis overall across all age groups is *S aureus*.

ETIOLOGY

- Neonates: *S aureus*, group B strep
- Children and adolescents: *S aureus*, *Haemophilus*
- Adults age < 50 years: *Neisseria, gonorrhoeae, S aureus*
- Adults age > 50 years: *S aureus, Escherichia coli*
- IV drug users: *Pseudomonas aeruginosa*

EPIDEMIOLOGY

- Two peaks: In children and the elderly
- Males affected twice as often

RISK FACTORS

- Rheumatoid arthritis (RA)
- Osteoarthritis (OA)
- Risky sexual behavior (*N gonorrhoeae*)
- Immunocompromised states: Alcoholism, liver or kidney disease, diabetes, cancer

The most common joint involved is the knee, followed by hip, shoulder, and wrist.

SIGNS AND SYMPTOMS

- Fever, chills.
- Acute joint pain.
- Joint stiffness.
- Recent urethritis, salpingitis, or hemorrhagic vesicular skin lesions (*N gonorrhoeae*).
- Maculopapular or vesicular rash (*N gonorrhoeae*).
- Tenosynovitis → migratory polyarthritis → oligoarthritis (*N gonorrhoeae*).
- Pain with passive motion of the involved joint.
- Joint is warm, tender, and swollen, with evidence of effusion.

DIAGNOSIS

- Via arthrocentesis (see Procedures chapter).
- A WBC count of > 50,000 in the joint fluid with 75% granulocytosis is diagnostic.
- Erythrocyte sedimentation rate (ESR) and C-reactive protein often elevated (but not 100% sensitive and poor specificity), blood cultures usually positive.
- Plain radiographs of joint looking for underlying osteomyelitis or joint disease.
- If *N. gonorrhoeae* is suspected, culture the cervix, anus, and/or eye.

TREATMENT

- IV antibiotics.
- Splinting of joint.
- Analgesia.
- Surgery is recommended in children and for joints with loculated effusions.
- Shoulder and hip septic arthritis are drained openly in the operating room due to risk of avascular necrosis (AVN).

Osteomyelitis

DEFINITION

Inflammation or infection of bone.

ETIOLOGY

- *S aureus*
- *Streptococcus* spp.
- *Pseudomonas aeruginosa* (especially in IV drug users and foot puncture wounds)

EPIDEMIOLOGY

More common in males.

RISK FACTORS

- Trauma (including surgery)
- Immunocompromise (diabetes, sickle cell disease, alcoholism, etc)
- Soft-tissue infection

SIGNS AND SYMPTOMS

- Pain, swelling, and warmth of bone or joint
- ↓ range of motion (ROM)
- Fever

DIAGNOSIS

- Bone scan will detect osteomyelitis within 48 hours.
- Radiograph will demonstrate periosteal elevation within 10 days (see Figure 13-3).
- Blood cultures will demonstrate causative organism in 50% of cases.
- ESR and C-reactive protein support presence of inflammation.

Patients with sickle cell disease and asplenism can get *Salmonella* osteomyelitis, though *S aureus* is still the most common cause.

A 42-year-old male athlete steps on a nail through his sneaker. Two weeks later, he presents to the ED with pain and swelling of his left foot. *Think: Osteomyelitis due to* Pseudomonas.

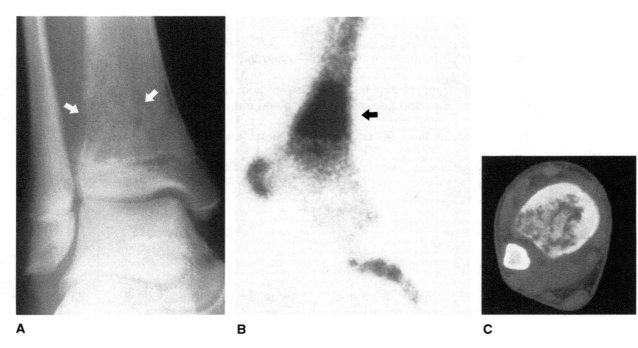

A   **B**   **C**

FIGURE 13-3. Osteomyelitis of the distal tibia.

A. Plain film of tibia demonstrating slight lucency at arrow. **B.** Bone scan of the same tibia demonstrating increased uptake. **C.** Computed tomography scan (cross-section) demonstrating mottled appearance of the bony cortex. (Reproduced, with permission, from Schwartz DT, Reisdorff EJ. *Emergency Radiology*. New York: McGraw-Hill, 2000: 23.)

TREATMENT

- Antibiotics for 6 weeks (some bugs may need shorter courses)
- Splinting of joint

NONINFECTIOUS CONDITIONS

Carpal Tunnel Syndrome

A 37-year-old secretary presents with pain and numbness in her right wrist and fingers, accompanied by a tingling sensation. The pain awakens her from sleep, and she is no longer able to perform her duties at work. Both Tinel's and Phalen's tests are abnormal. What is causing this and what can be done for her in the ED?

She has carpel tunnel syndrome. She can receive a removable wrist splint for support, and should follow up as an outpatient with orthopedics regarding possible need for surgical management.

Carpal tunnel syndrome is the most common entrapment neuropathy.

DEFINITION

Compression of the median nerve, resulting in pain along the distribution of the nerve.

ETIOLOGY

- Tumor (fibroma, lipoma).
- Ganglion cyst.
- Tenosynovitis of flexor tendons due to RA or trauma.
- Edema due to pregnancy or thyroid or amyloid disease.
- Trauma to carpal bones.
- Tendon inflammation from repetitive wrist movements.

RISK FACTORS

Repetitive hand movements.

EPIDEMIOLOGY

More common in women 3:1.

SIGNS AND SYMPTOMS

- Pain and paresthesia of volar aspect of thumb, digits 2 and 3, and half of digit 4.
- Activity and palmar flexion aggravate symptoms.
- Thenar atrophy: Uncommon but irreversible and indicates severe long-standing compression.
- Sensory deficit (two-point discrimination > 5 mm).

DIAGNOSIS

- **Tinel's sign:** Tapping over median nerve at wrist produces pain and paresthesia (see Figure 13-4).
- **Phalen's test:** One minute of maximal palmar flexion produces pain and paresthesia (see Figure 13-4).
- Consider ESR, thyroid function tests, serum glucose, and uric acid level to look for underlying cause.

Twenty to 50% of the population normally have a positive Phalen's test and Tinel's sign.

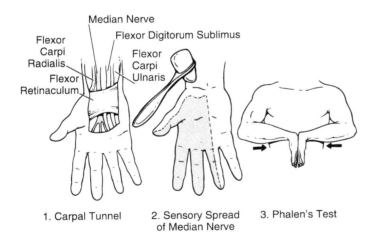

1. Carpal Tunnel 2. Sensory Spread of Median Nerve 3. Phalen's Test

FIGURE 13-4. Carpal tunnel syndrome.

1. The flexor retinaculum in the wrist compresses the median nerve to produce hyperesthesia in the radial 3.5 digits. 2. Tinel sign: Percussion on the radial side of the palmaris longus tendon produces tingling in the 3.5 digit region. 3. Phalen's test: Hyperflexion of the wrist for 60 seconds may produce pain in the median nerve distribution, which is relieved by extension of the wrist. (Reproduced, with permission, from DeGowin RL, Brown DD. *DeGowin's Diagnostic Examination*, 7th ed. New York: McGraw-Hill, 2000: 720.)

TREATMENT

- Treat underlying condition.
- Rest and splint.
- Nonsteroidal anti-inflammatories (NSAIDs) for analgesia.
- Surgery for crippling pain, thenar atrophy, and failure of nonoperative management.

Ganglion Cyst

DEFINITION

A synovial cyst, usually present on radial aspect of wrist.

ETIOLOGY

Idiopathic.

SIGNS AND SYMPTOMS

- Presence of mass that patient cannot account for.
- May or may not be painful.
- Pain aggravated by extreme flexion or extension.
- Size of ganglia ↑ with ↑ use of wrist.
- Compression of median or ulnar nerve may occur (not common).

DIAGNOSIS

Radiographs to ascertain diagnosis; since a ganglion cyst is a soft-tissue problem only, no radiographic changes should be noted.

TREATMENT

- Reassurance for most cases
- Wrist immobilization for moderate pain
- Aspiration of cyst for severe pain
- Surgical excision for cases involving median nerve compression and cosmetically unacceptable ganglia

Trigger Finger

DEFINITION

Stenosis of tendon sheath flexor digitorum → nodule formation within the sheath.

RISK FACTORS

- RA
- Middle-aged women
- Congenital

SIGNS AND SYMPTOMS

Snapping sensation or click when flexing and extending the digit (Figure 13-5).

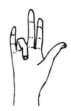

FIGURE 13-5. Trigger finger.

Usually involves third or fourth digit. Flexion is normal, but extension involves a painful "snap." (Reproduced, with permission, from DeGowin RL, Brown DD. *DeGowin's Diagnostic Examination*, 7th ed. New York: McGraw-Hill, 2000: 701.)

TREATMENT

- Splinting of metacarpophalangeal (MCP) joint in extension
- Injection of corticosteroid into tendon sheath
- Surgical repair if above fail

LOW BACK PAIN

Leading Causes of Lower Back Pain

- Fracture
- Abdominal aortic aneurysm
- Cauda equina syndrome
- Tumor (cord compression)
- Other (OA, severe musculoskeletal pain, other neurological syndromes)
- Infection (eg, epidural abscess)
- Disk herniation/rupture

OA can → osteophytes and hypertrophy of spinal facets, which compress nerve roots.

Lumbar Disk Herniation

DEFINITION

- Disk herniation is a common cause of chronic lower back pain.
- L4–5 and L5–S1 are the most common sites affected.
- Herniation occurs when the nucleus pulposus prolapses posteriorly through the annulus fibrosis.
- More common in men.

The nucleus pulposus is a thick gel. Herniation of the nucleus pulposus is like toothpaste being squeezed out of the tube.

SIGNS AND SYMPTOMS

- Limited spinal flexion.
- Pain and paresthesia with a dermatomal distribution.
- Specific signs depend on nerve root involved:
  - L4: ↓ knee jerk, weakness of anterior tibialis.
  - L5: Weakness of extensor hallucis longus, ↓ sensation over lateral aspect of calf and first web space.
  - S1: ↓ ankle jerk, ↓ plantar flexion, ↓ sensation over lateral aspect of foot.

Vertebral Compression Fracture

- Most common manifestation of osteoporosis.
- Also seen in patients on long-term steroids and in patients with lytic bony metastases.
- The thoracic spine is the most common site affected.

SIGNS AND SYMPTOMS

- Height loss
- Sudden back pain after mild trauma
- Local radiation of pain—the extremities are rarely affected (unlike a herniated disk)

DIAGNOSIS

Plain radiographs of lumbosacral spine will not show compression fracture until there is loss of 25–30% of bone height.

TREATMENT

- Symptomatic relief with NSAIDs, acetaminophen, opioids for short-term pain control.
- Intranasal calcitonin may ↓ pain in acute fractures.
- Treatment of osteoporosis prevents compression fractures:
  - Recommend weight-bearing exercises
  - Estrogen replacement therapy
  - Calcium supplementation
  - Calcitonin inhibits bone resorption
  - Bisphosphonates ↑ bone mass by inhibiting osteoclast activity

Epidural Abscess

A 33-year-old male is brought in by EMS to the ED with back pain that began 2 weeks ago. He has a history of polysubstance and injection drug use (IDU). He has been taking opioids with minimal improvement. He has not had a bowel movement in 3 days. He has had some numbness and "giving out" in his legs for 2 days and today was unable to walk. His temperature is 37.8°C (100.0°F) and pulse 100 bpm. What diagnosis must be considered and what diagnostic test is now indicated?

Spinal epidural abscess. He has concerning symptoms with his back pain and IDU, borderline fever, fecal retention, and new neurologic deficits. He needs to undergo an emergent thoracic and lumbar magnetic resonance imaging (MRI).

- Spinal abscesses are most commonly found in the immunosuppressed, IV drug users, and the elderly.
- An abscess can form anywhere along the spinal cord, and as it expands, it compresses against the spinal cord and occludes the vasculature.

ETIOLOGY

- The infection is generally spread from the skin or other tissue.
- S *aureus*, gram-negative bacilli, and tuberculosis bacillus are the leading organisms involved.

SIGNS AND SYMPTOMS

- Triad of pain, fever, and progressive weakness.
- The pain develops over the course of a week or two, and the fever is often accompanied by an elevated WBC count.

DIAGNOSIS AND TREATMENT

- MRI can localize the lesion. Lumbar puncture is not required unless meningitis is suspected.
- Emergent decompressive laminectomy can prevent permanent sequelae. This should be followed up with long-term antibiotics.

Spinal Cord Compression

Please also see "Spinal Cord Compression" in Hematology/Oncology chapter.

Spinal cord compression is an oncologic emergency. Missed diagnosis can → permanent paralysis.

DEFINITION

Malignancy metastasizing to and destroying vertebral bodies and extending into the epidural space causing thecal sac or cord impingement.

ETIOLOGY

Most common malignancies: prostate, breast, lung.

DIAGNOSIS

MRI is the preferred imaging technique.

Any cancer patient who develops back pain should be evaluated for cord compression.

TREATMENT

- Rapid treatment is essential as duration of symptoms is inversely proportional to chances of recovery. Pretreatment neurologic status is most important prognostic factor (ie, the best chance of walking out is for those who walk in).
- High-dose steroids to control inflammation/edema.
- Surgery is superior for patients with single area of compression, radioresistant tumors (renal cell, melanoma, prostate cancer) or have mechanical cause such as a posterior protuberant bone from a pathologic fracture.
- Radiation for patients with multiple areas of compression, poor prognosis, or radiosensitive tumor (small cell lung cancer, myeloma).

Cauda Equina Syndrome

DEFINITION

Compression of the lumbar and sacral nerve roots that comprise the cauda equina.

ETIOLOGY

- Tumor
- Midline disk herniations (rare)
- Congenital narrowing of the lumbar canal

SIGNS AND SYMPTOMS

- Low back pain, radicular pain.
- Saddle anesthesia.
- Weakness of foot plantar flexion, loss of ankle reflexes, and sensory and motor disturbances of the lower extremities can occur.
- ↓ anal sphincter tone, bowel and bladder incontinence or retention.

TREATMENT

- Malignant etiology:
  - An oncologic emergency
  - Steroids
  - Consult spine surgery, radiation oncology
  - Definitive treatment with either radiation or surgical decompression
- Nonmalignant etiology:
  - Bed rest and analgesia
  - Neurosurgical evaluation for potential laminectomy

Saddle anesthesla: Loss of sensation over the buttocks, perineum, and proximal thighs. Frequently seen in cauda equina syndrome.

SYSTEMIC PROBLEMS

Osteoarthritis (OA)

DEFINITION

- OA is the result of mechanical and biological factors that destabilize articular cartilage and subchondral bone.
- There is softening, ulceration, and loss of articular cartilage, eburnation (sclerosis) of subchondral bone, osteophytes, and subchondral cysts.
- Cause is unclear but is probably multifactorial.

EPIDEMIOLOGY

- Most common form of arthritis.
- Affects males and females equally.
- Peak age is 45–55 years, but after 55 years is more common in women.
- Fifty percent of people over 65 years have radiographic changes in the knees.
- Obesity correlates with OA of the knees.
- Weight-bearing joints, including the lumbosacral spine, hips, knees, and feet, are most commonly involved.
- Cervical spine and proximal interphalangeal (PIP) and distal interphalangeal (DIP) joints are frequently involved.
- Elbows and shoulders are effected only when involved in trauma or overuse.

SIGNS AND SYMPTOMS

- Pain and stiffness in and around the joint.
- Limitation of function.
- Insidious onset.
- Worse with activity, relieved by rest.
- Worse in rainy, damp, and cool weather.
- Gel phenomenon (stiffness after periods of rest) that resolves within several minutes.
- Knee instability and buckling.
- Hip-gait disturbance and pain in groin or radiation to anterior thigh and knee.

OA can cause morning stiffness but is usually short lived (in contrast to RA).

OA affects the outer joints on the hand—the DIPs. RA affects the inner joints— MCPs and PIPs.

- Hands: PIP (Bouchard's nodes) and DIP (Heberden's nodes) (Figure 13-6).
- Facet joints of cervical spine and lumbosacral spine cause neck and low back pain.
- Symptoms are localized, and limitation of function is secondary to osteophytes, cartilage loss, and muscle spasm.
- Locking of joint is secondary to loose bodies.
- Crepitation is present in 90%.

DIAGNOSIS

- Osteophytes and spurs at joint margin
- Asymmetric joint space narrowing
- Subchondral cysts and bone remodeling later on in the disease

TREATMENT

- Goals of treatment: Relieve symptoms, limit disability, improve function.
- Physical and occupational therapy for ROM and strengthening exercises and providing assistive devices.
- Weight loss.
- Nonopioid analgesics (acetaminophen).

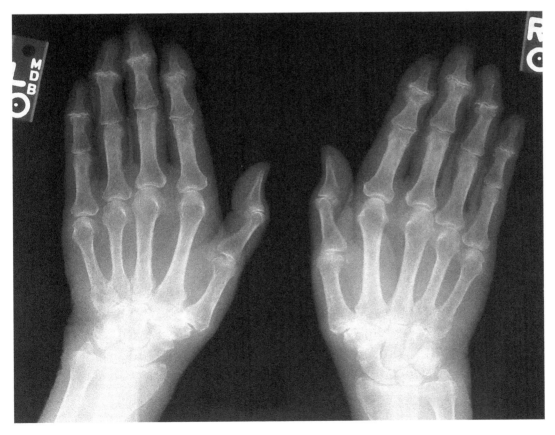

FIGURE 13-6. OA of the hands.

Note the bony swelling at the base of the thumb and Heberden's nodes at the DIPs. (Reproduced, with permission, from Simon RR, Koenigsknecht SJ. *Emergency Orthopedics: The Extremities*, 4th ed. New York: McGraw-Hill, 2001: 43.)

- NSAIDs (↑ risk of GI bleeding).
- Topical analgesics (capsaicin).
- Intra-articular steroid injections.
- Surgical intervention: Arthroscopic debridement and lavage, osteotomy, and arthroplasty.

Rheumatoid Arthritis (RA)

DEFINITION

- RA is a chronic, inflammatory, systemic disease that is manifested in the diarthrodial and peripheral joints.
- Etiology is still unknown; may be infectious.
- A combination of genetic and environmental factors control the progression.
- Disease process ranges from self-limited to progressively chronic with severe debilitation.

EPIDEMIOLOGY

- All ethnic groups affected; may be higher in Native Americans.
- Worldwide distribution.
- Affects all ages, prevalence ↑ with age, and peak incidence is between the fourth and sixth decades.
- Females affected more commonly than males (2:1).
- Associated with HLA-DR4 and HLA-DRB1 genes.

SIGNS AND SYMPTOMS

Common deformities:

- **Ulnar deviation** of the digits.
- **Boutonniere deformity**—hyperextension of the DIP and flexion of the PIP (Figure 13-7).
- **Swan-neck deformity**—flexion of the DIP and extension of the PIP.

DIAGNOSIS

Diagnosis is based on a constellation of findings over several weeks to months or longer.

- Rheumatoid factor (RF) is present in 70% of patients.
- ESR correlates with the degree of inflammation and is useful in following the course of the disease.
- C-reactive protein can monitor inflammation.

CRITERIA FOR CLASSIFICATION OF RA

At least four of the following seven criteria must be present to diagnose RA; criteria 1–4 must have been present for ≥ 6 weeks.

1. Morning stiffness for ≥ 1 hour.
2. Arthritis of ≥ three joint areas.
3. Arthritis of hand joints (see Figure 13-7).
4. Symmetric arthritis.

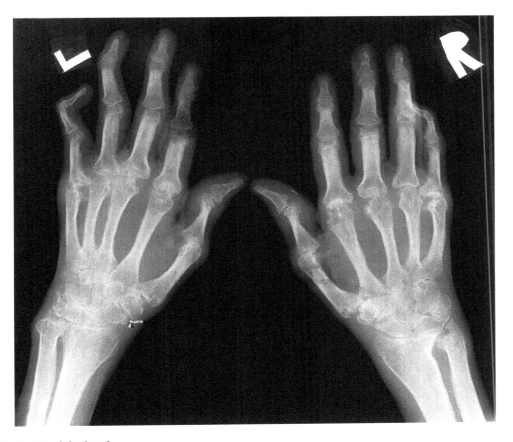

FIGURE 13-7. RA of the hands.

Note inflammation and fusion of the PIP and metacarpointerphalangeal joints with relative sparing of the DIP joint, and the boutonniere deformities on the fifth digits. (Reproduced, with permission, from Simon RR, Koenigsknecht SJ. *Emergency Orthopedics: The Extremities*, 4th ed. New York: McGraw-Hill, 2001: 50.)

5. Rheumatoid nodules.
6. Positive serum RF.
7. Radiographic changes: Erosions or bony decalcifications on posteroanterior hand and wrist.

TREATMENT

- Fifty percent of patients are refractory to treatment and display systemic disease.
- Physical and occupational therapy to maintain strength and flexibility and splinting of inflamed joints.
- NSAIDs.
- Corticosteroids.
- Disease-modifying antirheumatic drugs: Gold compounds, hydroxychloroquine (Plaquenil) penicillamine, methotrexate, azathioprine (Imuran), sulfasalazine, cyclophosphamide (Cytoxan), cyclosporine.

Most arthritis patients (regardless of the type of arthritis) have taken NSAIDs for long periods of time. This places them at high risk for ulcers and GI bleeding.

Gout:
- *Small* joints
- *Negative* birefringence

Pseudogout:
- *Large* joints
- *Positive* birefringence

Gout

A 65-year-old man presents with acute onset of severe pain and redness at the metatarsophalangeal (MTP) joint of his right great toe. He has never had anything like this before and wonders if he now has an infection of his foot. He denies any trauma. His past medical history is significant for hypertension, for which he takes hydrochlorothiazide (HCTZ). He has an average of 1–2 alcoholic beverages per day. His physical exam reveals a warm, red, swollen first MTP joint on the right. Does he have an infection of his foot or is there another explanation?

His symptoms are classic for podagra, a painful condition of the great toe secondary to gout. This is not an infection, and antibiotics have no role. No lab tests are indicated. If the diagnosis of gout is less clear (eg, acute swelling and redness of a knee), then arthrocentesis of the joint would be helpful to rule out a septic joint. He can be treated with indomethacin +/– colchicine. He should probably discontinue his HCTZ, limit his alcohol intake, and follow up closely with his primary care provider.

DEFINITION

A disorder in purine metabolism, resulting in the deposition of urate crystals in joint spaces, resulting in joint inflammation and exquisite pain.

EPIDEMIOLOGY

Seen most commonly in middle-aged men.

RISK FACTORS

- Age
- Hyperuricemia
- Alcohol consumption
- Drugs (eg, thiazide diuretics)

SIGNS AND SYMPTOMS

- Acute onset of extreme pain in small joints, accompanied by redness and swelling.
- **Tophi** are aggregates of gouty crystals and giant cells. They can erode away tissue.
- **Podagra** is inflammation of the first MTP joint, which presents in 50–75% of all patients as an exquisitely painful nodule on the medial aspect of the foot.

The most common and frequent manifestation of gout is podagra.

DIAGNOSIS

- Presence of negatively birefringent crystals in synovial fluid.
- Elevated serum uric acid levels between attacks (may be low or normal during an acute attack so limited utility in the ED).

TREATMENT

- ED:
  - Indomethacin to ↓ inflammation is first line.
  - Colchicine to inhibit chemotaxis is second line.

- Steroids (eg, prednisone 40 mg PO × 5 days) if NSAIDs contraindicated.
- Outpatient:
  - Allopurinol, a xanthine oxidase inhibitor, used as prophylaxis. Do not give in acute phase as it may induce an attack.
  - Uricosuric agents (probenecid).

Pseudogout

DEFINITION

Deposition of calcium pyrophosphate dihydrate (CPPD) crystals in joint spaces.

Pseudogout: Mostly large joints such as shoulder, wrist, and knee are involved.

ETIOLOGY

- Acute inflammatory reaction to the deposition of CPPD in joint spaces.
- Changes related to age that make the synovial fluid environment more hospitable to CPPD growth.

SIGNS AND SYMPTOMS

The most common presentation is erythema and swelling of the knee.

DIAGNOSIS

Presence of **positively birefringent crystals** in synovial fluid.

TREATMENT

- Splint joint.
- Aspiration is both diagnostic and therapeutic.
- NSAIDs.

Polymyositis and Dermatomyositis

DEFINITIONS

Connective tissue diseases that result in proximal muscle weakness. Dermatomyositis differs only in that there is a rash, typically affecting the face, neck, and shoulders. There is also a significant risk of an occult malignancy associated with dermatomyositis.

Polymyositis and dermatomyositis are both more common in women.

ETIOLOGY

Etiology unknown. Many viruses including *Toxoplasma*, influenza, and coxsackie have been implicated. Family history of autoimmune disease or vasculitis is a risk factor.

SIGNS AND SYMPTOMS

- Symmetrical proximal muscle weakness.
- Dysphagia.
- Difficulty getting out of a chair, climbing or descending stairs, kneeling, raising arms.

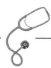

Polymyositis and dermatomyositis can be distinguished from myasthenia gravis by the lack of ocular involvement (ptosis).

Both azathioprine and methotrexate suppress the bone marrow. Azathioprine is also hepatotoxic.

DIAGNOSIS

- In the ED:
  - Proximal muscle weakness
  - Elevated CPK (from necrotic muscle fibers)
- At outpatient follow-up:
  - Low-amplitude action potentials and fibrillations on electromyography (EMG).
  - ↑ muscle fiber size on muscle biopsy.

LABORATORY

- Positive antinuclear antibody.
- Elevated CPK, lactic dehydrogenase, serum glutamic oxaloacetic transaminase, aldolase.
- ESR is elevated in only 50% of cases.
- Abnormal EMG.
- Biopsy shows inflammatory infiltrates.
- One-fifth of patients have myositis-specific antibodies (Anti-Jo-1).
- Chest x-ray may show interstitial pulmonary disease.

PROGNOSIS

Presentation is usually insidious and progresses slowly, but disease can be fatal. Seventy-five percent survival at 5 years with long-term corticosteroid therapy.

TREATMENT

- ROM exercises.
- Daily steroids.
- If refractory to steroids, azathioprine or methotrexate is given.

UPPER EXTREMITY TRAUMA

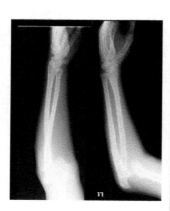

FIGURE 13-8. Posterior elbow dislocation.

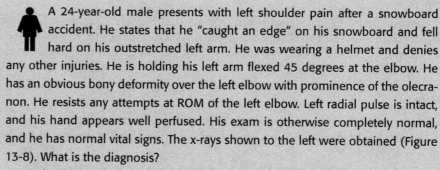

A 24-year-old male presents with left shoulder pain after a snowboard accident. He states that he "caught an edge" on his snowboard and fell hard on his outstretched left arm. He was wearing a helmet and denies any other injuries. He is holding his left arm flexed 45 degrees at the elbow. He has an obvious bony deformity over the left elbow with prominence of the olecranon. He resists any attempts at ROM of the left elbow. Left radial pulse is intact, and his hand appears well perfused. His exam is otherwise completely normal, and he has normal vital signs. The x-rays shown to the left were obtained (Figure 13-8). What is the diagnosis?

He has sustained a posterior elbow dislocation secondary to a fall on an extended extremity. Associated injuries such as elbow or forearm fractures, ulnar or median nerve injuries, or brachial artery injuries can occur. ED treatment involves sedation, closed reduction, and immobilization.

Anterior Shoulder Dislocation

ETIOLOGY

- Forcible external rotation and abduction of the arm
- 95–97% of all shoulder dislocations

SIGNS AND SYMPTOMS

- Shoulder pain.
- Patient maintains shoulder in elevated position.
- Resists internal rotation of arm.
- Axillary nerve palsy:
  - ↓ sensation over deltoid.
  - ↓ ability to abduct shoulder.

DIAGNOSIS

See Figure 13-9.

TREATMENT

- Closed reduction under conscious sedation.
- Sling and swathe for 4 weeks.
- ROM exercises.
- Surgical repair for nonreducible dislocations (uncommon).

COMPLICATIONS

Associated fractures (occur about 40% of the time):

- Bankart: Fracture of glenoid margin
- Hill-Sachs: Fracture of humeral head

Posterior Shoulder Dislocation

RISK FACTORS

- Lightning injury.
- Seizures.
- Anterior blow to shoulder or fall on outstretched hand.

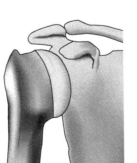
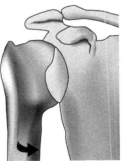
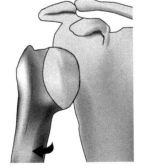

A   B   C

FIGURE 13-9. **Anatomy of shoulder dislocations.**

A. Anterior dislocation. **B.** Normal shoulder. **C.** Posterior dislocation.

> Posterior shoulder dislocations account for only 2% of all dislocations.

SIGNS AND SYMPTOMS

Arm is internally rotated and adducted.

DIAGNOSIS

Lightbulb sign: Lightbulb appearance of internally rotated proximal humerus (Figure 13-10).

TREATMENT

- Closed reduction under conscious sedation.
- Sling and swathe for 4 weeks.
- ROM exercises.
- Surgical repair for nonreducible dislocations.

Clavicle Injuries

- Fractures:
  - Common
  - Rarely require more than sling for support
- Acromioclavicular (AC) separation:
  - Tenderness over AC joint.
  - X-rays may be normal in partial tear of AC ligament. May show separation with upward displacement of clavicle.
  - Most are managed conservatively with a sling for support.
  - Severe injuries may require surgical management.

Scapular Fracture

- Requires severe mechanism of injury
- Commonly associated with other significant injuries

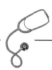

Posterior shoulder dislocations are frequently missed. Surgical fixation is necessary when the diagnosis is delayed for 2 weeks or more.

Inferior dislocations (luxatio erecta) are rare. Patient will present with arm fully abducted above head and elbow flexed.

Always look for other, more serious injuries if scapular fracture present.

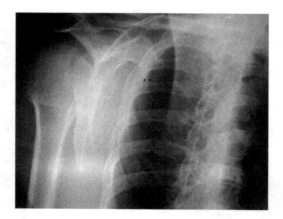

FIGURE 13-10. Posterior shoulder dislocation.

Note the "ice cream cone sign," so named because of the characteristic appearance of the neck and head of the humerus. (Reproduced, with permission, from Simon RR, Koenigsknecht SJ. *Emergency Orthopedics: The Extremities*, 4th ed. New York: McGraw-Hill, 2001: 325.)

Humeral Fracture

- Proximal fractures:
  - Most commonly seen in the elderly after falls.
  - Most often treated with shoulder immobilization and orthopedic follow-up.
  - Severe fractures with significant displacement need emergent orthopedic consultation and may require surgical repair.
- Midshaft fractures:
  - Sustained after direct blow to arm or after a fall.
  - Can be associated with radial nerve injury and subsequent wrist drop.
  - Treatment is usually nonoperative, with immobilization with a coaptation or sugar tong splint.

Supracondylar Humeral Fracture

- Common in children
- Fall on outstretched hand (FOOSH)

CLINICAL FEATURES

- Deformity and tenderness
- Joint effusion on x-ray
- Presence of anterior or posterior fat pad on lateral radiograph

TREATMENT

- Associated with compartment sydrome (Volkmann's ischemia)
- Require emergent orthopedic consultation
- Surgery needed if displacement, angulation, or neurovascular deficit

Elbow Dislocation

- Most commonly posterior
- Associated with other injuries:
  - Fractures (eg, elbow and forearm)
  - Injuries to ulnar and median nerves
  - Brachial artery injury
- Anterior dislocations rare and associated with higher rate of vascular injury

Colles Fracture

- Distal radius fracture with dorsal angulation.
- Most commonly caused by fall on outstretched hand.
- "Dinner fork deformity" is classic.
- More common in elderly women.

TREATMENT

- Short arm cast 4–6 weeks with volar flexion and ulnar deviation
- Surgical repair for open fracture
- Comminuted fracture
- Intra-articular displaced fracture > 5 mm

Potential complication of any shoulder injury is adhesive capsulitis (frozen shoulder). May be prevented by early ROM exercises.

A child returns with increasing pain after sustaining a supracondylar fracture. *Think: Compartment syndrome.*

Colles fracture may need closed reduction in the ED.

Smith Fracture

- Distal radius fracture with volar angulation
- Most commonly caused by direct trauma to dorsal forearm
- Garden spade deformity

TREATMENT

Surgical repair needed for most cases.

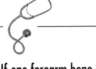

If one forearm bone is fractured, look for a fracture of dislocation in the other one.

Galeazzi Fracture

- Distal one-third radial fracture with dislocation of distal radioulnar joint
- Commonly caused by fall on outstretched hand with forearm in forced pronation or direct blow to back of wrist

TREATMENT

Surgical repair needed for most cases.

Monteggia Fracture

- Proximal one-third ulnar fracture with dislocation of the radial head
- Commonly caused by fall on outstretched hand with forearm in forced pronation or direct blow to posterior ulna
- May note injury of radial nerve

TREATMENT

- Surgical repair for adults
- Closed reduction for children (children can tolerate a greater degree of displacement)

If posterior fat pad is visible on x-ray, always assume radial head/neck fracture even if not visible.

Radial Head/Neck Fracture

- Fall on outstretched hand.
- Limited flexion and extension of elbow.
- Look for elbow effusion.
- Posterior fat pad visible on x-ray.

TREATMENT

- Collar and cuff if undisplaced.
- Displaced or comminuted fractures may need surgery.

Gamekeeper's thumb is commonly associated with ski pole injury.

Gamekeeper's Thumb

DEFINITION

Avulsion of ulnar collateral ligament of first metacarpophalangeal (MCP) joint (Figure 13-11).

ETIOLOGY

- Forced radial abduction of the thumb
- Can be associated with an avulsion fracture of the metacarpal base

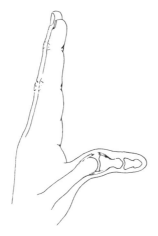

FIGURE 13-11. Gamekeeper's thumb.

(Reproduced, with permission, from Scaletta TA, et al. *Emergent Management of Trauma.* New York: McGraw-Hill, 1996: 220.)

SIGNS AND SYMPTOMS

Inability to pinch.

DIAGNOSIS

Application of valgus stress to thumb while MCP joint is flexed will demonstrate laxity of ulnar collateral ligament.

TREATMENT

- Rest, ice, elevation, analgesia
- Thumb spica cast for 3–6 weeks for partial tears
- Surgical repair for complete tears

Mallet Finger

DEFINITION

Rupture of extensor tendon at its insertion into base of distal phalanx (Figure 13-12).

ETIOLOGY

- Avulsion fracture of distal phalanx
- Other trauma

SIGNS AND SYMPTOMS

Inability to extend DIP joint.

TREATMENT

Splint finger in extension for 6–8 weeks.
Surgery may be required for large avulsions of distal phalanx and for injuries that were not splinted early.

If left untreated, mallet finger results in permanent boutonniere deformity.

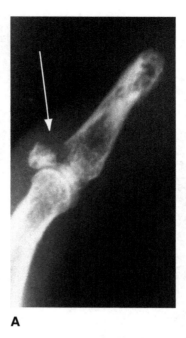
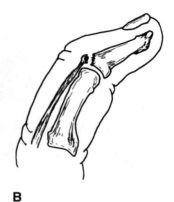

A   **B**

FIGURE 13-12. Mallet finger.

A. Radiograph of an avulsion fracture of the base of the distal phalanx (arrow), which is often associated with mallet finger. **B.** Avulsion of the extensor tendon. (Reproduced, with permission, from Schwartz DT, Reisdorff EJ. *Emergency Radiology.* New York: McGraw-Hill, 2000: 40.)

High-Pressure Hand Injury

ETIOLOGY

High-pressure injection of fluid or air, such as with paint or grease guns.

SIGNS AND SYMPTOMS

- Small injection site
- Often deceptively normal physical exam

DIAGNOSIS

- Based on history.
- X-ray may reveal degree of spread, if material is radiopaque.

TREATMENT

Emergent hand surgery consultation for operative care.

Common Hand and Wrist Injuries

See Table 13-1 for more upper extremity problems.

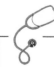

All wrist injuries with snuff box tenderness should be treated with a splint for occult scaphoid fracture.

356

TABLE 13-1. Common Hand and Wrist Injuries

INJURY	DESCRIPTION	TREATMENT

Boxer's fracture	Fracture of neck of fifth metacarpal sustained in a closed-fist injury	▪ Ulnar gutter splint/cast for 3–6 weeks
		▪ Reduction or surgical repair for:
		  ▪ Any rotational deformity
		  ▪ Angulation of fourth > 20°/fifth metacarpal > 40°
		  ▪ Angulation of second/third metacarpal > 10°–15°

Bennett fracture	Fracture-dislocation of base of thumb	▪ Initially immobilization in thumb spica cast ▪ Definitive treatment is with surgical fixation
Rolando fracture	Comminuted fracture of the base of the thumb	▪ Initially immobilization in thumb spica cast ▪ Definitive treatment is with surgical fixation
Scaphoid fracture	▪ Most commonly caused by fall on outstretched hand ▪ Snuffbox tenderness is classic	▪ Immobilization in thumb spica cast with wrist in neutral position for 12 weeks ▪ May take up to 2 weeks to be seen on radiographs

Nightstick fracture	Isolated fracture of the ulnar shaft	▪ Long arm cast for 3–6 weeks
		▪ Surgical repair for:
		  ▪ Angulation > 10°
		  ▪ Displacement > 50%

Lunate dislocation	▪ Often missed ▪ Fall on outstretched hand ▪ Pain and swelling anteriorly over wrist	Surgical repair

LOWER EXTREMITY TRAUMA

See Table 13-2 for lower extremity injuries.

Pelvis Fracture

▪ Requires high-impact injury to fracture pelvis (eg, motor vehicle accident)
▪ Usually one of multiple injuries

Consider x-ray of the pelvis in all patients with significant multisystem trauma.

CLINICAL FEATURES

▪ Pain
▪ Crepitus, bruising
▪ Pelvic instability
▪ May → extensive blood loss due to disruption of blood vessels, especially with open fractures

HIGH-YIELD FACTS

Musculoskeletal Emergencies

357

TABLE 13-2. Common Leg and Foot Injuries

INJURY	DESCRIPTION	TREATMENT
Lisfranc fracture	▪ Fracture through base of second metatarsal ▪ The second metatarsal is the stabilizing force of the tarsometatarsal joint	Surgical fixation (can be open or closed)

Maisonneuve fracture	Malleolar (ankle) and proximal fibula fracture with disruption of the medial deltoid ligament	▪ Long leg cast for 6–12 weeks
		▪ Surgical fixation for:
		  ▪ Medial malleolar fracture
		  ▪ Widened medial joint space

Baker cyst	▪ Cyst in the medial popliteal fossa ▪ Associated with arthritis and joint trauma ▪ Rupture of cyst can mimic symptoms of deep vein thrombosis	▪ Treat underlying cause (adults) ▪ Symptomatic relief with NSAIDs
Calcaneal fracture	▪ Most frequently injured foot bone ▪ Usually occurs due to fall from a height with patient landing on his feet	▪ Posterior splint for nondisplaced fractures ▪ Surgical repair for displaced fractures
Jones fracture	▪ Fracture of diaphysis of fifth metatarsal ▪ Usually occurs due to force applied to ball of foot, as in pivoting or dancing ▪ Often complicated by nonunion	▪ Short leg cast for nondisplaced fractures ▪ Surgical repair for displaced fractures

Hip fractures have a high mortality rate — ~30% die within 1 year as a result of the fracture.

TREATMENT

- Aggressive resuscitation with IV fluids and blood as required.
- Stabilize fracture with bed sheet or external fixation device.
- Consult orthopedic team early.
- Interventional radiology for bleeding site embolization.

Hip Fracture

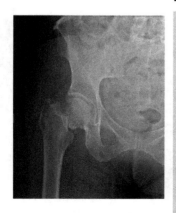

FIGURE 13-13. Right femoral neck fracture.

An 81-year-old woman was found by her husband on the floor of her home after she fell while trying to answer the phone. She denies any other injuries. She and her husband live in their own home. She denies any other injuries, and her husband found her just after the fall. She was not able to get up, so EMS was contacted and brought her to the ED. Her right leg is shortened and externally rotated. She resists active or passive ROM of the hip secondary to pain. The remainder of her exam is normal. An AP x-ray is shown to the left (Figure 13-13). What is the diagnosis?

Right femoral neck fracture. The x-ray also reveals evidence of osteopenia. She will require orthopedic consultation in the ED and hospital admission. The long-term affects of this injury may be significant and she will likely require at least a temporary stay in a nursing home.

- Incidence ↑ with age.
- Male-to-female ratio is 1:3.
- Twenty to 30% of elderly patients die in the first year after hip fracture.

CLINICAL FEATURES

- History of fall
- Inability to bear weight
- Leg shortened and externally rotated (may be internally rotated with intertrochanteric fractures)

DIAGNOSIS

- Anteroposterior (AP) and lateral x-rays of hip.
- Classified as intracapsular or extracapsular.

TREATMENT

- Intracapsular fractures are at risk of avascular necrosis of femoral head and often receive primary arthroplasty if displaced.
- Extracapsular fractures are usually treated by internal fixation.

Hip Dislocation

- Result of high-energy trauma.
- Associated with other injuries.
- Ninety percent are posterior dislocations. Also called "dashboard dislocations."
- At risk of AVN if left untreated for longer than 6 hours.

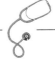

Check for sciatic nerve damage: Dorsiflexion of foot and sensation below knee.

DIAGNOSIS

- Posterior dislocation causes shortening, adduction, and internal rotation of extremity.
- Anterior dislocation leaves hip flexed and extremity abducted and externally rotated.

TREATMENT

Early closed reduction.

Femoral Shaft Fracture

- Very high-energy injury
- Often occurs in association with hip dislocation or pelvis fracture

CLINICAL FEATURES

- Deformity
- Shortened, externally rotated leg
- Can be associated with significant blood loss and hemorrhagic shock

TREATMENT

- Can be associated with marked blood loss.
- Resuscitate as appropriate.
- Splint with Thomas splint or other traction device.
- Orthopedic consultation.

There are five primary sites of bleeding that can cause hemorrhagic shock after trauma:
- Externally
- Long bones (primarily femur)
- Thorax
- Abdomen
- Pelvis

Proximal Tibial Fracture

- Also known as "bumper fracture"
- Fall onto extended leg or pedestrian hit by car bumper

CLINICAL FEATURES

- Swollen knee
- Tenderness over proximal tibia

TREATMENT

- Immobilize in long leg cast.
- Orthopedic consultation.

Common Leg and Foot Injuries

See Table 13-2 for more lower extremity injuries.

Ankle Fracture and Dislocation

- One of the most common orthopedic injuries.
- Classified as unimalleolar, bimalleolar, and trimalleolar.
- Unimalleolar fractures are stable, requiring only splinting.
- Bimalleolar and trimalleolar fractures usually require open reduction and internal fixation (ORIF).
- **Ottawa Rules:**
  - See Tables 13-3 and 13-4 and Figure 13-14.
  - The rule cannot be applied to patients who are intoxicated or who have an altered mental status.

Ankle dislocations are orthopedic emergencies requiring urgent reduction to prevent neurovascular compromise.

PEDIATRIC MUSCULOSKELETAL PROBLEMS

Legg-Calvé-Perthes Disease

DEFINITION

- Also called coxa plana, juvenile osteochondrosis
- Childhood hip disorder that involves AVN of femoral head (Figure 13-15)
- Bilateral in 10–15% of patients

EPIDEMIOLOGY

- Occurs in 1 in 1200 children ages 3–10 years.
- Peak incidence at age 6 years.

TABLE 13-3. Ottawa Ankle Rule

CRITERIA FOR ANKLE RADIOGRAPH

- Inability to bear weight immediately after injury and in emergency department
- Bony tenderness at posterior edge of distal 6 cm or tip of medial or lateral malleolus

TABLE 13-4. Ottawa Foot Rule

CRITERIA FOR FOOT RADIOGRAPH

- Bony tenderness at base of fifth metatarsal
- Bony tenderness over navicular
- Inability to bear weight immediately and in emergency department

- More common in males by factor of 4:1, but when it affects females, there is more extensive involvement of the epiphysis.

ETIOLOGY

Etiology is unknown but may be due to chronic synovitis, repeated trauma to hip in athletic children, infection, or congenital anomaly.

SIGNS AND SYMPTOMS

- Antalgic gait.
- May or may not identify history of trauma or strenuous activity followed by sudden onset of limping and pain in the anterior groin, anterior thigh or knee, making diagnosis difficult.
- Hip is held in external rotation and is limited in internal rotation. Muscle spasm may also be present.
- Buttock and thigh atrophy may be present on the affected side.

DIAGNOSIS

- Stage 1: No findings to slight widening of the joint space and lateral displacement of the head.

A 7-year-old boy presents with a limp and complains of groin and hip pain. Radiographs demonstrate a slight widening of the joint space. *Think: Legg-Calvé-Perthes disease.*

An **antalgic gait** is one that results from pain on weight bearing in which the stance phase of the gait is shortened on the affected side.

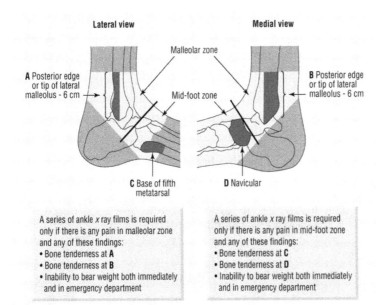

FIGURE 13-14. Ottawa ankle rules.

(Reproduced, with permission, from Bachman LM et al. *BMJ* 2003 Feb 22;326(7386):417.)

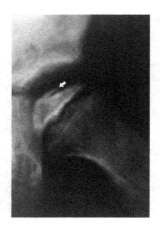

FIGURE 13-15. **AP view of pelvis demonstrating subchondral lucency of femoral head secondary to avascular necrosis.**

This is known as the "crescent sign" of Caffey. (Reproduced, with permission, from Schwartz DT, Reisdorff EJ. *Emergency Radiology.* New York: McGraw-Hill, 2000: 238.)

- Stage 2: Radiolucent and radiodense areas with epiphyseal fragmentation: This is the stage when most children present.
- Stage 3: Areas of radiolucency secondary to resorption of necrotic bone; this stage may last for several years in older children as new bone grows.
- Stage 4: Normal-appearing radiograph; however, femoral neck and epiphysis may remain widened. This is the healed phase.

TREATMENT

- Depends on the severity of the disease.
- Most cases are self-limited and no intervention is required.
- If ROM is limited, an abduction cast is applied. Traction may be used to relax adductor spasm and to maintain 45 degrees of abduction and slight internal rotation, which is the best position to center the femoral head to facilitate normal growth.
- The child may be mobilized using crutches and partial weight bearing with the cast. Cast should be removed periodically to mobilize the knee and ankle.
- Surgical intervention may be required for severe cases.

Slipped Capital Femoral Epiphysis (SCFE)

DEFINITION

Condition in which the femoral head maintains its position in the acetabulum but the femoral neck is displaced anteriorly.

EPIDEMIOLOGY

- Occurs between the ages of 10 and 15 years
- Male-to-female ratio 2:1
- Bilateral in 15–20%

An 11-year-old obese boy presents with thigh and knee pain that worsens when he plays sports. He is walking with a limp and holds his hip in slight external rotation. *Think: SCFE.*

ETIOLOGY

Cause is unclear, may involve:

- History of trauma
- Weakened physis
- Obesity
- Endocrine disorder

SIGNS AND SYMPTOMS

- Antalgic gait that may have been present for months or may have occurred acutely.
- Hip, medial thigh, or knee pain intermittently worsened with activity.
- Hip may be held in external rotation, and internal rotation is limited.

DIAGNOSIS

AP radiograph of the pelvis (Figure 13-16) and lateral and frogleg views (if no acute slippage) to look for:

- Irregular widening of the epiphyseal plate
- Globular swelling of the joint capsule
- Posterior and inferior displacement of the femoral head (if slippage)

TREATMENT

Surgical stabilization.

Osgood-Schlatter Disease

EPIDEMIOLOGY

- A cause of adolescent knee pain.
- Cause is uncertain but may be due to:
  - Apophysitis at the insertion of the patellar tendon at the tibial tuberosity.

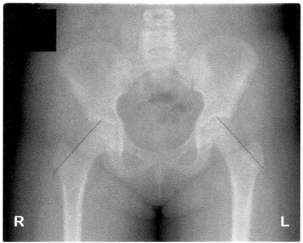

ANTEROPOSTERIOR (AP) VIEW

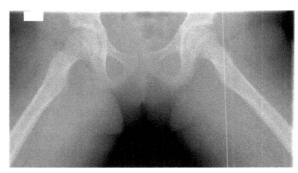

FROG LEG VIEW

FIGURE 13-16. Hip radiographs in a 13-year-old girl with mildly slipped capital femoral epiphysis (SCFE) on the right.

Note on the AP view that a line drawn along the superior border of the femoral neck (Klein line) shows less femoral head superior to the line on the right than it does in the normal hip on the left.

A 12-year-old boy presents complaining of knee pain for 2 weeks. Physical exam demonstrates a prominent tibial tubercle. *Think: Osgood-Schlatter disease.*

- Repeated quadriceps contraction resulting in tendonitis or partial avulsions at the tibial tubercle.
- Seen at ages 9–15 years, when the apophysis is most prone to injury.
- Males are affected more commonly than females.

SIGNS AND SYMPTOMS

- Pain at tibial tuberosity.
- Symptoms are worsened by palpation and knee extension against resistance.
- Prominent tibial tubercle.
- Soft-tissue swelling.

DIAGNOSIS

Radiographs demonstrate:

- Prominence of the tibial tubercle
- Heterotopic ossification, which appears as irregularities

TREATMENT

- Self-limited and usually resolves with complete ossification of the tibial tuberosity by age 15 years.
- NSAIDs.
- Cryotherapy.
- Stretching of the quadriceps.
- Limit activity to pain tolerance.
- Avoid kneeling, running, and jumping.

Pediatric Fractures

- Two important differences between children's bones and adults':
  - Presence of epiphyses.
  - They are softer, so it is more common to have a fracture than a significant ligament injury.
- Also unique to children are buckle fractures (incomplete fracture with buckling of cortex) and greenstick fractures (only one cortical surface breaks).
- Epiphyseal injuries: See Table 13-5.

ORTHOPEDIC COMPLICATIONS

General Complications of Orthopedic Trauma

- Compartment syndrome (see below)
- Rhabdomyolysis
- Malunion
- Nonunion
- AVN (see below)
- Fat embolism (especially with fracture of long bone)
- Hemorrhage (especially with pelvic fracture)
- Neurovascular injury

TABLE 13-5. Salter-Harris Fractures

CLASS	DEFINITION	TREATMENT
I	Fracture through epiphyseal plate	Closed reduction
II	Fracture of metaphysis with extension into epiphyseal plate Most common type of Salter-Harris fracture	Closed reduction
III	Intra-articular fracture of epiphysis with extension into epiphyseal plate	Open reduction
IV	Intra-articular fracture of epiphysis, metaphysis, and epiphyseal plate	Open reduction
V	Crush injury of epiphyseal plate	Open reduction

Compartment Syndrome

DEFINITION

- Compartment syndrome results when the pressure in a compartment exceeds the arterial perfusion pressure.
- This normally occurs at pressures > 20 mm Hg.
- Occurs at lower pressures when the arterial pressure is lower than normal, such as in prolonged systemic shock.
- Excess compartment pressure causes muscle and nerve necrosis due to ischemia.

ANATOMY

Major compartments include:

- Hand: Associated with crush injury
- Forearm: Associated with supracondylar fracture of the humerus
- Thigh: Associated with crush injury
- Leg: Associated with tibial fracture
- Foot: Associated with calcaneus fracture

RISK FACTORS

- Crush injuries
- Circumferential burns
- Constrictive devices (casts, clothing)
- Hemorrhage
- Edema
- Patients with altered mental status who cannot report compartment pain

SIGNS AND SYMPTOMS

- Earlier findings:
  - Pain out of proportion to the injury
  - Pain with passive flexion

Compartment syndrome is most common in the lower extremity.

6 **Ps** of compartment syndrome:
Pain on passive flexion (most reliable sign)
Paresthesia
Paralysis
Pallor
Pulselessness (very late finding)
Poikilothermia

The presence of pulses does *not* rule out compartment syndrome.

- ↓ two-point sensory discrimination
- Paresthesia or hypesthesia
- Tenseness of compartment
- **Late findings:**
  - Pallor of skin
  - Absence of pulses
  - Cold extremity

DIAGNOSIS

- Maintain high index of suspicion in those with high-risk injuries.
- Made by measuring compartment pressure, which can be done with a commercial device (the Stryker) or with an 18G needle connected to a manometer and a water piston via a three-way stopcock.

TREATMENT

- Remove any constricting devices.
- Fasciotomy for pressures > 30 mm Hg.

AVN of the Hip

ETIOLOGY

- The medial and lateral circumflex arteries supply the femoral head and then circle closely around the head of the femur, rendering them vulnerable.
- These arteries may become occluded as in sickle cell disease or during immobilization.
- AVN is also frequently a complication following fractures of the neck of the femur or dislocation of the head.
- May occur at any time postop up to 20 years later.

SIGNS AND SYMPTOMS

- Aching of joint early on
- Difficulty sitting for prolonged periods
- Weakness of hip
- Limp

DIAGNOSIS

- Radiographs may not show signs of the disease until it is more advanced so that the femoral head has started to flatten and become irregularly shaped.
- Later films show evidence of OA.

TREATMENT

- In less severe cases, physical therapy can provide a strengthening and mobility program and assistive devices for protective weight bearing.
- More severe cases require total hip replacement followed by physical therapy.
- There is a worse prognosis in older patients compared to the young who are still growing.

Endocrine Emergencies

The most common cause of adrenal crisis is abrupt withdrawal of steroid therapy.

DEFINITION

Acute life-threatening emergency that occurs secondary to cortisol and aldosterone insufficiency.

ETIOLOGY

- Autoimmune
- Infections (tuberculosis [TB], fungal)
- Metastatic cancer
- Adrenal hemorrhage (trauma, burns, sepsis, coagulopathy)
- Drugs
- Withdrawal of steroid therapy

SIGNS AND SYMPTOMS

- Shock
- Anorexia
- Nausea, vomiting
- Abdominal pain
- Fatigue
- Confusion, coma
- Fever
- Hyperpigmentation (seen in long-standing primary adrenal insufficiency)

Adrenal insufficiency is low serum cortisol, diagnosed by inadequate response to ACTH stimulation test, or 24-hour urine cortisol level.

DIAGNOSIS

- Blood draw for electrolytes, cortisol, adrenocorticotropic hormone (ACTH).
- Low serum cortisol level and inadequate serum cortisol response 30 or 60 minutes after ACTH stimulation test (cosyntropin stimulation test).
- Electrolyte abnormalities: Hyperkalemia and hyponatremia.
- Computed tomographic (CT) scan of the abdomen may show hemorrhage in the adrenals, calcification of the adrenals (seen with TB), or metastasis.
- Electrocardiogram (ECG) may show elevated peaked T waves indicating hyperkalemia.

TREATMENT

- Aggressive rehydration with normal saline (NS) or 5% dextrose in NS (D_5NS).
- Steroid replacement with dexamethasone (will not affect stimulation test).
- Identification and treatment of precipitating cause.
- Long-term glucocorticoid and mineralocorticoid replacement.
- An ACTH stimulation test may be helpful to confirm a diagnosis of adrenal insufficiency. However, it is not indicated in the emergency department (ED), and it should not delay timely treatment of patients in adrenal crisis.

DEFINITION

- Most common endocrine disorder in the world (up to 3% of population).
- Type 1: Autoimmune pancreatic beta-cell destruction with resulting insulin deficiency.
- Type 2: Genetically influenced disease characterized by impairment in insulin secretion and/or action (incidence is increasing in North America).
- Fasting plasma glucose > 126 mg/dL on two occasions in the presence of symptoms of hyperglycemia.
- Absolute or relative deficiency of insulin.

PATHOPHYSIOLOGY

- Insulin is a major anabolic hormone with inhibitory effects on ketogenesis, glycogenolysis, lipolysis, and proteolysis.
- Inhibits ketogenesis, glycogenolysis, lipolysis, gluconeogenesis.

SIGNS AND SYMPTOMS

- Usually presents with symptomatic hyperglycemia or diabetic ketoacidosis (DKA) (discussed below)
- Polyuria
- Polydipsia
- Weight loss
- Dehydration
- Blurred vision
- Fatigue

TREATMENT

- Insulin injections for Type 1 DM
- Oral hypoglycemic agents alone or in combination with insulin for Type 2 DM

DAWN PHENOMENON

Early morning hyperglycemia from decreasing insulin concentration and increasing insulin requirement from surge in counterregulatory hormones (eg, growth hormone [GH]).

SOMOGYI EFFECT

- Characterized by nighttime hypoglycemia followed by a dramatic ↑ in fasting glucose levels and ↑ plasma ketones.
- The morning hyperglycemia is a rebound effect.
- Intermediate-acting insulin administration at bedtime (rather than earlier in the evening) can prevent this effect (try to avoid peaking of insulin effect in the middle of the night).

A patient presents with persistent morning hyperglycemia, despite steadily increasing his nighttime NPH insulin dose. Further, he complains of frequent nightmares. His wife brings him now because she witnessed him having a seizure in the middle of the night. *Think: Somogyi effect.*

A 13-year-old boy presents with vomiting and not feeling well for 2 days. He reports several days of malaise and fatigue. He appears pale and diaphoretic. He is afebrile but tachycardic to 120 with a BP of 105/70 mm Hg. His blood sugar is 590. His Na is 127 mEq/L, Cl 97 mEq/L, bicarbonate 8 mEq/L, and K 5.8 mEq/L. He has no significant past medical history and takes no medications. On questioning, he does note that he has had some polydipsia and polyuria for the past several weeks. What is the cause of his symptoms?

He has DKA, as the first presentation of diabetes mellitus. He has an anion gap (22) metabolic acidosis, consistant with DKA. Serum ketones are also elevated. The initial goal of therapy is aggressive fluid rehydration. His hyponatremia is secondary to the elevated glucose, and his hyperkalemia will correct with insulin therapy.

DEFINITION

- State of absolute or relative insulin deficiency and counterregulatory excess resulting in hyperglycemia, dehydration, acidosis, and ketosis.
- More common in Type 1 diabetics.

ETIOLOGY

Most common causes:

- Infection
- Discontinuation of insulin replacement
- New-onset DM

PATHOPHYSIOLOGY

- Insulin deficiency and counterregulatory hormones cause severe hyperglycemia.
- Hyperglycemia → osmotic diuresis and depletion of Na, K^+, PO_4, water.
- Counterregulatory hormones enhance lipolysis and free fatty acid generation. Beta oxidation of free fatty acid produces ketones.
- Ketosis and anion gap metabolic acidosis.
- Acetone, a volatile ketone, produces the fruity odor typical of DKA.

SIGNS AND SYMPTOMS

- Symptomatic hyperglycemia (polyuria, polydipsia, nocturia).
- Weakness, nausea, vomiting.
- Confusion, coma.
- Signs of dehydration are present, and patients may be hypotensive and tachycardic.
- Kussmaul respirations (slow deep breaths) may be present.
- Acetone (fruity) odor may be present on the patient's breath.
- Fever suggests underlying infection.
- Cerebral edema primarily affects children; mortality is 20–40%.

DIAGNOSIS

- Hyperglycemia.
- Hyperketonemia.
- **Anion gap metabolic acidosis** (ketones are unmeasured ions).
- Usually, the diagnosis can be presumed at the bedside if patient's urine is strongly positive for ketones and the fingerstick glucose is high.
- Glucose is usually between 400 and 800 mg/dL.
- Initially, potassium is high due to acidosis but drops with treatment, so it is important to replace it.
- Blood urea nitrogen (BUN) may be ↑ because of prerenal azotemia.

TREATMENT

- Rapid administration of intravenous (IV) fluids (initially NS) should begin promptly (usual deficit is 3–6 L); fluid rehydration should be the first priority.
- Insulin infusion to control hyperglycemia and reverse ketosis: Infuse at 0.1 U/kg/h; an initial bolus of 0.1 U/kg can be given, but is not necessary.
- Continue insulin infusion until glucose is < 250 *and* ketoacidosis (anion gap) is resolved (change intravenous [IV] fluid to ½ NS when glucose is < 250).
- Monitor glucose every hour and electrolytes every 2–4 hours.
- Bicarbonate (to reverse acidosis) is not recommended:
  - Side effects include lowering intracellular pH, hypokalemia, and shifting O_2 dissociation curve.
  - Use of bicarbonate may ↑ the risk of developing cerebral edema in children.
  - If used, it should be reserved for selected patients with pH < 6.9 or severe hyperkalemia.
- A "normal" potassium in a patient with DKA is low and needs replacement. Remember, K^+ moves intracellularly with correction of acidosis.
- Frequent monitoring and replacement of serum potassium is essential. Add potassium to IV fluids when K^+ < 4.5; a normal K^+ can become critically low as treatment progresses.
- Replace other electrolytes (eg, phosphate) as needed.
- Identify and treat precipitating cause aggressively.

DKA treatment goals:
- Replacement of fluid losses
- Correction of metabolic derangements
- Reversal of ketosis
- Treatment of precipitating causes
- Restoration of normal diabetic regimen

Causes of DKA —
5 I's
Infection
Ischemia (cardiac, mesenteric)
Infarction
Ignorance (poor control)
Intoxication (alcohol)

HYPEROSMOLAR HYPERGLYCEMIC STATE (HHS)

DEFINITION

- Otherwise known as nonketotic hyperosmolar coma (NKHC), hyperosmolar nonketotic state (HNS), or hyperosmolar nonketotic coma (HONKC).
- Syndrome of marked hyperglycemia without ketoacidosis.
- Insulin action is inaedequate to prevent hyperglycemia. Small amounts of insulin are present that are enough to protect against lipolysis and subsequent ketoacid generation.
- Absence of ketosis → dramatic hyperglycemia (glucose > 800–1000).
- More common in Type 2 diabetics (who produce small amounts of insulin) and the elderly.

A 73-year-old woman who is a known diabetic is brought in due to altered mental status. The home health aide states the patient ran out of her medicines 4 days ago. Her fingerstick glucose is > 1000. *Think: HHS.*

Endocrine Emergencies

CAUSES

- Infection
- Myocardial infarction (MI)
- Stroke
- Gastrointestinal (GI) bleed
- Pancreatitis
- Uremia
- Drugs (steroids, thiazide diuretics)

SIGNS AND SYMPTOMS

- Symptomatic hyperglycemia and pronounced osmotic diuresis.
- Seizures, coma.
- ↓ skin turgor.
- Hypertonicity of serum.
- More pronounced K, Mg, PO_4 losses than DKA.
- Abdominal pain is usually not a presenting symptom.

TREATMENT

- Replacement of fluid losses (usually deficit is 8–10 L) with NS solution.
- May switch to ½ NS with potassium when $K^+ < 4.5$.
- Insulin requirements may be less than in DKA, but dosing is similar (0.1 U/kg/h).
- Identify and treat precipitating factor.

Rapid correction of hyperosmolar state may → cerebral edema (high mortality).

Even patients with heart failure will require aggressive fluid resuscitation in DKA and HHS.

HYPOGLYCEMIA

DEFINITION

Low plasma glucose (< 60 mg/dL).

CAUSES

Multiple.

SIGNS AND SYMPTOMS

- Low plasma glucose
- Neuroglycopenic symptoms (confusion, irritability)
- Sympathetic activation symptoms (sweating, palpitations, anxiety)

DIAGNOSIS

- Low blood sugar.
- Symptoms of hypoglycemia.
- Reversal of symptoms with restoration of blood glucose.

TREATMENT

- Oral replenishment with fast-acting carbohydrate (glucose tablet, candy, sweetened juice) is appropriate for patients with intact mental status.
- Obtunded patients who cannot tolerate PO should receive IV dextrose:
  - Adults: 25–50 g of 50% dextrose (D50).
  - Pediatrics: 0.25 g/kg (2.5 mL/kg) bolus of 10% dextrose. D50 is irritating to small veins and can cause rebound hypoglycemia from exaggerated insulin response.

Causes of hypoglycemia—
I NEED SUGAR
Insulin/sulfonylurea excess
Neoplasms
Endocrine (Dawn, Somogyi)
Exercise
Dieting/starvation
Sepsis Unreal (factitious)
GI (alimentary/ postprandial)
Alcohol (inhibits gluconeogenesis)
Renal failure

- Patients with adrenal insufficiency may require hydrocortisone in addition to dextrose.
- Patients who require prolonged monitoring of blood sugar (overdose of long-acting insulin or oral hypoglycemics) or are unable to maintain adequate oral glucose intake should be admitted.
- Intramuscular (IM) glucagon can reverse hypoglycemia in 10–15 minutes. Useful when IV access is a problem in obtunded patients.

Hypoglycemia due to certain oral hypoglycemic agents can last up to 24 hours, so it cannot be corrected quickly. Patients with long-acting oral hypoglycemic agent overdose should be admitted to the hospital for 24-hour monitoring and continuous glucose administration.

PARATHYROID DISORDERS

Parathyroid Physiology

- Parathyroid hormone (PTH), calcitonin (from thyroid), and vitamin D work in concert to regulate calcium.
- PTH ↑ serum calcium by three mechanisms:
  1. Increasing resorption of calcium (and phosphate) from bone.
  2. Decreasing renal excretion of calcium (and increasing phosphate excretion).
  3. Stimulating kidneys to produce calcitriol, a potent vitamin D metabolite that enhances intestinal absorption of calcium.

Hyperparathyroidism

CAUSES

- Primary hyperparathyroidism is most common: Parathyroid adenoma, hyperplasia, carcinoma.
- Multiple endocrine neoplasia types I and IIA both feature parathyroid neoplasms as part of the syndrome.
- Milk-alkali syndrome.
- Granulomatous.

Signs of hyperparathyroidism are secondary to hypercalcemia: "Stones, bones, abdominal groans, and psychic moans"

SIGNS AND SYMPTOMS

- Kidney stones
- Bone pain
- Fatigue, confusion, stupor
- Depression
- Abdominal pain (ulcers, pancreatitis)
- Can also be asymptomatic

TREATMENT

- Volume expansion with saline followed by loop diuretics to induce urinary Ca^{2+} loss.
- Identify and treat underlying cause of hypercalcemia.

Hypoparathyroidism

DEFINITION

Syndrome of ↓ calcium, ↑ phosphate, or ↓ PTH.

CAUSES

- Most commonly seen as a complication of thyroid/parathyroid surgery (inadvertent excision).
- Less common causes: Autoimmune, congenital (DiGeorge's), infiltrative (Wilson's hemochromatosis).

SIGNS AND SYMPTOMS

- Perioral and digital paresthesias
- ↓ myocardial contractility
- Chvostek and Trousseau signs

TREATMENT

Treat hypocalcemia.

PHEOCHROMOCYTOMA

> A 35-year-old woman presents to the ED with a sensation of anxiety, palpitations, nausea, and a headache that began 1 hour ago. She has had similar episodes over the past few months, but they seem to be getting worse and the frequency is increasing. She was seen previously for a similar episode and diagnosed with a panic attack. She is noted to be diaphoretic. Her vital signs are significant for a temperature of 37°C (98.6°F), BP of 188/120 mm Hg, and pulse of 120 bpm. What is the cause of her symptoms?
>
> She has hypertension, palpitations, headache, and diaphoresis with prior similar episodes. This is concerning for pheochromocytoma. A CT scan may show signs of an adrenal mass. A formal diagnosis will require urine or plasma metanephrine testing. Her hypertension can be treated with alpha blockade, such as phentolamine or phenoxybenzamine.

DEFINITION

Catecholamine-secreting tumor of neural crest cells, most often found in adrenal medulla.

EPIDEMIOLOGY

- Equal incidence in men and women.
- Tumors in women are three times as likely to be malignant.

CAUSES

Episodes precipitated by abdominal movement, trauma, drugs, or idiopathic.

SIGNS AND SYMPTOMS

Clinical presentation is of catecholamine excess:

- Hypertensive crisis with headaches, chest pain, palpitations, shortness of breath, sweating.
- Sequelae may include arrhythmias, MI, renal failure, lactic acidosis, cerebrovascular accident (CVA), and death.
- Hallmark of disease is marked hypertension (sustained or paroxysmal).

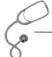

Rule of 10s for pheochromocytoma:
10% are extra-adrenal
10% are bilateral
10% are malignant
10% are familial
10% are pediatric
10% calcify
10% recur after resection

DIAGNOSIS

- Family history in familial disease.
- Elevated urinary catecholamine excretion (vanillylmandelic acid and metanephrines).
- CT or magnetic resonance imaging (MRI) scan of abdomen/pelvis.
- Metaiodobenzylguanidine (MIBG) scan to detect tumors not seen on CT/MRI.

TREATMENT

- Control of hypertension with alpha blockade (phenoxybenzamine).
- Tachycardia may be controlled with beta blockers (propranolol, esmolol) after alpha blockade.
- Avoid use of beta blockers alone (unopposed alpha activity may → paradoxical ↑ in BP).
- Acute hypertensive crisis can be controlled by nitroprusside or phentolamine.

6 H's:
Headache
Hypertension
Hot (diaphoretic)
Heart (palpitations)
Hyperhidrosis
Hyperglycemia

PITUITARY DISORDERS

Pituitary Physiology

- Pituitary gland sits in sella turcica (near optic chiasm and cavernous sinus).
- Anterior pituitary produces thyroid-stimulating hormone (TSH), ACTH, GH, follicle-stimulating hormone (FSH), luteinizing hormone (LH), and prolactin.
- Posterior pituitary stores and releases oxytocin and vasopressin (antidiuretic hormone).
- Tumors of pituitary gland (most commonly prolactinoma) may present with visual field defects (most commonly bitemporal hemianopsia) or cranial nerve palsies (III, IV, V, VI) from local compression.

Pituitary Apoplexy

- Sudden hemorrhage into the pituitary, often into a preexisting adenoma.
- Sudden, severe headache; diplopia; and hypopituitarism.
- May cause life-threatening hypotension.
- Prompt neurosurgical decompression is required.

Sheehan Syndrome

- Rare cause of hypopituitarism
- Postpartum pituitary necrosis
- Failure to lactate and menstruate after delivery

Panhypopituitarism

Hormone loss follows typical sequence: GH (first) → LH/FSH → TSH → ACTH → prolactin (last).

Thyroid Physiology

- Thyroid function controlled by hypothalamus (thyrotropin-releasing hormone) → pituitary (TSH) → thyroid (T_3, T_4).
- Thyroxine (T_4) is converted to triiodothyronine (T_3) (more potent) in peripheral tissues.

Causes of Hyperthyroidism

- Graves disease (autoimmune stimulation of TSH receptors)
- Toxic multinodular goiter
- Toxic adenoma
- Thyroiditis (autoimmune or viral)

Thyroid Storm

A 41-year-old woman with known hyperthyroidism is brought in by her family, who state that she has had days of diarrhea and has now started acting "crazy" with labile mood. She is febrile to 38.9°C (102°F), has a pulse of 140 bpm, a BP of 148/80 mm Hg, and has rales on auscultation. What is the likely diagnosis and first steps in therapy?

This patient appears to have thyroid storm, which is a clinical diagnosis. Given her fever, infectious etiologies (urine, blood, GI, central nervous system [CNS], skin, etc) need to be ruled out and could also have caused her to go into thyroid storm. She can receive acetaminophen for the fever. Propylthiouracil (PTU) or methimazole is given to block new thyroid production. Propranolol will block the adrenergic effects. She can receive iodine in the ED (or during hospital admission), but it should be given at least 90 minutes after the PTU. She will require admission to an intensive care unit setting.

DEFINITION

Life-threatening hypermetabolic state resulting from hyperthyroidism.

EPIDEMIOLOGY

Mortality is high (20–50%) even with the correct treatment. Incidence has ↓ with the advent of a preoperative preparation before thyroid surgery.

ETIOLOGY

- Infection
- Trauma and major surgical procedures
- DKA
- MI, stroke, pulmonary embolism
- Withdrawal of antihyperthyroid medications, iodine administration, thyroid hormone ingestion
- Idiopathic
- Iodine-containing contrast (eg, for CT)

Overactivated sympathetic nervous system causes most of the signs and symptoms of this syndrome:

- Fever > 101°F (38.5°C).
- Tachycardia (out of proportion to fever) with a wide pulse pressure.
- High-output congestive heart failure and volume depletion.
- Exhaustion.
- GI manifestations: Diarrhea, abdominal pain.
- Continuum of CNS alterations (from agitation to confusion when moderate, to stupor or coma with or without seizures).
- Jaundice is a late and ominous manifestation.

DIAGNOSIS

- This is a clinical diagnosis, and since most patients present in need of emergent stabilization, treatment is initiated empirically.
- Patients may have untreated hyperthyroidism.
- May also occur in the setting of unintentional or intentional toxic ingestion of synthetic thyroid hormone.

In initial stabilization of thyroid storm, cooling blankets can be applied to treat hyperpyrexia, if present.

TREATMENT

- Primary stabilization:
  - Airway protection.
  - Oxygenation.
  - Assess circulation (pulse/BP) and continuous cardiac monitoring.
  - IV hydration.
- Definitive treatment:
  - Beta-blocker therapy (eg, propranolol) to block adrenergic effects.
  - Treat fever with acetaminophen (not aspirin, which would displace T_4 from thyroid-binding protein).
  - PTU or methimazole to block synthesis of new thyroid hormone.
  - Iodine to ↓ release of preformed thyroid hormone. Do not give iodine until the PTU has taken effect (1.5 hours).
  - Treat any possible precipitating factors that may be present.
  - Radioiodine administration to destroy thyroid gland once patient is stable and euthyroid.

Treatment with iodine prior to giving PTU or methimazole could worsen symptoms.

Methimazole does not block conversion of T_3 to T_4.

Causes of Hypothyroidism

- Hashimoto thyroiditis (most common cause).
- Iodine deficiency or excess.
- Radiation therapy to neck (from other malignancy).
- Medications (lithium is most common).
- Secondary causes include pituitary tumor, tuberculosis, and Sheehan syndrome.

Myxedema Coma

DEFINITION

Life-threatening complication of hypothyroidism, with profound lethargy or coma usually accompanied by hypothermia: Mortality is 20–50% even if treated early.

Hypothermia may be missed by regular thermometers. Use a rectal or bladder probe if profound hypothermia is present.

Differential diagnosis of myxedema coma:

- **Severe depression or primary psychosis**
- **Drug overdose or toxic exposure**
- **CVA**
- **Liver failure**
- **Hypoglycemia**
- **CO_2 narcosis**
- **CNS infection**

ETIOLOGY

- Sepsis
- Prolonged exposure to cold weather
- CNS depressants (sedatives, narcotics)
- Trauma or surgery

SIGNS AND SYMPTOMS

- Profound lethargy or coma is obvious.
- Hypothermia: Rectal temperature < 35°C (95°F).
- Bradycardia or circulatory collapse.
- Delayed relaxation phase of deep tendon reflexes, areflexia if severe (this can be a very important clue).
- Hyponatremia.
- Hypoglycemia.
- Hypoventilation.

DIAGNOSIS

- History of hypothyroidism.
- Exclude other causes of coma.
- Complete blood count with differential.
- Blood and urine cultures.
- Serum electrolytes, blood urea nitrogen (BUN) and creatinine, blood glucose.
- Urine toxicology screen.
- Serum transaminases and lactic dehydrogenase.
- Arterial blood gas to rule out hypoxemia and CO_2 retention.
- Cortisol level.
- Carboxyhemoglobin.
- Thyroid function testing.
- CT scan and chest radiograph are also commonly ordered because myxedema coma is often a diagnosis of exclusion.

TREATMENT

- Airway management with mechanical ventilation is often necessary.
- Prevent further heat loss but do not initiate active rewarming unless cardiac dysrhythmias are present, as peripheral vasodilation can → hypotension.
- Monitor patient in an intensive care setting.
- Do not let lab results delay therapy.
- Pharmacologic therapy:
  - IV levothyroxine (oral absorption may be impaired).
  - Glucocorticoids (until coexisting adrenal insufficiency is excluded).
  - IV hydration (avoid hypotonic fluids).
  - Rule out and treat any precipitating causes (antibiotics for suspected infection).

Dermatologic Emergencies

Shapes

- Annular: Ring-shaped
- Arcuate: Arc-shaped
- Circinate: Circular
- Confluent: Coalescence of lesions
- Discoid: Coin- or disc-shaped
- Guttate: Scattered
- Gyrate: Coiled and winding
- Herpetiform: Creeping
- Linear: Line-shaped
- Retiform: Net like
- Serpiginous: Wavy linear lesions
- Target: Concentric rings (like a target sign)

Definitions

Flat Lesions

- **Macule:** Nonpalpable, discrete area of change in color. Generally < 10 mm diameter (Figure 15-1).
- **Erythema:** Nonpalpable, diffuse redness, blanchable.
- **Patch:** Nonpalpable, discrete area of change in color > 10 mm diameter. Macule with secondary skin changes like wrinkling, scaling.
- **Telangiectasia:** Small blanchable, visibly dilated blood vessel at skin surface.
- **Petechiae:** Nonblanching purple spots < 2 mm.
- **Purpura:** Nonblanching purple spots > 2 mm (can be palpable in some conditions). Extravasated blood from disruption of dermal vessels.

Raised, Solid Lesions

- **Papule:** Solid, raised lesion < 5 mm diameter (Figure 15-2).
- **Nodule:** Solid, raised lesion > 5 mm diameter (Figure 15-3).
- **Tumor:** Solid, palpable lesion > 10 mm.
- **Induration:** Raised "hardening" of the skin.
- **Cyst:** Nodule with fluid-containing material (Figure 15-4).
- **Wheal:** Transient localized skin edema with peripheral erythema (Figure 15-5).
- **Scale:** Flake of keratinized epidermal cells on top of skin surface (Figure 15-6).
- **Plaque:** Flat-topped lesion of induration (Figure 15-7). Confluence of papules > 5 mm.
- **Crust:** Dried serous/serosanguinous exudate (Figure 15-8).
- **Hyperkeratosis:** Thickened stratum corneum.
- **Lichenification:** Indurated and thickened skin caused by excessive scratching and chronic inflammation.
- **Filiform/Warty:** Flesh-colored, circumscribed hypertrophy of epidermal papillae.

Raised, Fluid-Filled Lesions

- **Vesicle:** Blister < 5 mm diameter (Figure 15-9).
- **Bulla:** Blister > 5 mm diameter.
- **Pustule:** Vesicle with pus (yellow, white, or green in color) (Figure 15-10).

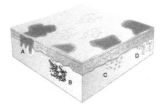

FIGURE 15-1. Macule.

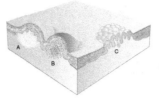

FIGURE 15-2. Papule.

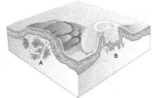

FIGURE 15-3. Nodule.

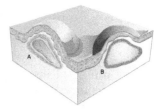

FIGURE 15-4. Cyst.

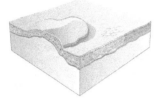

FIGURE 15-5. Wheal.

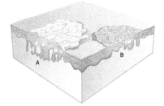

FIGURE 15-6. Scale.

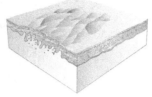

FIGURE 15-7. Plaque.

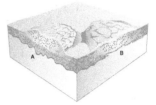

FIGURE 15-8. Crust.

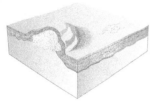

FIGURE 15-9. Vesicle.

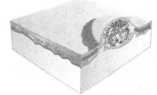

FIGURE 15-10. Pustule.

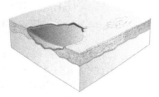

FIGURE 15-11. Erosion.

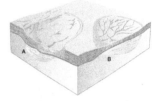

FIGURE 15-12. Atrophy.

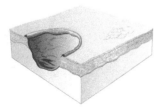

FIGURE 15-13. Ulcer.

Also see Color Insert. (Figures 15-1 to 15-13 are reproduced, with permission, from Wolff K, Johnson RA. *Fitzpatrick's Color Atlas and Synopsis of Clinical Dermatology*, 6th ed. New York: McGraw-Hill, 2009: xxi–xxix.)

- **Comedone:** Collection of sebum and keratin in a blocked, dilated sebaceous duct.
- **Abscess:** Tender, fluctuant pocket of pus with surrounding inflammation deep to skin.

Depressed Lesions
- **Erosion:** Localized epidermal loss (Figure 15-11).
- **Atrophy:** Thinning of skin from layer loss (Figure 15-12).
- **Excoriation:** Abraded or scratched skin.
- **Ulcer:** Localized dermal and epidermal loss (can be deeper) (Figure 15-13).
- **Fissure:** Cleft-shaped ulcer.

Color

Black, white, yellow, red, flesh, brown, hyper- or hypopigmented, blanchable, or nonblanchable.

Distribution

Flexor/extensor surfaces, sun-exposed, dermatomal, clothing-covered, intertriginous, discrete/scattered/grouped.

Size (Does Matter)

- Planar dimensions: Circular—average diameter, oblong—length and width.
- Height/depth: If raised or depth discernible, or if biopsied.
- Large lesions: Estimate body surface area involved (see Environmental Emergencies chapter).

Use the "Rule of 9s" to estimate body surface area. Remember palm of hand is 1%. See Figure 18-2.

GENERAL DIAGNOSIS

History of Present Illness

- Signs and symptoms (painless, itching, burning, etc).
- How long present?
- Where are lesions?
- Evolutionary changes?
- Systemic complaints?
- Exposures (chemicals, foods, animals, plants, medications, etc)?
- Allergies?
- Ever have this before?
- Partially treated?

Examination

See above.

Dermatologic physical exam: Look everywhere.

Diagnostic Procedures

See Table 15-1.

TABLE 15-1. Diagnostic Procedures Used in Dermatology

	DEFINITIONS
Diascopy	Pressing of a glass slide firmly against a red lesion will determine if it is due to capillary dilatation (blanchable) or to extravasation of blood (nonblanchable).
KOH preparation	Used to identify fungus and yeast. Scrape scales from skin, hair, or nails. Treat with a 10% KOH solution to dissolve tissue material. Septated hyphae are revealed in fungal infections, and pseudohyphae and budding spores are revealed in yeast infections.
Tzanck preparation	Used to identify vesicular viral eruptions. Scrape the base of a vesicle and smear cells on a glass slide. Multinucleated giant cells will be identified in herpes simplex, herpes zoster, and varicella infections.
Scabies preparation	Scrape skin of a burrow between fingers, side of hands, axilla, or groin. Mites, eggs, or feces will be identified in scabies infection.
Wood's lamp	Certain conditions will fluoresce when examined under a long-wave ultraviolet light ("black" lamp). Tinea capitis will fluoresce green or yellow on hair shaft.
Patch testing	Detects type IV delayed hypersensitivity reactions (allergic contact dermatitis). Nonirritating concentrations of suspected allergen are applied under occlusion to the back. Development of erythema, edema, and vesicles at site of contact 48 hours later indicates an allergy to offending agent.
Biopsy	Type of biopsy performed depends on the site of lesion, the type of tissue removed, and the desired cosmetic result. Shave biopsy is used for superficial lesions. Punch biopsy (3–5 mm diameter) can remove all or part of a lesion and provides tissue sample for pathology. Elliptical excisions provide more tissue than a punch biopsy and are used for deeper lesions or when the entire lesion needs to be sent to pathology.

Top Dermatologic Problems in Emergency Medicine

(These are the problems you'll most likely be tested on, not necessarily the ones you'll see most frequently in the emergency department).

- Decubitus ulcer
- Abscess
- Cellulitis
- Erysipelas
- Necrotizing infection
- Herpes zoster
- Erythema multiforme (EM)
- Henoch-Schönlein purpura (HSP)
- Purpura
- Urticaria
- Pemphigus
- Staphylococcal scalded syndrome
- Stevens-Johnson syndrome (SJS)
- Toxic epidermal necrolysis (TEN)

Top 12 Causes of Rash with Fever

- Rubella
- Measles
- Staphylococcal scalded skin syndrome
- Toxic shock syndrome
- Scarlet fever
- Meningococcemia
- Disseminated gonococcal infection
- Bacterial endocarditis
- Rocky Mountain spotted fever (RMSF)
- Kawasaki's disease
- Erythema nodosum
- Hypersensitivity vasculitis

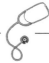

Rashes that can be seen on palms and soles —
MRS. HEP
Meningococcemia
RMSF
Syphilis
Hand, foot, and mouth disease
EM
Psoriasis

GENERAL TREATMENTS

Initial Modalities

- Astringents (drying agents): Domeboro solution
- Emollients (moisturizers): Eucerin cream, lotion

Antihistamines

For pruritic (itchy) disorders:

- Diphenhydramine: Adult, 25–50 mg PO q6h; child, 4–6 mg/kg/24 hr ÷ q6–8 (max 200 mg). Also available as a topical (lotion).
- Hydroxyzine: Adult, 25–100 mg PO q8h; child, 2–4 mg/kg/24 hr ÷ q8–12 (max 200 mg).
- Cetirizine/loratadine/fexofenadine.

If it's wet — dry it.
If it's dry — wet it.
If present, remove offending agent.

Antibacterials (Topical)

- Mupirocin: Used for impetigo
- Bacitracin: Used for burns and cuts
- Neomycin/polymixin B: Used for cuts
- Silver sulfadiazine: Used for burns

Absorption of topical antihistamines is unpredictable.

Antifungals (Topical)

- Polyenes: Nystatin, amphotericin B 3%.
- Imidazoles: Ketoconazole 1%, clotrimazole 1%, miconazole 2%, econazole 1%.

Antiparasitics (Topical)

- Lindane (for age > 1 year):
  - Lice: 1% shampoo 30 mL for 4 minutes, then rinse thoroughly; again after 5 days.
  - Scabies: Lotion 30–60 mL and wash after 8 hours.

Warn patients about drowsiness associated with antihistamines.

Dermatologic Emergencies

Lindane can induce seizure if overused.

The thicker the skin, the more potent steroid needed.

Topicals are first-line agents for treatment of acne.

Tretinoin and isotretinoin are teratogenic.

Exposure to sun while on tetracycline or doxycycline can cause a rash.

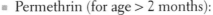

- Permethrin (for age > 2 months):
  - Lice: 1% rinse—wash after 10 minutes, again after 5 days for next generation.
  - Scabies: 5% cream all over and wash thoroughly after 8–12 hours.

Antivirals

Topical
- Acyclovir: 5% ointment q3h × 7 days.
- Used for herpes (varicella, zoster, simplex, and genitalis).

Oral
- Acyclovir:
  - Genitalis: 400 mg PO tid × 10 days
  - Zoster: 800 mg PO 5/day × 7 to 10 days
  - Varicella: 20 mg/kg PO qid × 5 days—max 800 mg
- Famciclovir:
  - Genitalis: 250 mg PO tid × 10 days
  - Zoster: 500 mg PO tid × 7 days
- Valacyclovir:
  - Genitalis: 1 g PO bid × 10 days
  - Zoster: 1 g PO tid × 7 days

Corticosteroids (Topical)

- Potency graded on ability to vasoconstrict: High potency, group I; low potency, group VII.
- Avoid using groups I, II, III, and IV in pregnancy, infancy, face, genitalia, flexure creases, and intertriginous areas.
- Bid–tid therapy for 1–2 weeks (potent), or 2–4 weeks (less potent).

Acne

Topical
- Benzoyl peroxide: Many preparations
- Clindamycin: 10 mg/mL bid
- Tretinoin: Many preparations
- Erythromycin: 1.5–2% bid

Oral
- Tetracycline: 250 mg PO qid
- Doxycycline: 100 mg PO bid
- Isotretinoin: 0.5 mg/kg PO bid

CUTANEOUS BACTERIAL INFECTIONS

Abscess

- **Location:** Back, buttocks, axillae, groin, and anywhere pus can accumulate (acne, wounds).
- **Definition:** Pocket of pus from skin flora.
- **Signs and symptoms:** Red, hot, swollen, and tender.
- **Treatment:** Incise, drain, pack, wound check (see Procedures chapter).

Cellulitis

> A 55-year-old diabetic man presents with a right lower extremity that is red, warm, and tender to the touch. The rash has poorly demarcated borders and has been spreading over the last day. He is febrile to 38.3°C (101°F). What is his most likely diagnosis?
>
> This patient most likely has cellulitis. The borders of the erythema should be marked with a skin marker to assess whether it is receding after therapy. Treatment consists of an antibiotic that targets the causative organism. Usually, this is *Staphylococcus aureus* or other skin flora. Patients should also be advised to keep the area clean. Note in this patient who is diabetic, the risk for his cellulitis becoming systemic sepsis is higher.

- **Location:** Commonly lower extremities (diabetics and peripheral vascular disease), but can be anywhere.
- **Definition:** Superficial skin and subcutaneous tissue infection from skin flora *(S aureus, Streptococcus pyogenes)*.
- **Signs and symptoms:** Red, hot, swollen, and tender.
- **Treatment:** Outpatient oral antibiotics in the young and healthy (first-generation cephalosporin) or inpatient intravenous (IV) antibiotics in the frail/elderly. Consideration should also be given for MRSA coverage (eg, TMP/SMX), especially in communities with high rates of MRSA.

Erysipelas, erysipeloid, and necrotizing fasciitis are variants of cellulitis.

Impetigo

- **Definition:** Bacterial superinfection of epidermis from broken skin. Bullous *(S aureus)* and nonbullous (group A beta-hemolytic strep [GAS]).
- **Location:** Face (usually), can be anywhere (Figure 15-14).
- **Age group:** Preschool children with predisposing atopic dermatitis.
- **Signs and symptoms:**
  - Slow evolving pustules.
  - Initial lesion is a transient erythematous papule or thin-roofed vesicle that ruptures easily and forms a "honey-colored" crust.

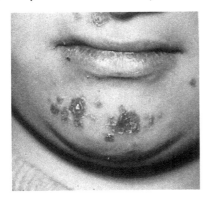

FIGURE 15-14. Impetigo.

(Reproduced, with permission, from Pantell R, et al. *The Common Symptom Guide*, 4th ed. New York: McGraw-Hill, 1996.)

- Lesions can be discrete and scattered or become confluent, forming a superficial crusted plaque.
- Pruritic but not painful.
- Lymph nodes—enlarged.
- Contagious.
- Investigations: Gram staining after removal of the crust.
- **Treatment:**
  - Remove crusts by soaking in warm water.
  - Antibacterial washes (benzoyl peroxide).
  - Topical antibiotic if disease is limited (mupirocin).
  - Oral antibiotics (eg, first-generation cephalosporin or erythromycin).
  - For bullous impetigo–penicillinase-resisitant penicillins like dicloxacillin/erythromycin.
- **Complications:** Post–pyodermal acute glomerulonephritis.

Erysipelas

- **Definition:** An acute onset of superficial spreading cellulitis, arising in inconspicuous breaks in skin; involves dermis and epidermis. Pathogens include *S aureus*, GAS, and occasionally *Haemophilus influenzae*.
- **Location:** Leg (most often), face, arm (Figure 15-15).
- **Age group:** Very young or very old.
- **Signs and symptoms:**
  - An erythematous, shiny area of warm and tender skin with a well-demarcated and indurated advancing border.
  - Less edematous than cellulitis, but margins are more sharply demarcated and elevated.
  - Can affect any area, especially sites of chronic edema.
  - Painful.
- **Treatment:** Same as for cellulitis, including elevation, IV antibiotics (penicillin G or amoxicillin), with care taken if orbital involvement to consult ophthalmologist.

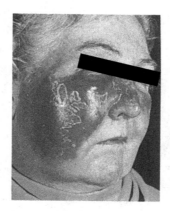

FIGURE 15-15. Erysipelas.

Also see Color Insert. (Reproduced, with permission, from Fauci AS et al. *Harrison's Principles of Internal Medicine*, 17th ed. New York: McGraw-Hill, 2009: Figure e5-15.)

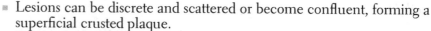

Lyme Disease

- Most common vector-borne disease in the United States.
- **Definition:** Chronic multisystem infection with spirochete *Borrelia burgdorferi* transmitted through *Ixodes* ticks in Atlantic and Northeast states. Rash is erythema chronicum migrans (ECM), a spreading, annular, macular erythema seen 2–20 days from site of tick bite.
- **Location:** Usually affects the groin, popliteal folds, axillary folds, earlobes.
- Viral prodrome followed by neurologic cardiac or joint manifestations followed by chronic joint and neurologic abnormality.

SIGNS AND SYMPTOMS

- Stage 1:
  - Within weeks of exposure.
  - Fever, malaise, headache.
  - Rash: Erythema migrans characterized by target lesions. A target lesion is a red annular lesion with a central clearing.
- Stage 2:
  - Weeks to months after exposure.
  - Neurologic symptoms: (encephalitis, cranial neuropathy [Bell's palsy]).
  - Myocarditis.
- Stage 3:
  - Chronic infection, months to years after exposure.
  - Migratory oligoarthritis.
  - Subtle neurologic symptoms.

DIAGNOSIS

- Clinical suspicion
- Serologic testing

TREATMENT

Doxycycline 100 mg PO bid × 21 days (or clarithromycin, amoxicillin, cefuroxime).

Rocky Mountain Spotted Fever (RMSF)

A 7-year-old boy presents with a high fever, myalgias, and a rash of 2 days that consists of 2- to 6-mm pink, blanchable macules that first appear peripherally on wrists, forearms, ankles, palms, and soles, then spread to the trunk. He complains that his calves hurt. He just returned from a camping trip in Oklahoma a few days ago. What infection are you worried about?

Rocky Mountain spotted fever. RMSF is potentially life-threatening disease secondary to a tick bite. The infected tick adheres to vascular endothelium, resulting in vascular necrosis and extravasation of blood. Highest incidence occurs in children aged 5–10 years, with 95% cases occurring from April to September. This child should be treated promptly with antibiotics, even if diagnosis is not fully confirmed. Some patients develop long-term sequelae lasting > 1 year, including paraparesis, hearing loss; peripheral neuropathy; bladder/bowel incontinence; and cerebellar, vestibular, and motor dysfunction.

Lyme disease can cause Bell's palsy (CNVII dysfunction).

A 39-year-old woman presents with a rash on her right leg that she initially thought was an insect bite. It is an erythematous annular plaque with a central clearing. *Think: ECM.*

- **Definition:** A potentially life-threatening disease caused by *Rickettsia rickettsii* transmitted by a tick bite (*Dermacentor* tick).
- **Location:** Wrists and ankles (acral rash), then spreads to trunk (Figure 15-16).
- **Age groups:** 5- to 10-year-olds.
- Ninety-five percent of cases occur from April through September.
- Occurs only in the Western hemisphere, primarily in southeastern states and most often in Oklahoma, North and South Carolina, and Tennessee.
- Zoonotic hosts: Deer, rodents, horses, cattle, cats, dogs.
- Rarely occurs in the Rocky Mountains.
- Only 60% of patients report a history of a tick bite.

SIGNS AND SYMPTOMS

- *R rickettsii* through tick bite invades bloodstream and causes blanching, maculopapular lesions that become petechial and can coalesce and become ecchymotic or gangrenous.
- Sudden onset of high **fever,** myalgia, severe headache, rigors, nausea, and photophobia within first 2 days of tick bite.
- Classic triad: Fever, rash with history of tick bite.
- Fifty percent develop rash within 3 days. Another 30% develop the rash within 6 days.

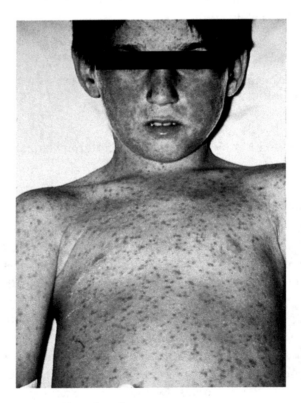

FIGURE 15-16. Late manifestation of RMSF.

Also see Color Insert. Note disseminated macules and papules. Initial lesions were noted on the palms and soles, wrists, and ankle and extended centripetally. (Reproduced, with permission, from Wolff K, Johnson RA. *Fitzpatrick's Color Atlas and Synopsis of Clinical Dermatology*, 6th ed. New York: McGraw-Hill, 2009: 765.)

- Rash consists of 2- to 6-mm pink **blanchable macules** that first appear peripherally on wrists, forearms, ankles, palms, and soles.
- Within 6–18 hours the exanthem spreads centrally to trunk, proximal extremities, and face.
- Within 1–3 days, the macules evolve to deep red papules, and within 2–4 days, the exanthem is hemorrhagic and no longer blanchable.
- Up to 15% have no rash.

DIAGNOSIS

- Indirect fluorescent antibody (IFA) assay.
- Titer > 1:64 is diagnostic.
- Most sensitive and specific test.
- Other, less sensitive tests include indirect hemagglutinin, Weil-Felix, complement fixation, and latex agglutination tests.
- Biopsy would demonstrate necrotizing vasculitis.
- Laboratory analysis typically demonstrates neutropenia with thrombocytopenia with hyponatremia and elevated liver function tests (LFTs).
- In real time, RMSF is a clinical diagnosis (because current diagnostic tests aren't back fast enough). It is important not to delay treatment.

Many patients with RMSF have exquisite tenderness of the gastrocnemius muscle.

TREATMENT

- Doxycycline 100 mg PO bid × 7 days.
- Use chloramphenicol for pregnant patients and children under age 8. (*Note:* Chloramphenicol is contraindicated for children < 2 years.)

Scarlet Fever

- **Definition:** An erythrogenic toxin-mediated disease caused by Group A or C β-hemolytic streptococci.
- **Location:** Neck, axillae, groin.

SIGNS AND SYMPTOMS

- Fever, abdominal pain, sore throat.
- Pain precedes rash and follows fever.
- A finely punctate pink-scarlet exanthem first appears on upper trunk 12–48 hours after onset of fever.
- As the exanthem spreads to extremities, it becomes confluent and feels like sandpaper and fades within 4–5 days, followed by desquamation.
- Linear petechiae evident in body folds (Pastia's sign).
- Facial flush and circumoral pallor.
- Pharynx is beefy red and tongue is initially white, but within 4–5 days, the white coating sloughs off and tongue becomes bright red ("strawberry tongue").
- Hemorrhagic spots are noted on the soft palate.
- Desquamation happens post 2 weeks.

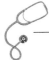

The sandpaper rash is typical of scarlet fever.

Complications of untreated scarlet fever include:
- Acute rheumatic fever
- Acute glomerulonephritis
- Erythema nodosum

TREATMENT

Oral penicillin or erythromycin, acetaminophen.

Gonococcemia

A 20-year-old college student has a low-grade fever, chills, and migratory polyarthralgias accompanied by a tender rash. The rash initially consisted of erythematous macules that have now evolved into hemorrhagic pustules. What diagnosis are you concerned about? Disseminated gonococcal infection.

- **Definition:** Emboli of disseminated *Neisseria gonorrhoeae*, usually in menstruating or peripartum females. Looks like multiple papular, vesicular, and pustular petechial lesions with erythematous base that become hemorrhagic; associated fever and arthralgias.
- **Location:** Anywhere.
- **Risk factors:** Third-trimester pregnancy, postpartum period, 7 days within menses onset.
- **Signs and symptoms:** Painful.
- **Treatment:** IV ceftriaxone or ciprofloxacin.

Meningococcemia

- **Definition:** Infectious vasculitis from emboli of disseminated *Neisseria meningitidis*.
- **Location:** Extremities and trunk (anywhere) (Figure 15-17). Mucous membrane involvement is present.
- **Age group:** < 20 years.
- Often occur in epidemics, aerosol transfer.

Complications of meningococcemia include meningitis and Waterhouse-Friderichsen syndrome (fulminant meningococcemia with adrenal hemorrhage).

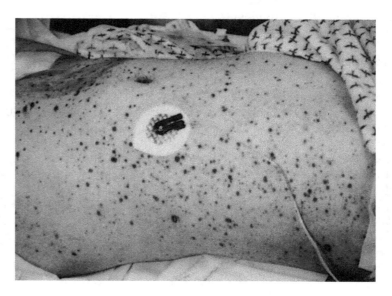

FIGURE 15-17. Meningococcemia.

Also see Color Insert. (Photo contributed by Kevin J. Knoop, MD. Reproduced, with permission, from Knoop KJ, Stack LB, Storrow AB, Thurman RJ. *The Atlas of Emergency Medicine*, 3rd ed. New York: McGraw-Hill, 2010: 423.)

- Petechia, urticaria, hemorrhagic vesicles, macules, and papules with surrounding erythema.
- Associated with fever, altered mental status and vitals, headache, arthralgias, and stiff neck.
- Petechiae transform into papules with grey necrotic central areas.

TREATMENT

IV ceftriaxone, add vancomycin for cephalosporin-resistant pneumococcus. Admit to the hospital.

Toxic Shock Syndrome

- **Definition:** Severe, life-threatening, multisystem syndrome arising because of *S aureus* toxic shock syndrome toxin (TSST-1) in menstruating women using tampons, or enterotoxins B and C also from *Staphylococcus* but unrelated to tampon use.
- **Location:** Diffuse or just extremities/trunk.

SIGNS AND SYMPTOMS

- Nonpruritic, tender erythroderma.
- **Fever, hypotension,** diffuse organ pathology, erythroderma followed by desquamation, mucosal hyperemia (three of four must be present).
- Staphylococcal—painless; streptococcal—may present with local tenderness.
- Erythema may resolve in 3–5 days with subsequent desquamation of hands and feet in 5–14 days.
- In addition to major criteria, there must be evidence of multisystem involvement such as altered mental status, heart failure, adult respiratory distress syndrome (ARDS), diarrhea, renal insufficiency, thrombocytopenia, or arthralgias.

TREATMENT

Hospital admission, aggressive IV fluid resuscitation, IV oxacillin or cefazolin, vancomycin if penicillin allergic.

Patients with circulatory insufficiency, WBC < 10,000, and coagulopathy are at higher risk of systemic involvement and death.

FUNGAL INFECTIONS

Candida

- **Definition:** *Candida albicans,* normally a nonpathogenic colonizer of moist skin and mucosa, causes painful, raised, whitish plaques that detach and leave red erosions.
- **Location:** Can be on mucous membranes (palate, pharynx, tongue, vagina) or can be cutaneous (intertriginous, groin, under fat pannus).
- **Risk factors:** Obesity, systemic antibiotics, corticosteroid or chemotherapy, urinary or fecal incontinence, and immunocompromised states.
- **Signs and symptoms:** Painful, pruritic in vagina.
- **Treatment:** Oral nystatin swish and swallow 5 mL tid for oral lesions; topical nystatin or clotrimazole cream for cutaneous and vaginal types. Fluconazole 150 mg PO single dose for both oral and vaginal types.

Tinea Infection

- Tinea are fungal infections caused by *Trichophyton* and *Microsporum* species and are named according to the part of the body they are on:
  - Tinea cruris: Groin, gluteal cleft.
  - Tinea pedis: Feet, in between toes (athlete's foot).
  - Tinea versicolor: On trunk, multiple-colored lesions that do not tan with surrounding skin in sunlight.
  - Tinea corporis: See Figure 15-18.
  - Tinea capitis: Invade hair shafts and surrounding skin; causes red, circular patches with raised edges, sometimes swollen, boggy, and crusted, with loss of hair:
  - **Treatment:** Griseofulvin 7.5 mg/kg PO bid × 6 weeks.

PARASITIC INFECTIONS

Pediculosis (Lice)

- **Definition:** *Phthirus capitis* mite lives on scalp and lays eggs (nits) on hair shafts; lives on human blood.
- **Location:** *P capitis* on scalp and neck. *Phthirus pubis* (crabs) in pubic hair.
- **Signs and symptoms:** Severe itch.
- **Treatment:** Permethrin, then lindane, fine-toothed comb to manually remove nits.

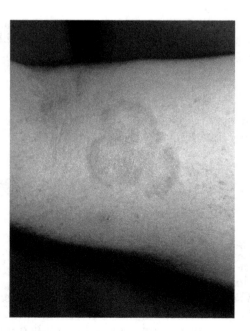

FIGURE 15-18. Tinea corporis.

Also see Color Insert. (Reproduced, with permission, from Kane KS et al. *Color Atlas and Synopsis of Pediatric Dermatology*, 2nd ed. New York: McGraw-Hill, 2009: 393.)

Scabies

- **Location:** Flexural creases, hands, feet.
- **Definition:** *Sarcoptes scabiei*, the "itch mite," burrows into the skin and lays its eggs.
- **Signs and symptoms:** Intense itch and mild burning; excoriations and pruritic red papules (Figure 15-19).
- **Treatment:** Lindane or permethrin.

VIRAL INFECTIONS

Varicella-Zoster (Shingles)

- **Definition:** An acute dermatomal viral infection caused by reactivation of latent varicella-zoster virus that has remained dormant in a sensory root ganglion. The virus travels down the sensory nerve, resulting initially in dermatomal pain, followed by skin lesions.
- **Location:** Commonly thoracic and facial dermatomes.
- **Risk factors:** Age, malignancy, immunosuppression, and radiation.

SIGNS AND SYMPTOMS

- Prodrome of pain, burning, itching, and paresthesia in affected dermatome precedes eruption by 3–5 days.
- Accompanied by fever, headache, and malaise, and heightened sensitivity to stimuli (allodynia).
- Maculopapular rash that quickly transitions to become a vesicular eruption.
- Grouped vesicles on an erythematous base distributed unilaterally along a dermatome (Figure 15-20).
- Crust formation within 5–10 days.
- Some vesicles may occur outside of involved dermatome.

A 27-year-old human immunodeficiency virus (HIV)-positive patient presents due to an intensely painful erythematous rash that is over his right flank in a dermatomal distribution. *Think: Varicella-zoster.*

Patients with zoster can infect nonimmune contacts with chickenpox. Exposed nonimmune contacts should be treated with varicella-zoster immune globulin.

Varicella-zoster infection of cranial nerve VIII is called Ramsay Hunt syndrome and results in hearing loss, vertigo, and tinnitus.

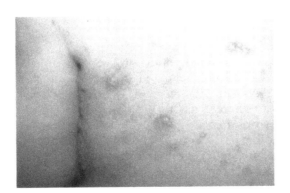

FIGURE 15-19. Scabies.

Notice the papulovesicular nature of the rash, which tends to occur in places where mites can burrow, such as the web spaces of the digits and the axilla, as shown here. (Reproduced, with permission, from Rudolph A, et al. *Rudolph's Pediatrics*, 20th ed. Stamford, CT: Appleton & Lange, 1997.)

HIGH-YIELD FACTS

Dermatologic Emergencies

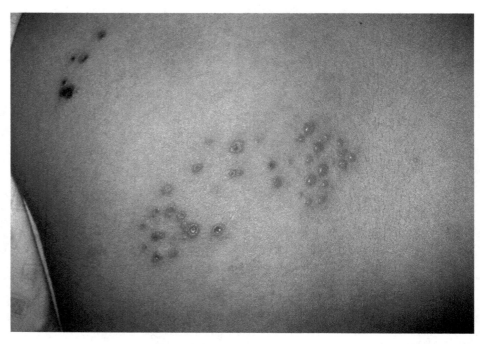

FIGURE 15-20. Varicella-zoster infection.

Also see Color Insert. Note dermatomal distribution (T8–10) to rash. (Reproduced, with permission, from Kane KS et al. *Color Atlas and Synopsis of Pediatric Dermatology*, 2nd ed. New York: McGraw-Hill, 2009: 431.)

Varicella-zoster infection of V₁ (ophthalmic branch of trigeminal nerve) can be vision threatening. Ophthalmic consultation should be obtained for these cases.

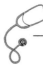

Hutchison sign:
Tip of nose lesions — suborbital ophthalmic branch of CN V being involved.
Be wary of development of herpes zoster ophthalmicus.

TREATMENT

- Moist and cool compresses to affected dermatome.
- Oral acyclovir, valacyclovir, or famciclovir (accelerate healing of lesions and ↓ duration of pain if started within 3 days of infection).
- Analgesics.

Molluscum Contagiosum

- **Definition:** A self-limited contagious poxvirus infection transmitted by direct contact and characterized by an umbilicated "pearly" papule; commonly seen with HIV.
- **Location:** Anywhere, typically head and neck.
- **Signs and symptoms:**
  - Mild pruritus.
  - Shiny, umbilicated, slightly translucent skin or flesh-colored papules (Figure 15-21); slow growing, < 10 mm diameter, sometimes grouped.
- **Treatment:** Cryotherapy, surgical excision, or wait it out; resolves in 12–18 months.

Verruca (Warts)

- **Definition:** Human papillomavirus (common warts—hard, rough, skin-colored papules) and others (plantar warts—bottom of foot; plane warts, also called flat warts; mosaic warts) caused by different viruses.
- **Location:** Anywhere, typically hands.

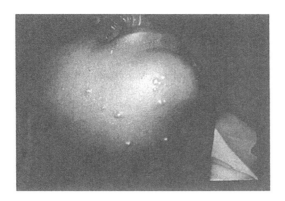

FIGURE 15-21. Molluscum contagiosum.

(Reproduced, with permission, from Seltzer V, Pearse WH. *Women's Primary Health Care: Office Practice and Procedures*, 2nd ed. New York: McGraw-Hill, 2000.)

SIGNS AND SYMPTOMS

- Initial lesion is skin colored with a smooth surface.
- As lesion enlarges with time, the surface becomes roughened and papillomatous.
- Several types of warts exist and are named according to their location.

TREATMENT

- Cryotherapy with liquid nitrogen or carbon dioxide (requires multiple treatments every 2–3 weeks and is painful).
- Topical application of keratolytic agents (salicylic acid and lactic acid) and destructive agents (podophyllin or cantharidin).
- Curettage and desiccation.
- Topical imiquimod (an immune response modifier that stimulates the immune system to fight the virus).
- Or wait it out; resolves in 2–3 years.

There is an ↑ incidence of verrucae in atopic and immunocompromised patients.

IMMUNOGENIC CUTANEOUS DISORDERS

Angioedema

- Definition:
  - Immunologic (associated with food, cold, insect venom, pollen) mechanism is immunoglobulin E (IgE)–antigen complex triggered massive histamine release.
  - Nonimmunologic (associated with angiotensin-converting enzyme [ACE] inhibitors, contrast dye) mechanism not well understood.
- **Location:** Face (tongue, lips, larynx, more), anywhere.
- **Signs and symptoms:** Warm; itchy; difficulty breathing, talking, and swallowing due to airway edema.

Remember:
Hereditary angioedema:
C1 esterase deficiency

TREATMENT

- Airway, breathing, circulation (ABCs).
- For stridor, wheezing, or low SaO_2:
  - Subcutaneous (SQ) epinephrine.
  - Albuterol nebulizer.

- Consider early intubation (patient's airway can be rapidly lost due to significant airway edema).
- IV methylprednisolone.
- IV diphenhydramine (H_1 blocker).
- Some people give IV H_2 blocker (thought to provide some cross-reactive antihistamine benefit).
- Admit for observation.

Urticaria

- **Definition:** An immunologic reaction that results in mast-cell degranulation of histamine, causing localized capillary and postcapillary venule leak of proteinaceous fluid that is gradually resorbed. Histamine also causes vasodilation, giving localized erythema and classic wheal appearance. Types include immune type I (IgE) and type III immune-complex IgG and IgM (drugs, pollen, dust, animal dander) and non–immune mediated (cold, pressure, heat, cholinergic, dermatographism, strawberries).
- **Location:** Anywhere.

Signs and Symptoms

- Characterized by **wheals:** An abrupt development of transient, edematous, pink papules and plaques that may be localized or generalized and are usually pruritic.
- Wheals may develop after exposure to circulating antigens (drugs, food, insect venom, animal dander, pollen), hot and cold temperatures, exercise, and pressure or rubbing (dermatographism).
- Wheals usually last < 24 hours and may recur on future exposure to the antigen.

Treatment

- Antihistamines (H_1 and H_2 blockers).
- SQ epinephrine if anaphylactic/impending associated airway compromise.
- PO or IV corticosteroids if severe.
- Observation.
- Supportive therapy.

Bullous Pemphigoid

- **Definition:** Autoimmune disorder with immunoglobulin G (IgG) antibodies to the dermoepidermal junction giving vesicles and bullae that lyse and yield erosions.
- **Location:** Anywhere (skin and mucosa—usually oral).
- **Age group:** Elderly.

Signs and Symptoms

- Occasional pruritus and tenderness/burning sensation.
- Large, erythematous urticarial plaques may precede bullae by months.
- Multiple, intact, tense bullae become crusted after rupturing.
- Bullae can be localized or generalized, primarily distributed on intertriginous areas, flexural areas of axilla, groin, medial thighs, forearms, and lower legs (Figure 15-22).

Pemphigus Vulgaris vs. Bullous Pemphigoid
In pemphigus vulgaris the bullae are intraepidermal whereas in bullous pemphigoid they are subepidermal. Since the lesions are below the basement membrane, bullae in bullous pemphigoid are more tense.

Remember: Nikolsky's sign is positive in pemphigus vulgaris.

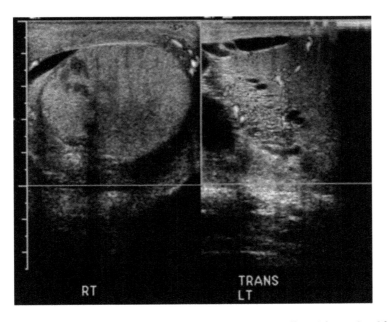

FIGURE 9-2. Doppler ultrasound of bilateral testes shows swollen right testis with hypoechoic areas within and reduced arterial signal suggesting testicular torsion with necrosis *(left panel).* This is compared to the left testis, which has normal flow *(right panel).*

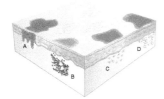

FIGURE 15-1. Macule.

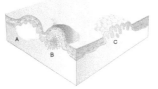

FIGURE 15-2. Papule.

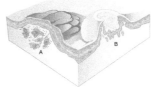

FIGURE 15-3. Nodule.

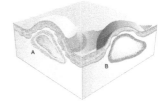

FIGURE 15-4. Cyst.

(Figures 15-1 to 15-4 are reproduced, with permission, from Wolff K, Johnson RA. *Fitzpatrick's Color Atlas and Synopsis of Clinical Dermatology,* 6th ed. New York: McGraw-Hill, 2009: xxvii–xxxiii.)

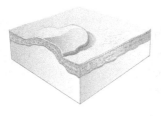

FIGURE 15-5. Wheal.

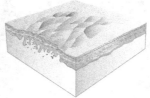

FIGURE 15-6. Scale.

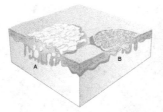

FIGURE 15-7. Plaque.

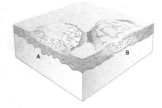

FIGURE 15-8. Crust.

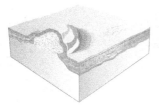

FIGURE 15-9. Vesicle.

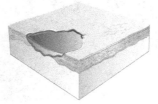

FIGURE 15-10. Pustule.

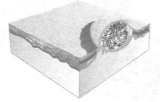

FIGURE 15-11. Erosion.

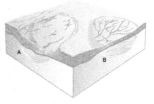

FIGURE 15-12. Atrophy.

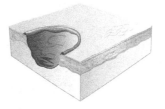

FIGURE 15-13. Ulcer.

HIGH-YIELD FACTS

High-Yield Images

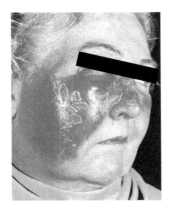

FIGURE 15-15. Erysipelas.

(Reproduced, with permission, from Fauci AS et al. *Harrison's Principles of Internal Medicine*, 17th ed. New York: McGraw-Hill, 2009: Figure e5-15.)

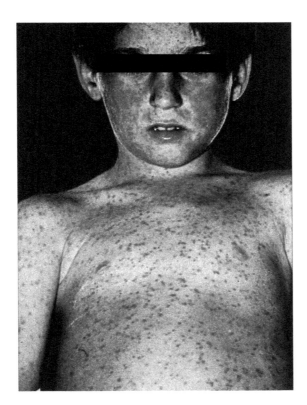

FIGURE 15-16. Late Manifestation of RMSF.

Note disseminated macules and papules. Initial lesions were noted on the palms and soles, wrists, and ankle and extended centripetally. (Reproduced, with permission, from Wolff K, Johnson RA. *Fitzpatrick's Color Atlas and Synopsis of Clinical Dermatology*, 6th ed. New York: McGraw-Hill, 2009: 765.)

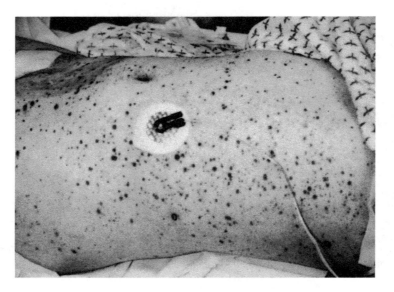

FIGURE 15-17. **Meningococcemia.**

(Photo contributed by Kevin J. Knoop, MD. Reproduced, with permission, from Knoop KJ, Stack LB, Storrow AB, Thurman RJ. *The Atlas of Emergency Medicine*, 3rd ed. New York: McGraw-Hill, 2010: 423.)

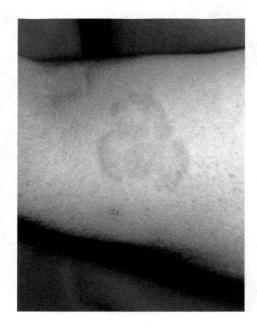

FIGURE 15-18. **Tinea corporis.**

(Reproduced, with permission, from Kane KS et al. *Color Atlas and Synopsis of Pediatric Dermatology*, 2nd ed. New York: McGraw-Hill, 2009: 393.)

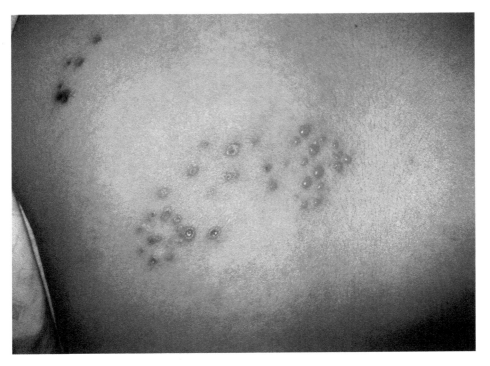

FIGURE 15-20. Varicella-zoster infection.

Note dermatomal distribution (T8–10) to rash. (Reproduced, with permission, from Kane KS et al. *Color Atlas and Synopsis of Pediatric Dermatology*, 2nd ed. New York: McGraw-Hill, 2009: 431.)

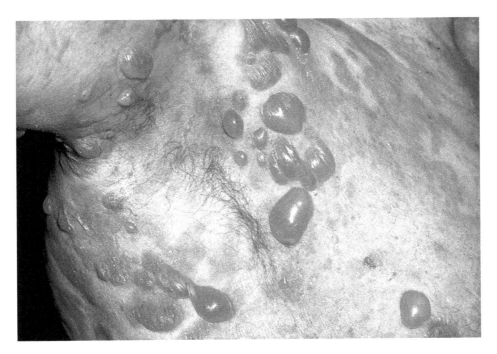

FIGURE 15-22. Bullous pemphigoid.

(Reproduced, with permission, from Wolff K, Johnson RA. *Fitzpatrick's Color Atlas and Synopsis of Clinical Dermatology*, 6th ed. New York: McGraw-Hill, 2009: 113.)

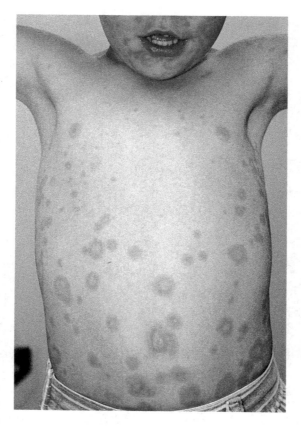

FIGURE 15-24. Erythema multiforme.

Note the many different-sized lesions. Photo contributed by Michael Redman, PA-C. (Reproduced, with permission, from Knoop KJ, Stack LB, Storrow AB, Thurman RJ. *The Atlas of Emergency Medicine*, 3rd ed. New York: McGraw-Hill, 2010: 346.)

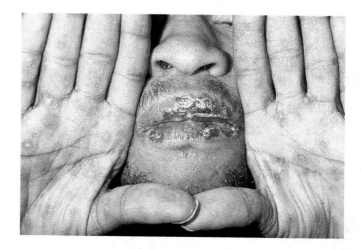

FIGURE 15-25. Stevens-Johnson syndrome.

Note involvement of oral mucous membranes. (Photo contributed by Alan B. Storrow, MD. Reproduced, with permission, from Knoop KJ, Stack LB, Storrow AB, Thurman RJ. *The Atlas of Emergency Medicine*, 3rd ed. New York: McGraw-Hill, 2010: 344.)

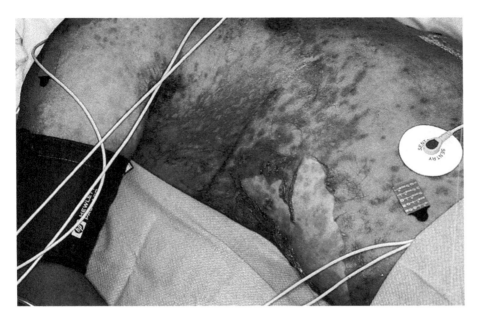

FIGURE 15-26. Toxic epidermal necrolysis.

Note the generalized macular eruption and large denuded erosive area. (Photo contributed by Keith Batts, MD. Reproduced, with permission, from Knoop KJ, Stack LB, Storrow AB, Thurman RJ. *The Atlas of Emergency Medicine*, 3rd ed. New York: McGraw-Hill, 2010: 345.)

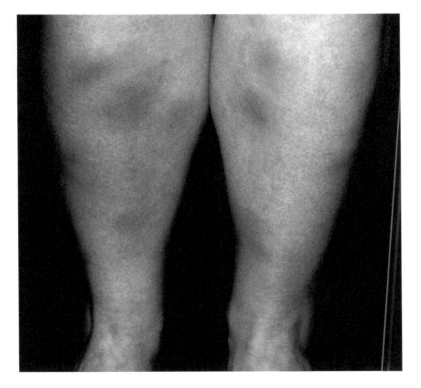

FIGURE 15-27. Erythema nodosum.

Note indurated, very tender inflammatory nodules mostly over pretibial region. Palpable as deep nodules. (Reproduced, with permission, from Wolff K, Johnson RA. *Fitzpatrick's Color Atlas and Synopsis of Clinical Dermatology*, 6th ed. New York: McGraw-Hill, 2009: 153.)

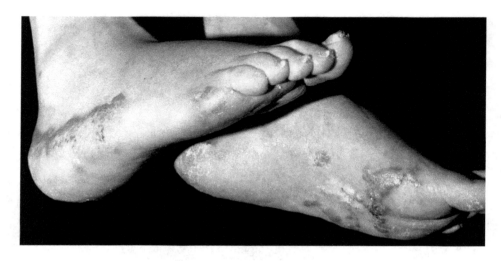

FIGURE 15-31. Kaposi's sarcoma.

Note multiple purplish confluent papules, often mistaken for bruising. (Reproduced, with permission, from Wolff K, Johnson RA. *Fitzpatrick's Color Atlas and Synopsis of Clinical Dermatology*, 6th ed. New York: McGraw-Hill, 2009: 541.)

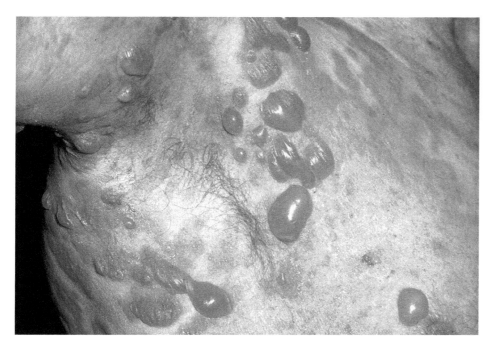

FIGURE 15-22. Bullous pemphigoid.

Also see Color Insert. (Reproduced, with permission, from Wolff K, Johnson RA. *Fitzpatrick's Color Atlas and Synopsis of Clinical Dermatology*, 6th ed. New York: McGraw-Hill, 2009: 113.)

- Only one-third of patients have oral involvement. Oral lesions heal without scarring and hence are easy to miss!

TREATMENT

Oral/IV steroids; consult dermatologist for management.

Eczema

- **Definition:** Also called dry skin; from loss of epidermal lipids by excessive washing or ↓ in production (elderly), causing flaking and cracking.
- *Eczema* is a broad term used to describe several inflammatory skin reactions and is used synonymously with dermatitis. Eczema is an inherited skin condition with a discrete classification system (atopic, contact, allergic, stasis, or seborrheic).
- **Location:** Extremities (usually).

SIGNS AND SYMPTOMS

- Lesions can be described as acute or chronic.
- Acute lesions are red, blistery, and oozy.
- Chronic lesions are thickened, lichenified, and pigmented.

TREATMENT

↓ frequency of washing or use moisturizer after each washing.

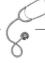

Areas involved in eczema—
FACE
Flexor surfaces = Adults
Children = Extensor surfaces

Psoriasis is worse in winter.

A 35-year-old man has salmon-colored papules covered with silvery white scales on his scalp, elbows, and knees. *Think: Psoriasis.*

Psoriasis

- **Definition:** Inherited disorder in which the keratinocyte life cycle is shortened (ie, rapid cell turnover) looking like erythema, scaly silvery plaques, fissures, and nail plate separation from nail bed with pitting of nails. Variant exists with pustules on palms and soles, minimal scale.
- **Location:** Palms, soles of feet, dorsum of hand and feet.

SIGNS AND SYMPTOMS

- Well-demarcated, thick, "salmon-pink" **plaques** with an adherent silver-white scale (Figure 15-23).
- Distributed bilaterally over **extensor surface** of extremities, often on elbows, knees, trunk, and scalp.
- Nails are commonly involved: Pitting of nails, oil spots (yellow-brown spots under nail plate), onycholysis (separation of distal nail plate from nail bed), subungual hyperkeratosis (thickening).
- Can occur at site of injury (Koebner phenomenon).
- Pinpoint capillary bleeding occurs if scale is removed (Auspitz sign).

TREATMENT

Tar emulsion (1 tsp in quart of water) applied bid followed by topical steroid cream, moisturizer creams.

Erythema Multiforme (EM)

- **Definition:** Immune complex–mediated (IgM, C3) vasculitis of blood vessels at dermo-epidermal junction that give rise to multiple pink-red, target-shaped bullae and papules of varying sizes; most commonly due to drugs, infections, x-ray therapy, malignancy, rheumatologic disease, pregnancy, and unknown etiology.
- **Location:** Palms, soles, extremities, anywhere.
- **Age group:** Most commonly seen in 20- to 40-year-old age group.

SIGNS AND SYMPTOMS

- Viral-like prodrome may precede eruption.
- Lesions itch and burn, may lyse yielding erosions.
- Although characterized by target lesions, multiforme refers to the wide variety of lesions that may be present, including papules, vesicles, and bullae (Figure 15-24).
- Ocular involvement in 10% of cases.

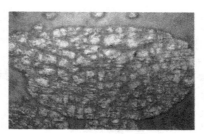

FIGURE 15-23. Psoriasis.

(Reproduced, with permission, from Rudolph A, et al. *Rudolph's Pediatrics*, 20th ed. Stamford, CT: Appleton & Lange, 1997.)

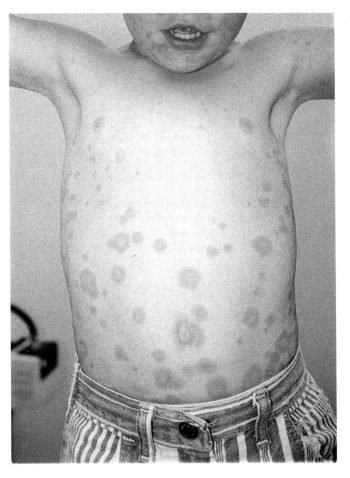

FIGURE 15-24. Erythema multiforme.

Also see Color Insert. Note the many different-sized lesions. Photo contributed by Michael Redman, PA-C. (Reproduced, with permission, from Knoop KJ, Stack LB, Storrow AB, Thurman RJ. *The Atlas of Emergency Medicine*, 3rd ed. New York: McGraw-Hill, 2010: 346.)

TREATMENT

- Cessation of medication (if possible).
- Antihistamines for itch.
- Wet-to-dry dressings with topical bacitracin for erosions.
- Look for underlying cause.
- Supportive care.

Stevens-Johnson Syndrome (SJS)

- **Definition:** Bullous variant of EM most often secondary to medication (sulfonamides, barbiturates, phenytoin, carbamazepine, thiazide diuretics, penicillins) or infection (upper respiratory infections, gastroenteritis, mycoplasma, herpes simplex virus).
- **Location:** Mucous membranes, conjunctiva, respiratory tract, various areas of skin.

Fifty percent of cases are idiopathic, but herpes simplex virus accounts for most cases of recurrent EM.

SIGNS AND SYMPTOMS

- Viral-like prodrome precedes skin and mucosal lesions, which are itchy, burning, red-pink, target-shaped bullae, lysing to give erosions (Figure 15-25).
- Bullous target lesions often less than 10% of epidermis.
- High morbidity and mortality.
- Ocular involvement present in 75% of cases.

TREATMENT

- Hospital admission may be required.
- Antihistamines for the itch.
- Corticosteroid (IV/oral) use is controversial, with most favoring its use.
- Removal of offending medication if possible.
- Soft/liquid diet.
- Eroded lesions treated with wet-to-dry dressings and topical bacitracin.

> SJS and toxic epidermal necrolysis are severe variants of EM that are potentially life threatening.

Toxic Epidermal Necrolysis (TEN)

- **Definition:** EM variant that is a true emergency from lysis of 30–100% of epidermis at dermal junction caused by similar things that cause EM/SJS; mortality high.
- **Location:** Everywhere, with mucosal involvement.

SIGNS AND SYMPTOMS

- Prodrome of fever and influenza-like symptoms.
- Pruritus, pain, tenderness, and burning.
- Classic target-like lesions symmetrically distributed on dorsum of hands, palms, soles, face, and knees.
- Initial **target lesions** can become confluent, erythematous, and tender, with bullous formation and subsequent loss of epidermis.
- Epidermal sloughing may be generalized, resembling a second-degree burn, and is more pronounced over pressure points (Figure 15-26).

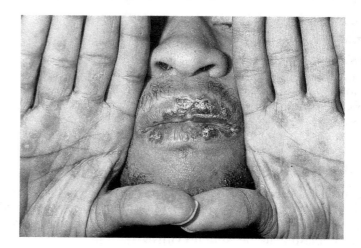

FIGURE 15-25. Stevens-Johnson syndrome.

Also see Color Insert. Note involvement of oral mucous membranes. (Photo contributed by Alan B. Storrow, MD. Reproduced, with permission, from Knoop KJ, Stack LB, Storrow AB, Thurman RJ. *The Atlas of Emergency Medicine,* 3rd ed. New York: McGraw-Hill, 2010: 344.)

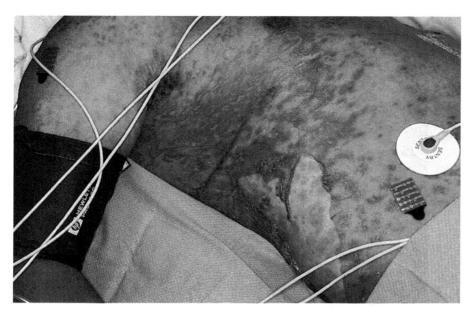

FIGURE 15-26. Toxic epidermal necrolysis.

Also see Color Insert. Note the generalized macular eruption and large denuded erosive area. (Photo contributed by Keith Batts, MD. Reproduced, with permission, from Knoop KJ, Stack LB, Storrow AB, Thurman RJ. *The Atlas of Emergency Medicine*, 3rd ed. New York: McGraw-Hill, 2010: 345.)

- Positive Nikolsky sign.
- Ninety percent of cases have mucosal lesions—painful, erythematous erosions on lips, buccal mucosa, conjunctiva, and anogenital region.

TREATMENT

- Hospital admission (usually to burn unit).
- Wounds treated as second-degree burns.
- Avoid steroid use.
- Studies suggest that plasmapheresis or exchange, hyperbaric O_2, and cyclosporine can ↓ extent of disease and facilitate healing.

PROGNOSIS

- Mortality rate as high as 30%.
- Typical causes of death include hypovolemia, infection, and electrolyte disturbances (as would be expected for widespread burns).

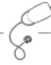

Nikolsky sign: Sloughing of epidermis with light pressure over lesion.

Erythema Nodosum

- **Definition:** Hypersensitivity vasculitis of venules in subcutaneous tissue from drugs (sulfonamides, oral contraceptives), infections (tuberculosis, *Streptococcus* spp., coccidioidomycosis), or systemic disease (sarcoidosis, inflammatory bowel disease, lymphoma, leukemia) and look like red subcutaneous nodules with surrounding erythema; can last 6 weeks.
- **Location:** Shins, lower extremities (Figure 15-27).
- **Signs and symptoms:** Painful and tender lesions accompanied by fever, malaise, and arthralgias; +/− regional adenopathy.
- **Treatment:** Cessation of medication (if possible), nonsteroidal anti-inflammatory drugs for pain, look for underlying etiology.

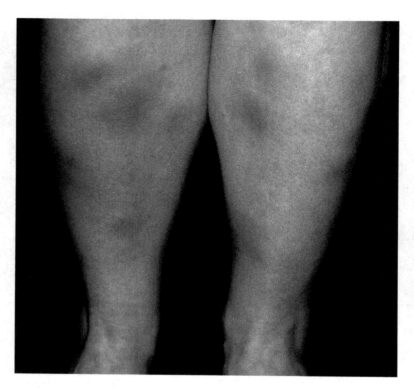

FIGURE 15-27. Erythema nodosum.

Also see Color Insert. Note indurated, very tender inflammatory nodules mostly over pretibial region. Palpable as deep nodules. (Reproduced, with permission, from Wolff K, Johnson RA. *Fitzpatrick's Color Atlas and Synopsis of Clinical Dermatology*, 6th ed. New York: McGraw-Hill, 2009: 153.)

A 5-year-old child presents with a palpable purpura over his buttocks and back of his legs and also complains of joint pains and nausea. *Think: HSP.*

Henoch-Schönlein Purpura (HSP)

- **Definition:** IgA immune complex vasculitis involving arterioles and capillaries caused by drugs, infections, foods, immunizations, and insect bites; usually a childhood disorder.
- **Location:** Lower legs and buttocks.

SIGNS AND SYMPTOMS

- Purplish raised papules and "palpable purpura."
- Arthralgias.
- Gastrointestinal complaints (nausea, vomiting, diarrhea, abdominal pain—70%).
- Renal involvement (hematuria, red blood cell [RBC] casts—50%).

TREATMENT

- Admit for IV steroids if renal involvement.
- Otherwise, discharge home on PO prednisone 1 mg/kg/day, and remove the offending agent if possible.

Systemic Lupus Erythematosus (SLE)

- **Definition:** Multisystem anti–double-stranded DNA autoantibody-mediated inflammatory disorder.
- **Location:** Face (malar rash), widespread (discoid) (Figure 15-28).

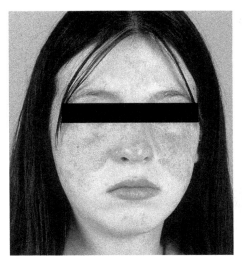
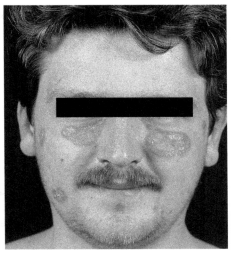

A   **B**

F I G U R E   1 5 - 2 8   **Malar (A) and discoid (B) rashes of systemic lupus erythematosus.**

(Reproduced, with permission, from Fitzpatrick TB, et al. *Color Atlas and Synopsis of Clinical Dermatology: Common and Serious Diseases*, 4th ed. New York: McGraw-Hill, 2001: 363, 364.)

- **Signs and symptoms:** Systemic symptoms include fever, arthralgia, pneumonitis, nephritis, pericarditis, and vasculitis.
- **Treatment:** Systemic steroids and immunosuppressive therapy for flare-ups.

MISCELLANEOUS RASHES

Pityriasis Rosea

- **Definition:** A common self-limiting eruption of a single herald patch followed by a generalized secondary eruption within 2 weeks.
- **Location:** Chest or back or both.
- **Age group:** 10–35 years.

SIGNS AND SYMPTOMS

- A 2- to 10-cm solitary, oval, erythematous "herald patch" with a collarette of scale precedes the generalized eruption in 80% of patients.
- Within days, multiple, smaller, pink, oval, scaly patches appear over trunk and upper extremities.
- Secondary eruption occurs in a Christmas tree distribution, oriented parallel to the ribs (Figure 15-29).

TREATMENT

Antihistamines for itch.

Seborrheic Dermatitis

- **Definition:** Waxy, erythematous scale possibly related to yeast *(Pityrosporum ovale)*; "cradle cap" in infancy.

A 21-year-old male presents with a pruritic, spotted rash on the trunk that began as one solitary larger patch. *Think: Pityriasis rosea.*

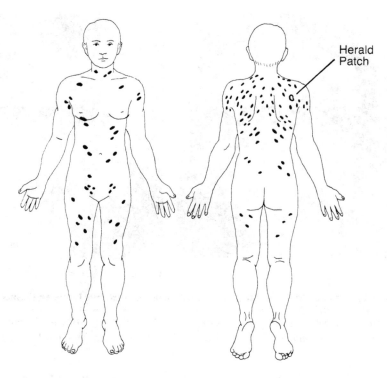

FIGURE 15-29. Distribution of pityriasis rosea.

Note "Christmas tree" pattern of rash and location of herald patch. (Reproduced, with permission, from Fitzpatrick TB, et al. *Color Atlas and Synopsis of Clinical Dermatology: Common and Serious Diseases*, 4th ed. New York: McGraw-Hill, 2001: 107.)

Stages of decubitus ulcers:

I—nonblanching erythema of intact skin

II—partial-thickness skin loss involving epidermis and/or dermis (superficial ulcer)

III—full-thickness skin loss involving epidermis and dermis (deep, crateriform ulcer); may involve damage to subcutaneous tissue, extending down to, but not through, fascia

IV—full-thickness skin loss with extensive damage to muscle, bone, or other supporting structures

- **Location:** Skin folds and hair-bearing areas of face, scalp, chest, groin.
- **Signs and symptoms:** Mild itch.
- **Treatment:** Zinc pyrethrin (Head & Shoulders), selenium sulfide (Selsun Blue), or tar (Neutrogena T-Gel) shampoo—lathered for 10 minutes, then rinsed, three times a week; 1–2.5% hydrocortisone cream for face.

Decubitus Ulcers

- **Definition:** Any pressure-induced ulcer that occurs secondary to external compression of the skin, resulting in ischemic tissue necrosis (ie, bedsore, pressure ulcer). Early ulcers have irregular, ragged borders, but chronic ulcers have smooth, well-demarcated borders. Infection is usually polymicrobial: *S aureus, Streptococcus, Pseudomonas, Enterococcus, Proteus, Clostridium,* and *Bacteroides.*
- **Location:** Over bony prominences (sacrum, ischial tuberosities, iliac crests, greater trochanters, heels, elbows, knees, occiput).
- **Signs and symptoms:** Painful, ulcerated.

TREATMENT

- **Prophylaxis:**
  - Mobilize patients as soon as possible.
  - Reposition patients every 2 hours.

406

- Pressure-reducing devices (foam, air, or liquid mattresses).
- Correction of nutritional status.
- **Local wound care:**
  - Proper cleansing with mild agents.
  - Moisturize to maintain hydration and promote healing.
  - Polyurethane, hydrocolloid, or absorptive dressings, and topical antibiotics for wound.
  - Necrotic tissue may require surgical debridement, flaps, and skin grafts.
  - Appropriate antibiotic therapy for infected ulcer.

MALIGNANT GROWTHS

Basal Cell Carcinoma (Rodent Ulcer)

- **Definition:** Slow-growing proliferation of basal keratinocytes.
- **Location:** Sun-exposed areas (forehead, nose).
- **Signs and symptoms:**
  - Asymptomatic, rarely painful.
  - Flesh-colored or hyperpigmented nodule with surface telangiectasia that expands outward leaving central ulcer and "rolled" raised edge (Figure 15-30).
- **Treatment:** Surgical excision.

Kaposi's Sarcoma

- **Definition:** Multisystem vascular neoplasm characterized by mucocutaneous violaceous lesions, commonly seen in AIDS patients.
- **Location:** Anywhere (skin and mucosa).
- **Signs and symptoms:** Cutaneous, nonblanching, reddish-purple macules, plaques, and nodules made of vasoformative tissue (spindle cells, vascular spaces, hemosiderin-stained macrophages, extravasated RBCs) (Figure 15-31).
- **Treatment:** Radiation therapy (if limited disease), chemotherapy, and radiation (if disseminated—palliative).

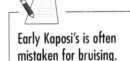

Early Kaposi's is often mistaken for bruising.

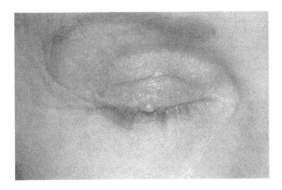

FIGURE 15-30. Basal cell carcinoma.

Note the translucent nature of the lesion. (Reproduced, with permission, from Seltzer V, Pearse WH. *Women's Primary Health Care: Office Practice and Procedures*, 2nd ed. New York: McGraw-Hill, 2000.)

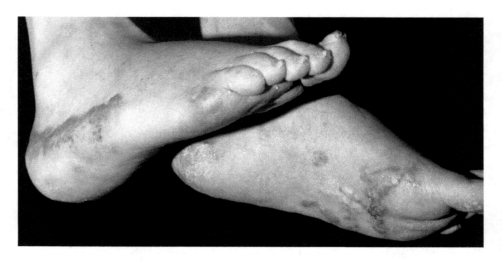

FIGURE 15-31. Kaposi's sarcoma.

Also see Color Insert. Note multiple purplish confluent papules, often mistaken for bruising. (Reproduced, with permission, from Wolff K, Johnson RA. *Fitzpatrick's Color Atlas and Synopsis of Clinical Dermatology*, 6th ed. New York: McGraw-Hill, 2009: 541.)

Melanoma

- **Definition:** A malignant proliferation of melanocytes (> 10 mm diameter, crusting or inflammation, change in size, color, contour, texture, or sensation) (Figure 15-32).
- **Location:** Anywhere.
- **Signs and symptoms:** May itch or lose sensation.
- **Treatment:** Wide surgical excision.

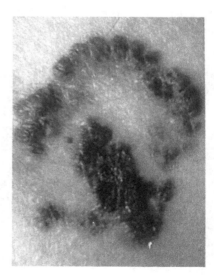

FIGURE 15-32. Melanoma.

(Reproduced, with permission, from Pantell R, et al. *The Common Symptom Guide*, 4th ed. New York: McGraw-Hill, 1996.)

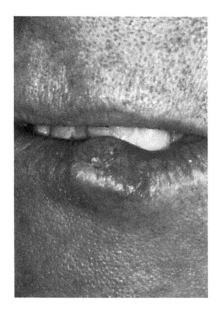

FIGURE 15-33. Squamous cell cancer.

(Reproduced, with permission, from Pantell R, et al. *The Common Symptom Guide*, 4th ed. New York: McGraw-Hill, 1996.)

Squamous Cell Carcinoma

- **Definition:** Malignant proliferation of epidermal keratinocytes, sometimes locally invasive; expanding nodular plaque, with indurated base and central ulcer with crust/scale (Figure 15-33).
- **Location:** Sun-exposed areas (face, neck, forearms).
- **Signs and symptoms:** A cut that won't heal, bleeds easily.
- **Treatment:** Surgical excision.

Dermatologic Emergencies

HIGH-YIELD FACTS

Dermatologic Emergencies

Procedures

- Procedures are a regular part of emergency medicine practice.
- This chapter describes some of the commonly performed procedures in the emergency department (ED).
- EM physicians may even be called on to perform procedures they have never done before (eg, lateral canthotomy, perimortem C-section, etc).
- One of the best references for EM procedures is: Roberts JR and Hedges JR, ed. *Clinical Procedures in Emergency Medicine*, 5th ed. Philadelphia: Saunders/Elsevier, 2010.

TUBE THORACOSTOMY

A 22-year-old man is dropped off in the ED by friends. He is diaphoretic and short of breath. The report is that he was assaulted by two unknown individuals outside a local bar. As you walk up to him, you notice several lacerations over his right arm. Primary survey reveals an intact airway but ↓ lung sounds on the right. He is becoming more short of breath, pale, obtunded, and you notice his O_2 sats are 78% and his blood pressure is 65/40. The x-ray tech arrives ready to obtain a chest x-ray (CXR). What should you do at this point?

He has a right-sided tension pneumothorax, likely from a stab wound. You should not wait to obtain a CXR, but need to act immediately. A needle decompression should be performed using a 14G angiocatheter in the second intercostal space, midclavicular line (or fourth intercostals space, midaxillary line). The angiocatheter should remain in place until a chest tube is placed.

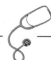

Needle decompression with a 14G angiocatheter at the second intercostal space, midclavicular line is the emergent treatment for a tension pneumothorax until a chest tube can be placed.

DEFINITION

Tube thoracostomy, commonly called a chest tube, is used to remove air or fluid from the pleural space.

INDICATIONS

- Pneumothorax (a small, spontaneous pneumothorax may be managed by observation or needle aspiration)
- Hemothorax
- Hemopneumothorax
- Open pneumothorax (sucking chest wound)
- Drainage of recurrent pleural effusion
- Empyema
- Chylothorax

The neurovascular bundle runs on the inferior margin of each rib.

RELATIVE CONTRAINDICATIONS

- Multiple adhesions
- Need for thoracotomy
- Recurrent pneumothorax requiring definitive treatment
- Severe coagulopathy

PROCEDURE (MIDAXILLARY LINE PLACEMENT)

1. Elevate the head of the bed at least 30 degrees to reduce the chances of injury to abdominal organs.
2. Identify the fourth intercostal space in the midaxillary line.
3. Prep and sterilize the area.
4. Anesthetize the skin, muscle, periosteum, and parietal pleura through which the tube will pass by utilizing a local anesthetic such as lidocaine. If time permits, do intercostal blocks above and below to provide better anesthesia.
5. Estimate the distance from incision to apex of the lung on the chest tube, ensuring that the distance is enough to allow the last drainage hole of the chest tube to fit inside the pleura. Place a clamp at this point of the chest tube.
6. Make a 2- to 4-cm skin incision over the rib below the one the tube will pass over (Figure 16-1A). The incision should be big enough for the tube and one finger to fit through at the same time. Use blunt dissection to penetrate down to the fascia overlying the intercostal muscles.
7. Insert a closed, heavy clamp over the rib and push through the muscles and parietal pleura. Spread the tips of the clamp to enlarge the opening.
8. Close the clamps and insert one finger next to the clamp into the pleural space. Sweep the finger around to ensure that you are in the pleural space and there are no adhesions. While leaving your finger in, remove the clamp and insert the chest tube by clamping the tip with a curved clamp and following the path of your finger (Figure 16-1B).
9. Remove the clamp and guide the chest tube in a superior and posterior direction.
10. Insert the tube until your previously placed marker clamp is against the skin.
11. Attach the tube to a water seal.
12. Secure the tube by using suture material to close the skin and then wrapping it around the chest tube tightly enough to prevent slipping (the two ends of the suture are wrapped in opposite directions [Figure 16-1C]). A purse-string stitch also works nicely.
13. Place an occlusive dressing over the area.
14. Chest tube placement should be confirmed by CXR.

When the clamp enters the pleura, a rush of air or fluid should be obtained.

Size of chest tube to use:
For adult large hemothorax: 36–40 French
For adult pneumothorax: 24 French
For children: Four times the size of appropriate endotracheal tube

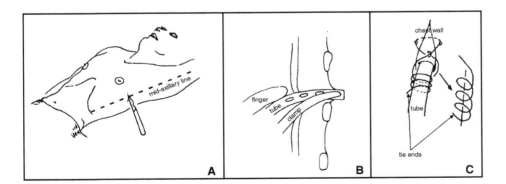

FIGURE 16-1. Procedure for tube thoracostomy.

A. An incision is made in the fourth or fifth intercostal space in the midaxillary line. B. Following finger exploration to confirm space, the tube is advanced, guided by the curved clamp. C. The tube is secured in place. (Modified, with permission, from Scaletta TA, Schaider JJ. *Emergent Management of Trauma.* New York: McGraw-Hill, 1996: 359–361.)

COMPLICATIONS

- Subcutaneous (SQ) rather than intrathoracic placement
- Bleeding from intercostal vessels
- Injury to intercostal nerves
- Infection
- Lung laceration
- Diaphragm injury
- Liver injury

PERICARDIOCENTESIS

DEFINITION

The drainage of fluid from the pericardium, which relieves tamponade (Figure 16-2).

PROCEDURE

1. If possible, ultrasound guidance or electrocardiographic (ECG) monitoring should be utilized by clamping one of the precordial leads to the needle.
2. After prepping the area, insert a 16 or 18G needle at a 30-degree angle into the left xiphocostal angle about 0.5 cm below the costal margin.
3. Advance the needle to the inner aspect of the rib cage.
4. Depress the needle to get under the ribs and point it toward the left shoulder.
5. Advance the needle as you aspirate until fluid is reached.

COMPLICATIONS

- Dry tap
- Dysrhythmias
- Air embolism
- Cardiac, vessel, or lung injury

Pericardiocentesis is usually performed with ultrasound guidance or under fluoroscopy. Blind pericardiocentesis should be performed only in the unstable patient or as part of cardiac arrest protocols when other modalities are not available. In this instance, the subxiphoid approach is recommended.

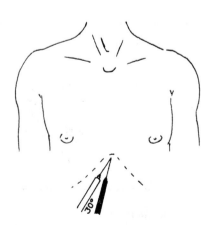

FIGURE 16-2. **Pericardiocentesis via subxiphoid approach.**

(Reproduced, with permission, from Scaletta TA, Schaider JJ. *Emergent Management of Trauma*, 2nd ed. New York: McGraw-Hill, 2001: 450.)

TABLE 16-1. **Commonly Used Local Anesthetic Agents**

AGENT	CONCENTRATION	ONSET OF ACTION	MAXIMUM DOSAGE
Lidocaine (Xylocaine)	1% or 2%	Immediate: 4–10 min Duration: 1–2 hr	4.5 mg/kg = 30 mL of 1% solution
Mepivacaine (Carbocaine)	1% or 2%	Immediate: 6–10 min Duration: 1.5–2.5 hr	5 mg/kg = 35 mL of 1% solution
Bupivacaine (Marcaine)	0.25%	Slower: 8–12 min Duration: 6–8 hr	3 mg/kg = 80 mL of 0.25% solution

LOCAL ANESTHESIA

- Local anesthesia is done by local infiltration into and around the wound or by regional block.
- Anesthetic is slowly injected adjacent to the wound edge in a sequential fashion or directly into the dermis and SQ tissue through the open wound edge using a small-gauge (25G) needle.
- Epinephrine may be added to provide vasoconstriction and prolong the action of the anesthetic.
- Commonly used local anesthetic agents are listed in Table 16-1. Topical preparations such as LET and EMLA are also options.

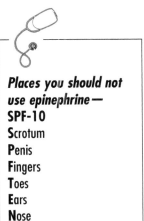

Places you should not use epinephrine—
SPF-10
Scrotum
Penis
Fingers
Toes
Ears
Nose

DIGITAL BLOCK

Indicated for any potentially painful procedure to the fingers or toes.

PROCEDURE

- A 27 or 30G needle is used to inject a local anesthetic (< 3 mL) at the base of the digit.
- Approach can be dorsal, volar, or single injection at metacarpal head.
- See Figure 16-3.

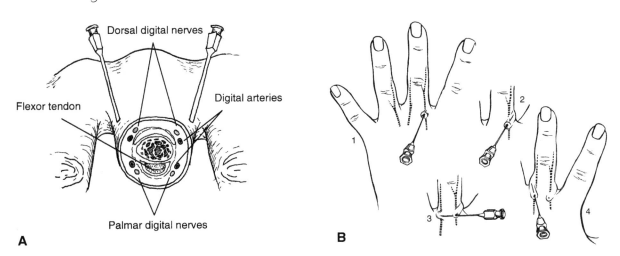

A

Dorsal digital nerves
Flexor tendon
Digital arteries
Palmar digital nerves

B

FIGURE 16-3. **Palmar digital nerves.**

(Reproduced, with permission, from Tintinalli JE, Kelen GD, Stapczynski JS. *Tintinalli's Emergency Medicine: A Comprehensive Study Guide*, 6th ed. New York: McGraw-Hill, 2004.)

INDICATIONS

- Diagnose acute, painful nontraumatic or traumatic joint disease by synovial fluid analysis.
- Therapeutic intervention to drain an effusion or hemarthrosis.

CONTRAINDICATIONS

Infection (ie, cellulitis or abscess) overlying affected joint.

PROCEDURE

1. Under sterile conditions, use povidone-iodine solution to prep skin, then wipe off with alcohol to prevent introduction of iodine into the joint space.
2. Apply sterile drape and anesthetize skin and overlying SQ tissue down to the joint capsule.
3. When joint space is entered (Figure 16-4), there will be an abrupt ↓ in resistance.
4. Remove anesthetizing needle and syringe and follow same track using an 18G needle, or catheter for large joints, with a 30-mL syringe so as to completely drain the joint space.
5. Once in joint space, gently aspirate. Then send fluid for analysis, which should include: Gram stain and culture, microscopy for crystals, complete blood count with differential, glucose, and protein.
6. Cover area with sterile dressing.

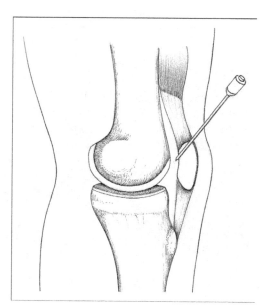

FIGURE 16-4. Knee arthrocentesis.

Viewing the patella as the face of a clock, the needle is inserted just behind the patella at either 10 or 2 o'clock (medially or laterally). (Reproduced, with permission, from Wilson FC, Lin PP. *General Orthopaedics.* New York: McGraw-Hill, 1997: 123.)

- **Septic:**
  - White blood cell (WBC) > 50,000
  - Polymorphonuclear neutrophil (PMN) > 85%
  - Glucose < 50 mg/dL
  - Gram stain positive in 65%
  - Culture positive (will be pending while in ED)
- **Gout/pseudogout:**
  - WBC 2500–50,000
  - PMN 40–90%
  - Urate crystals (gout)
  - Ca^{2+} pyrophosphate crystals (pseudogout)
- **Inflammatory:**
  - WBC 10,000–50,000
  - PMN 65–85%
- **Degenerative joint disease:**
  - WBC < 5000
  - PMN < 25%
- **Traumatic:**
  - Bloody
  - WBC < 1000
  - Fat droplets (with fracture)

- **Shoulder:** Patient sits upright with arm held in neutral position. Enter joint space anteriorly and inferiorly to the coracoid process.
- **Elbow:** Place elbow at 90 degrees of flexion with hand prone. Locate the radial head, lateral epicondyle, and lateral aspect of the olecranon tip (anconeus triangle). Needle enters at center of triangle, perpendicular to radius (Figure 16-5).

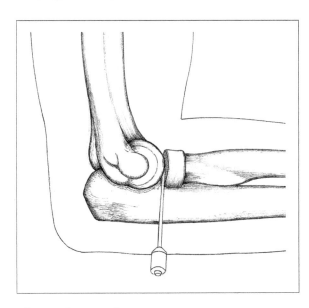

FIGURE 16-5. Elbow arthrocentesis.

(Reproduced, with permission, from Wilson FC, Lin PP. *General Orthopaedics*. New York: McGraw-Hill, 1997: 121.)

417

- **Knee:** With knee held in extension and slight flexion, enter joint space medially and inferior to the patella at its midpoint.
- **Ankle:** With the foot in plantar flexion, place needle just medial to the anterior tibial tendon at the anterior edge of the medial malleolus.
- **Fingers/toes:** With the digit flexed 15–20 degrees and traction applied, enter joint from the dorsal aspect medially or laterally to extensor tendon.
- **Wrist:** With the wrist held at 20–30 degrees of flexion and traction applied, place needle dorsal and ulnar to the extensor pollicis longus tendon.
- **Thumb:** With the thumb opposed, place the needle at the base of the first metacarpal on the palmar side of the abductor pollicis longus.

INTRAOSSEOUS ACCESS

INDICATIONS

- Whenever vascular access cannot be obtained through other means.
- Bone marrow acts like a noncollapsible vein.

SITES

- Proximal tibia (most common in children) puncture site is 1–3 cm below the tibial tuberosity, midline on the medial flat surface of the anterior tibia. Direct needle 15 degrees off the perpendicular away from the epiphysis (Figure 16-6).
- Distal tibia (common in adults) puncture site is the medial surface of the ankle proximal to the medial malleolus.
- Distal femur puncture site is on the dorsal surface where the condyle meets the shaft of bone.
- Sternum (high complication rate).

PROCEDURE

1. Using sterile technique, a battery-powered drill device may be used to guide the needle into position or a manual technique may be utilized.

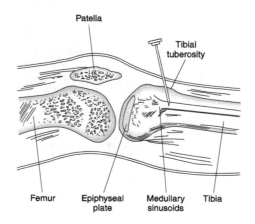

FIGURE 16-6. Intraosseous access.

(Reproduced, with permission, from Morgan G. *Clinical Anesthesiology*, 4th ed. New York: McGraw-Hill, 2006: 989.)

For the manual technique, an intraosseous infusion needle is grasped in the palm of the hand and a twisting motion is used to bore into the periosteum until the resistance ↓.

2. Proper placement is confirmed by bone marrow aspiration or successful infusion of several milliliters of normal saline (NS).

3. Local anesthesia is optional.

COMPLICATIONS

- Cellulitis
- Osteomyelitis ($< 1\%$)
- Fracture
- Fat embolism (rare)
- Growth plate injury
- Fluid extravasation

PROCEDURAL SEDATION

A 4-year-old girl suffered a 2-cm upper lip laceration through her vermillion border falling off playground equipment. She is otherwise doing well, but will not let the examiner thoroughly evaluate the wound, and it is clear she will not tolerate any attempt at a suture repair. What can be done at this point?

This patient has a wound that needs to be repaired carefully to reduce the cosmetic impact. She will require procedural sedation to perform this procedure well and safely. A good choice for this case (and for most pediatric EM procedures) is ketamine. It can be given either IM (4 mg/kg) or IV (2 mg/kg) and will allow ideal conditions to repair this wound.

INDICATIONS

- Painful procedures done in the ED.
- Uncooperative/anxious child who needs procedure or diagnostic test performed.
- Because of procedural sedation, many more procedures are now performed outside of the operating room (OR).

GOALS

- Place patients in a state where they can tolerate unpleasant procedures while maintaining an independent airway, reflexes, and stable cardiac and respiratory function.
- To allow patient to be discharged quickly and safely.

PATIENT SELECTION

- Relatively healthy individuals with minimal comorbidities.
- Minimal neurologic impairment.
- Fasting at least 4 hours from solid food or 2 hours from liquids (nonemergent cases only).

MONITORING

- Cardiac monitor and pulse oximetry throughout procedure.
- Use of capnography may detect hypoxic events earlier.
- O_2, intubation equipment, and medical reversal agents should be readily available.
- Initial set of vitals, vitals 10 minutes after administration, and every 15 minutes thereafter until patient is alert and oriented × 3 and can sit up (if previously able to sit up).

MEDICATIONS

- **Midazolam (Versed):**
  - Benzodiazapine.
  - Good sedation, anxiolysis, and amnesia, but no analgesia
  - 0.05–0.1 mg/kg IV, incremental dose at 2-minute intervals to desired effect (maximum cumulative dose 5 mg)
  - Onset: 1–2 minutes
  - Duration: 30–45 minutes
- **Fentanyl:**
  - Opioid; provides analgesia
  - When combined with midazolam (or other benzodiazapine), good sedation and analgesia
  - 1 μg/kg IV, incremental dose at 2-minute intervals to desired effect (maximum 4 μg/kg)
  - Onset: 1–3 minutes
  - Duration: 30–60 minutes
- **Ketamine (Ketalar):**
  - Dissociative hypnotic; allows painful procedures performed while maintaining sedation
  - 1–2 mg/kg IV, 3–4 mg/kg IM
  - Onset: 30–60 seconds
  - Duration: 15 minutes
  - ↑ blood pressure and intracranial pressure
  - May see emergence reaction, generally in patients > 15 years of age
- **Propofol:**
  - Sedation and anesthesia, not analgesia
  - 1 mg/kg IV loading dose followed by 0.5 mg/kg dosing every 3–5 minutes until desired effect
  - Onset within 40 seconds
  - Duration: 3–5 minutes
  - Lowers blood pressure, so not a good choice for hypotensive patients
- **Etomidate:**
  - Nonbarbiturate hypnotic
  - Anesthesia, not analgesia
  - 0.1–0.2 mg/kg IV
  - Onset: Within 60 seconds
  - Duration: 3–5 minutes
- **Nitrous oxide (N_2O):**
  - 50% N_2O/50% O_2 via inhalation
  - Onset: 2–5 minutes
  - Duration: 2–5 minutes
  - Must administer continuously
- **Naloxone:**
  - Opiate receptor antagonist
  - 0.2–2.0 mg IV
  - Onset: 30–90 seconds

Chest wall rigidity can occur with rapid IV administration of fentanyl and ketamine.

An emergence reaction is the occurrence of hallucinations and nightmares during the wearing off of ketamine. It is uncommon in children, but can occur in 10–20% of adults. Allowing the patient to recover in a dark, quiet room minimizes this phenomenon.

Propofol and midazolam/fentanyl ↓ blood pressure. Etomidate and ketamine do not and are preferred agents for hypotensive patients.

- Duration: 2–3 hours
- Can induce opioid withdrawal for those on chronic opioids
- **Flumazenil:**
  - Benzodiazepine antagonist
  - Rarely used as it may precipitate seizures in those on chronic benzodiazapines

INDICATIONS

- Fractures to be seen by orthopedics at a later date
- Dislocations that have been reduced

MATERIALS

Fiberglass or plaster.

PREPARATION

Plaster
1. Measure the length of the affected extremity with the plaster, then place the plaster roll on a flat surface and unroll the plaster back and forth on itself to a total of 12 layers.
2. Measure several layers of padding to be both longer and wider than the plaster.
3. Submerge the plaster in water and hold until the bubbling stops.
4. Strip excess water from plaster by holding plaster up in one hand and use the other hand to squeeze plaster between thumb and index finger from top to bottom.
5. Place plaster on flat surface and massage layers together.
6. Place padding on top, then apply to extremity with padding against skin and mold with palms, not fingers, to avoid creating pressure points.
7. Wrap with Ace bandage (over gauze) for compression.

Fiberglass
1. Cut material to desired length.
2. Do not submerge in water. Put one strip of water down center of splint then curl up splint in a towel to remove excess moisture.
3. Stretch outer padding over the ends of the fiberglass to avoid sharp edges and apply to extremity. Wrap with elastic bandage (Ace wrap).
4. Fiberglass will harden within 10 minutes, much more quickly than plaster.

Upper Extremity Splints

- **Reverse sugar tong** (Figure 16-7):
  - Indications: Forearm or Colles fracture.
  - Use 3- to 4-inch adult; cut splint in center, leaving small piece to overlie thumb.
- **Boxer splint** (Figure 16-8): Indications: Fourth and fifth metacarpal fracture.
- **Long arm ulnar gutter (elbow) splint** (Figure 16-9):
  - Indications: Supracondylar fracture, elbow sprain, radial head fracture.

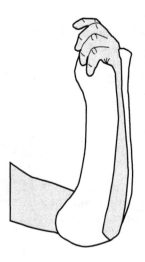

FIGURE 16-7. Reverse sugar tong splint.

- Elbow is held at 90 degrees. Splint extends from metacarpal heads to upper arm below axillary crease along ulnar surface.
- **Cock-up splint:**
  - Indications: Wrist sprain, carpal tunnel syndrome.
  - Wrist is in extension, splint extends from midforearm to metacarpophalangeal (MCP) on volar surface of hand.
- **Thumb spica** (Figure 16-10):
  - Indications: Navicular or scaphoid fracture, thumb dislocation, ulnar collateral ligament sprain, thumb proximal phalanx fracture, MCP fracture.
  - The wrist is in neutral position and the thumb in abduction; the splint extends from the ulnar aspect of forearm and comes radially over dorsum of wrist and hand to encompass thumb.

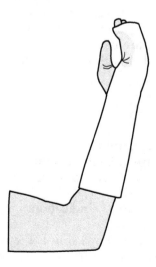

FIGURE 16-8. Boxer splint.

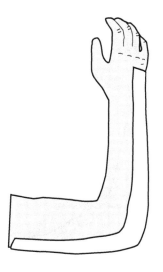

FIGURE 16-9. Elbow splint.

Lower Extremity Splints

- **Posterior leg (ankle) splint** (Figure 16-11):
  - Indications: Distal tibia and fibula fracture, ankle sprain, Achilles' tendon tear, metatarsal fracture.
  - The ankle is in neutral position, except for Achilles' tears in which the patient should be immobilized in plantar flexion. The splint extends from 2 inches posterior to knee to metatarsophalangeal heads.
- **Ankle stirrup** (Figure 16-12):
  - Indications: Ankle strain/sprain, shin splint, hairline fracture.
  - The splint extends from medial to lateral aspect of lower leg at mid-calf to encompass the calcaneus. This prevents inversion/eversion.
- **Long leg splint:**
  - Indications: Femoral fracture.
  - Apply like posterior leg splint, but superior aspect of splint extends to 3 inches below buttock.

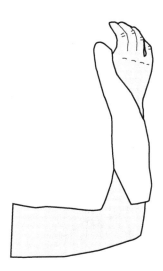

FIGURE 16-10. Thumb spica splint.

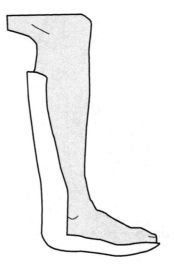

FIGURE 16-11. Posterior ankle splint.

- Knee immobilizer:
    - Indications: Knee sprain, postop knee surgery.
    - Usually ready-made device that wraps around posterior and sides of the lower extremities from upper thigh to lower leg above the ankle. It is held in place by anterior Velcro straps.

SUTURES

Types of Closure

- Primary:
    - Closure within 6–8 hours of any wound on body.
    - Face and scalp may be closed primarily up to 24 hours because of good vascular supply.

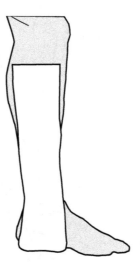

FIGURE 16-12. Ankle stirrup splint.

- **Secondary:** Wound heals by granulation alone (spontaneous healing).
- **Delayed primary closure:** Closure of a wound 3–5 days following injury.

Tetanus

- If unknown history or fewer than three doses, give Td (tetanus and diptheria) toxoid.
- If three doses given and within 7 years, no immunization necessary.
- If tetanus-prone wound (> 6 hours, avulsion, crush, > 1 cm depth, abrasion, contusion, contamination, devitalized tissue, or frostbite) and unknown tetanus history, give Td and tetanus immune globulin.

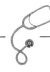

Give tetanus prophylaxis to anything that is CUT:
Contaminated wounds
Unknown tetanus history
Tetanus status expired

Prevent Infection

- Irrigation is the most important procedure required to clean a wound.
- Use tap water or saline, an 18G needle, and 30-cc syringe to irrigate wound with 8–10 psi.
- Antibiotics are not proven to be of prophylactic benefit. Reserve for grossly contaminated wounds.

Tap water is as effective as sterile saline for irrigation of a wound. The key is volume—irrigate with 500–1000 mL.

Suture Equipment

- Needles:
  - Cutting: Has two cutting edges for shallow bites.
  - Reverse cutting: Has three cutting edges for deeper bites.
- Needle holder:
  - Place at 90-degree angle.
  - One-third from swage.
  - Needle at tip of needle holder.
- Dissecting forceps: To gently evert skin edges.
- Skin hooks.
- Scissors.
- Local anesthetic.
- Suture material: See Tables 16-2 and 16-3. See Table 16-4 for closure recommendations by wound site.

TABLE 16-2. Suture Materials: Absorbable

MATERIAL	HALF-LIFE	TYPE	COMMENTS
Gut	5–7 days	Natural	Stiff, rapidly absorbed, used for mucosal closure only
Chromic gut	10–14 days	Natural	Used for intraoral lacerations
Polyglycolic acid (Dexon)	10–15 days	Synthetic multifilament	Used for SQ sutures, difficult to tie
Polyglactin 910 (Vicryl)	14–21 days	Synthetic multifilament	Use clear variety on face, easy workability, SQ
Polydioxanone (PDS II)	28 days	Synthetic monofilament	Very strong, low reactivity, large knot mass

TABLE 16-3. Suture Materials: Nonabsorbable

MATERIAL	TYPE	COMMENTS
Silk	Natural multifilament	Easiest to handle but poses greatest risk of infection, not used on face
Nylon (Ethilon and Dermalon)	Synthetic mono- or multifilament	Low tissue reactivity, most often used for cutaneous closure
Polypropylene (Prolene)	Synthetic monofilament	Stiffest sutures, requires five to six knots, tends to untie
Polyester (Mersilene)	Synthetic multifilament	Easy handling with excellent security, often used for vascular or facial wounds
Polybutester (Norafil)	Synthetic monofilament	Slight elasticity allows wound swelling

TABLE 16-4. Closure Recommendations by Wound Sites

LOCATION	MATERIAL	TECHNIQUE
Scalp	Staples or 3-0 or 4-0 nylon or polypropylene	Interrupted in galea, single tight layer in scalp, horizontal mattress if bleeding not well controlled
Pinna	5-0 Vicryl/Dexon in perichondrium	Close perichondrium with interrupted Vicryl and close skin with interrupted nylon
Eyebrow	4-0 or 5-0 Vicryl (SQ) 6-0 nylon	Layered closure
Eyelid	6-0 nylon	Single-layer horizontal mattress or simple interrupted
Lip	4-0 Vicryl (mucosa) 5-0 Vicryl (SQ or muscle) 6-0 nylon (skin)	If wound through lip, close three layers (mucosa, muscle, skin); otherwise, do two-layer closure. Must line up vermillion border carefully to minimize scar.
Oral cavity	4-0 Vicryl	Simple interrupted or horizontal mattress if muscularis of tongue involved
Face	6-0 nylon (skin) 5-0 Vicryl (SQ)	Simple interrupted for single layer, layered closure for full-thickness laceration
Trunk	4-0 Vicryl (SQ, fat) 4-0 or 5-0 nylon (skin)	Single or layered closure
Extremity	3-0 or 4-0 Vicryl (SQ, fat, muscle) 4-0 or 5-0 nylon (skin)	Single-layer interrupted or vertical mattress; apply splint if over a joint
Hands and feet	4-0 or 5-0 nylon	Single-layer closure with simple interrupted or horizontal mattress; apply splint if over a joint
Nail bed	5-0 Vicryl	Meticulous placement to obtain even edges, allow to dissolve

HIGH-YIELD FACTS

Procedures

Suturing Techniques

A 4-year-old girl suffered a 2-cm upper lip laceration through her vermillion border falling off playground equipment. She is now sedated with ketamine. What should you do next?

Irrigate the wound. She should then have the wound closed with simple interrupted sutures starting at the vermillion border (distinct area of demarcation between red of the lip and normal skin color). This area must be closed precisely, or the patient will have an obvious scar with any misalignment. 6-0 suture should be used. While nonabsorbable sutures are generally used on the face, special fast-absorbing sutures (eg, fast-absorbing chromic gut) may be used on the face. In this case, fast-absorbing sutures might be preferred as the patient would not be required to have the sutures out in 5 days like she will with nonabsorbable sutures.

- **Simple interrupted** (Figure 16-13): To close most simple wounds.
  - Edges should always be everted to prevent depression of scar. Do this by entering needle at 90 degrees to skin surface and follow curve of needle through skin.
  - Entrance and exit point of needle should be equidistant from laceration.
  - Do not place suture too shallow, as this will cause dead space.
  - Use instrument tie or surgeon's knot and place knot to one side of laceration, not directly over laceration.
- **Running suture** (Figure 16-14):
  - Not commonly used in the ED.
  - Disadvantage: One nicked stitch or knot means the entire suture is out.

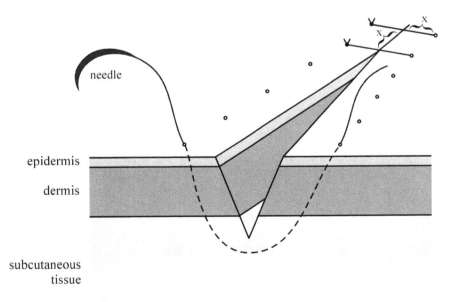

FIGURE 16-13. Simple interrupted suture.

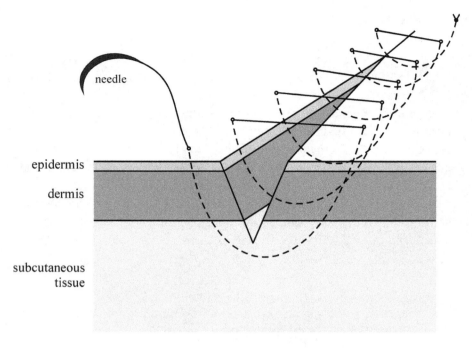

FIGURE 16-14. Running suture.

- Advantage: Done well with sturdy knots, it provides even tension across wound.
- **Vertical mattress** (Figure 16-15):
  - This suture helps in reducing dead space and in eversion of wound edges.
  - It does not significantly reduce tension on wound.

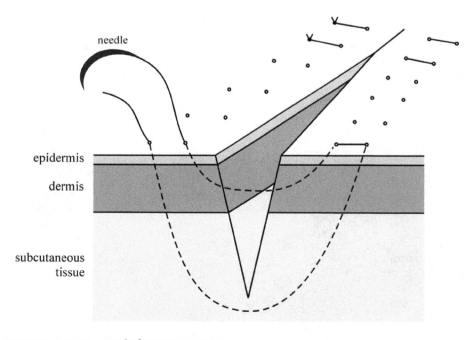

FIGURE 16-15. Vertical mattress suture.

- The needle enters the skin farther away (more lateral) from the laceration than the simple interrupted and also exits further away on the opposite side.
- It then enters again on the same side that it just exited from but more proximal to the laceration and exits on the opposite side (where it originally entered) proximally.
- **Horizontal mattress** (Figure 16-16):
  - This suture also assists in wound edge eversion and helps to spread tension over a greater area.
  - This stitch starts out like a simple interrupted suture; however, after the needle exits, it then enters again on the same side that it exited from only a few millimeters lateral to the stitch and equidistant from the wound edge and exits on the opposite side.
- **Deep sutures (absorbable):**
  - Used for multilayered closure.
  - Deep sutures are absorbable because you will not be removing them.
  - Use your forceps (pickups) to hold the skin from the inside of the wound.
  - The first stitch is placed deep inside wound and exits superficially in dermal layer on same side of wound.
  - Then it enters in the superficial dermal layer on the opposite side and exits deep.
  - Tie a square knot and cut the tail of the suture close to the knot, which is called a *buried knot*.
  - Now proceed with your superficial closure of the skin with nonabsorbable sutures.
- **Corner stitch** (Figure 16-17):
  - Used to repair stellate lacerations and help to preserve the blood supply to the tips of the skin.
  - The needle enters the epidermis of the nonflap or nontip portion of the wound.

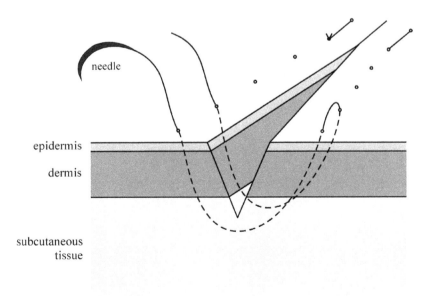

FIGURE 16-16. Horizontal mattress suture.

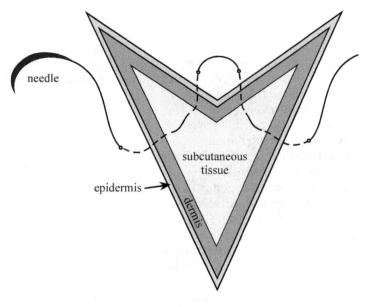

FIGURE 16-17. Corner stitch.

- It then enters the dermal layer of the skin tip on one side and proceeds through the dermal layer to exit the dermis on the other side of the tip (this portion will be buried).
  - It then enters and exits the other side of the stellate wound. It will appear as a simple interrupted suture.

Dressing

- Bacitracin ointment may be used over the repair.
- Cover the laceration with a single layer of nonadherent dressing, then cover that with gauze.
- For an extremity, wrap with gauze bandage (Kerlix) and take care not to tape circumferentially.
- The patient should come back for a wound check in 2–3 days for contaminated or deep wounds.
- The dressing should be changed every day and replaced with a Band-Aid or gauze.
- Keep area dry and look for signs of infection: ↑ warmth, swelling, increasing erythema, streaking, dehiscence, more-than-normal discharge from wound, and fever.
- See Table 16-5 for when to remove sutures.

TABLE 16-5. Suture Removal Times

Site	Days
Face, eyelid, ear, nose	3–5
Neck	5–7
Scalp, trunk	7–12
Arm, hand	8–12
Leg, foot, extensor surface of joints	10–14

CENTRAL VENOUS ACCESS

A 64-year-old woman with a history of liver failure appears to be septic. Her blood pressure is 88/34 and heart rate is 120 despite 4 L of IV normal saline. Phenylephrine is given in her peripheral IV, and a subclavian is attempted for access for further resuscitation. Labs are still pending. Venous appearing blood is obtained, but the guidewire meets resistance at about 8 cm. What should you do at this point?

The wire should never be forced, as that can cause significant injury or malposition. It should be withdrawn, and an additional attempt at gentle passage can be made. If still meeting resistance, it should be withdrawn and a new attempt made. In this case, consideration should be given to finding a new site, given her history of liver failure and possible ↑ International Normalized Ratio (INR). An ultrasound-guided IJ or a femoral line would be better choices in this case.

RELATIVE INDICATIONS

- In general, rate of line-related infections and order of preference for site is: subclavian (SC), internal jugular (IJ), and femoral vein.
- SC may be preferred if patient cannot lie flat.
- IJ and femoral will allow identification of vessels by ultrasound.
- Femoral may be preferred in cardiopulmonary arrest as it will not interfere with cardiopulmonary resuscitation (CPR).
- Coagulopathy: Femoral because more readily compressible.

RELATIVE CONTRAINDICATIONS

- **General (applies to all routes):**
  - Distorted anatomy
  - Overlying cellulitis or severe dermatitis
  - Prior scarring of vein
  - Significant coagulopathy
- **Subclavian:**
  - Contralateral pneumothorax
  - Chest wall deformity
  - Chronic obstructive pulmonary disease
  - Coagulopathy (noncompressible site)

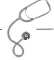

Subclavian vein cannulation can be via infraclavicular or supraclavicular approach.

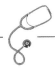

If patient has unilateral lung injury (eg, pneumothorax, effusion, etc), remember to place IJ or SC on this side to avoid injury to the "good" lung.

- **IJ:**
  - Carotid artery stenosis (dislodging of plaque may occur due to inadvertent carotid artery cannulation).
  - Coagulopathy (difficult to compress over carotid).
- **Femoral:**
  - Ambulatory patient
  - Groin trauma

> The Trendelenburg position is thought to prevent air embolism.

> The right subclavian is preferred over the left in order to avoid thoracic duct (on left) or lung injury (dome of right lung is lower).

PROCEDURE (CENTRAL VENOUS CANNULATION)

1. Use aseptic technique (hat, mask, sterile gown, glove, draping).
2. Place patient in Trendelenburg position.
3. Use ultrasound to identify and locate vessel for IJ and femoral.
4. Local anesthesia at point of needle entry.
5. Insert and aim needle on syringe as appropriate for approach with gentle negative pressure to the syringe.
6. Nonpulsatile free flow flashback of blood indicates good position. Pulsatile flow may indicate inappropriate arterial placement (if in doubt, consider transduction prior to dilating the vessel to rule out arterial stick).
7. Once within the vein, advance the guidewire through the needle (Seldinger technique).
8. Use scalpel to make small stab incision adjacent to guidewire and pass dilator to enlarge opening for catheter.
9. Pass catheter over guidewire. In most sets, removing the guidewire from the distal end of the catheter requires removal of the brown port.
10. NEVER let go of the guidewire.
11. Catheter should pass easily, without any forcing.
12. Once catheter is in to desired length, remove guidewire.
13. Check blood flow from catheter.
14. If not a triple lumen, connect catheter to IV tubing.
15. Suture catheter in place.
16. Place occlusive dressing over site.
17. Obtain chest x-ray for SC or IJ lines to confirm placement and to be certain no pneumothorax was caused by the procedure.

Landmarks for IC Subclavian

- Insert needle at junction of middle and proximal thirds of clavicle (Figure 16-18).
- Aim needle toward suprasternal notch.
- Vein entry at 4 cm.

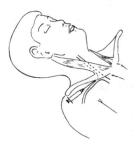

FIGURE 16-18. IC approach to subclavian vein cannulation.

(Reproduced, with permission, from Scaletta TA, Schaider JJ. *Emergent Management of Trauma*, 2nd ed. New York: McGraw-Hill, 2001: 441.)

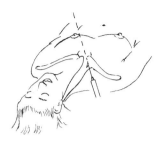

FIGURE 16-19. **Supraclavicular (SC) approach to subclavian vein cannulation.**

(Reproduced, with permission, from Scaletta TA, Schaider JJ. *Emergent Management of Trauma*, 2nd ed. New York: McGraw-Hill, 2001: 442.)

Landmarks for SC Subclavian
- Insert needle behind the clavicle, lateral to the clavicular head of the sternocleidomastoid (SCM) (Figure 16-19).
- Aim needle toward contralateral nipple.
- Vein entry at 3 cm.

Landmarks for IJ Cannulation, Central Approach
- Use ultrasound to confirm vessel anatomy (IJ compresses, carotid does not).
- Insert needle at junction of the two heads of the SCM.
- Aim needle toward ipsilateral nipple.
- Maintain needle at 30- to 45-degree angle.
- Vein entry at 1–1.5 cm.

Landmarks for IJ Cannulation, Anterior Approach
- Use ultrasound to confirm vessel anatomy (IJ compresses, carotid does not).
- Insert needle at medial edge of sternal head of SCM halfway up (Figure 16-20).
- Maintain needle at 30- to 45-degree angle.
- Aim needle toward ipsilateral nipple.
- Vein entry at 1.5 cm.

Landmarks for IJ Cannulation, Posterior Approach
- Use ultrasound to confirm vessel anatomy (IJ compresses, carotid does not).
- Insert needle at lateral edge of clavicular head of SCM, a third of the way up between the clavicle and the mastoid (Figure 16-21).
- Aim needle toward sternal notch.
- Vein entry at 5 cm.

Landmarks for Femoral Vein Cannulation
- Insert needle medial to pulsation of femoral artery.
- Maintain needle at 45-degree angle.
- Aim needle toward the head.
- Vein entry at 3 cm.

Remember **NAVEL** from lateral to medial: **N**erve, **A**rtery, **V**ein, **E**mpty space, **L**ymphatics; vein is medial to artery ("venous toward the penis").

COMPLICATIONS
- Infection
- Thrombosis
- Pneumothorax (not with femoral)
- SQ emphysema

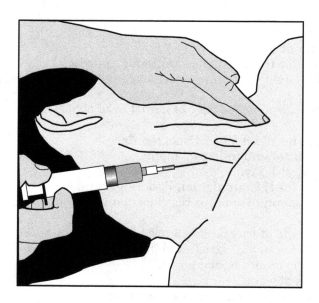

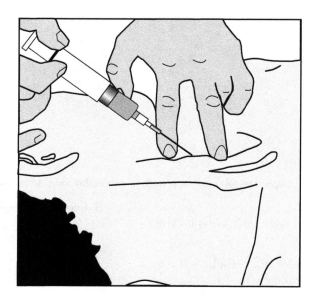

FIGURE 16-20. Anterior IJ cannulation.

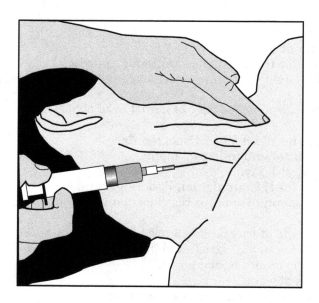

FIGURE 16-21. Posterior IJ cannulation.

The incision and drainage (I&D) of abscesses is a very common procedure performed in the ED. Most skin abscesses are uncomplicated and can be drained easily with local anesthetic. Larger abscesses or ones in exquisitely sensitive areas may require conscious sedation or, occasionally, drainage in the operating room under general anesthesia.

MOST COMMON SITES

- Axilla: 25%
- Buttock/perirectal: 25%
- Head/neck: 20%
- Extremities: 18%
- Inguinal area: 15%

PATHOGENS

Variety of aerobic and anaerobic. Most common:

- *Staphylococcus aureus*
- *Bacteroides fragilis*
- *Streptococcus viridans*

EQUIPMENT NEEDED

- Scalpel
- Hemostats
- Scissors
- Iodine solution
- Gauze
- Packing material—most commonly 1- or 2-inch plain or iodoform
- Dressing material
- Chucks
- Personal protective equipment
- Gloves
- Gown
- Eye protection
- Mask

PROCEDURE

After explaining the procedure and placing the patient in a comfortable position with adequate exposure and lighting with chucks to minimize the mess:

1. Clean the area and prepare it with iodine solution.
2. Anesthetize the skin with the lidocaine preparation.
3. Make an incision large enough to ensure adequate exposure and drainage. Err on the side of a larger incision.
4. Care must be taken with the incision in the face and breast due to cosmetic considerations.
5. In areas of cosmetic concern, cut along the natural wrinkle or crease lines to minimize scarring or consider needle aspiration with frequent rechecks.
6. Explore the cavity with the hemostats to break up any loculations and express remaining pus.
7. If the abscess is large enough, pack it as much as possible, leaving some packing outside of the cavity.

Immunocompromise is associated with recurrent abscesses (ie, diabetes, human immunodeficiency virus).

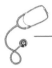

It is very difficult to completely anesthetize the abscess locally due to the acidic environment of abscesses. Use a regional block if possible. Use systemic medication or even conscious sedation when necessary.

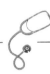

While this is not a sterile procedure, it should be a clean procedure. Care should be taken not to infect areas not involved with the abscess.

Antibiotics in healthy individuals are unnecessary. Consider antibiotics in immunocompromised individuals and in patients with valvular disease to prevent seeding due to transient bacteremia.

HIGH-YIELD FACTS

Procedures

8. Dress the area appropriately.
9. Patients should return in 24 hours for packing removal and wound check.

SPECIAL CONSIDERATIONS

- Perirectal abscesses require careful evaluation because they can extend deep into the perineum.
- Sebaceous cyst/abscesses can be excised with the shell intact, thus preventing recurrences.
- Cultures are generally unnecessary in first-time abscesses.

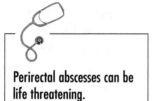

Perirectal abscesses can be life threatening.

NASOGASTRIC TUBE PLACEMENT

INDICATIONS

- **Therapeutic:**
  1. Gastric decompression prior to surgery or in trauma
  2. Recurrent vomiting as with intestinal obstruction or paralytic ileus
  3. Administration of medication/feeds
- **Diagnostic:**
  1. Lab analysis of gastric contents
  2. Determination of presence, volume of an upper GI hemorrhage
  3. Instillation of air to enhance visualization of free air under the diaphragm on an erect chest film in gut perforation

CONTRAINDICATIONS

- Facial fractures or cribriform plate injury (absolute)
- Esophageal strictures
- Esophageal weakening (eg, recent alkali exposure)
- Coagulopathy

PROCEDURE

1. Position the patient sitting upright against the bed/backrest.
2. After selecting tube type and size, estimate insertion depth by adding the distance from the tip of the nose to the earlobe plus the earlobe to the xiphoid.
3. Check patency of the nostrils by occluding each nostril separately and asking the patient to inhale.
4. Anesthetize nares and oropharynx with lidocaine jelly.
5. Lubricate the distal 6 mm of the nasogastric tube.
6. Insert at a 90-degree angle to the patient's face until it reaches the posterior nasal pharynx, where resistance will be encountered.
7. Gentle pressure helps turn the tube and advance it caudally. Have the patient sip water simultaneously to facilitate the passage of the tube until depth marked.
8. Secure using tape and confirm position a chest x-ray.

COMPLICATIONS

- Nasopharyngeal injury
- Pulmonary placement
- Pneumothorax, pneumomediastinum
- Oropharyngeal coiling

INDICATIONS

- Any unstable patient with tachyarrhythmia should be immediately treated with synchronized electrical cardioversion.
- Cardioversion can also be used in hemodynamically stable patients to restore sinus rhythm in conditions like:
  - Atrial fibrillation
  - Atrial flutter
  - Ventricular tachycardia
  - Supraventricular tachycardias

RELATIVE CONTRAINDICATIONS

- Known digitalis toxicity–associated tachydysrhythmia
- Sinus tachycardia caused by various clinical conditions

PROCEDURE

1. Procedural sedation.
2. Selection of synchronized mode on the cardioverter to synchronize the discharge and avoid cardioversion during repolarization. Synchronization should not be used in patients with ventricular fibrillation (VF) as it may delay delivery of shock.
3. Apply conductive gel pads in the anteroposterior or anterolateral position.
4. Energy is dialed up according to the indication and discharged until patient reverts to sinus rhythm.

Always use synchronized cardioversion unless patient is in VF arrest (then defibrillation).

ENERGY SETTINGS

Energy levels used depend on whether the defibrillator is monophasic or biphasic. Energy settings for common indications are given below (initial followed by subsequent attempts):

	MONOPHASIC (J OR WATT-SEC)	BIPHASICE (J OR WATT-SEC)
Atrial fibrillation	100, 200	75
Ventricular tachycardia	100, 200	50–100, 200
Ventricular fibrillation	360	120-200, 200, 360

Settings on biphasic defibrillators depend on the manufacturer recommendations for different brands (follow the manufacturer recommendations, if available).

COMPLICATIONS

- Arrhythmias and conduction abnormalities
- Embolization
- Myocardial necrosis or dysfunction
- Transient hypotension
- Pulmonary edema
- Painful skin burns from electrode placement

TABLE 16-6. Procedures Covered in Other Chapters

PROCEDURE	CHAPTER
Intubation, cricothyroidotomy (needle and surgical), laryngeal mask airway, Heimlich maneuver	Resuscitation
Interpretation of ECGs and imaging studies	Diagnostics
Reading a C-spine film, focused assessment with sonography for trauma, diagnostic peritoneal lavage, retrograde urethrogram, and cystogram	Trauma
Lumbar puncture	Neurologic Emergencies
Nasal packing	Head and Neck Emergencies
Testicular detorsion	Renal and Genitourinary Emergencies
Vaginal wet prep	Gynecologic Emergencies
Gastric lavage	Emergency Toxicology

OTHER PROCEDURES

See Table 16-6 for procedures covered in other chapters.

Emergency Toxicology

- Initial management of poisoned patient should emphasize supportive care:
  - Stabilize ABCs and abnormal vital signs.
  - Search to identify toxidromes.
  - Perform a focused diagnostic workup.
  - Decontamination, elimination, and antidotes as indicated.
  - Continuous reassessment is critical (patients may deteriorate rapidly).
- Clinical pictures of symptoms and physical findings that correlate with a specific toxin recognize that "classic" toxidromes may be obscured in the setting of a multidrug overdose (in which each toxin may cause competing signs/symptoms).
- Poison control:
  - Can be reached at: 1-800-222-1222.
  - Great resource for your patient and also provide epidemiologic data.

TOXIDROMES

Cholinergic

- Commonly seen with organophosphates and carbamates.
- Symptoms are due to excessive stimulation of nicotinic/muscarinic acetylcholine (ACh) receptors.
- Muscarinic effects: Bronchorrhea, miosis, bradycardia (SLUDGE).
- Nicotinic effects: Fasciculations, cramping, hyperreflexia, hypertension, tachycardia.
- **Treatment:** Use atropine +/– pralidoxime to reverse cholinergic excess.

Cholinergic toxidrome —
BAD SLUDGE
Bradycardia/**B**ronchorrhea
Anxiety
Delirium
Salivation
Lacrimation
Urination
Defecation
Gastrointestinal (GI) upset
Emesis

Anticholinergic

- Many potential agents: Scopolamine, amanita muscaria, monoamine oxidase inhibitors (MAOIs).
- Think of the following four "anti" groups of drugs: antidepressants, antihistamines, antipsychotics, antiparkinsonian.
- Clinical picture caused by antagonism/inhibition of ACh.
- Other findings: Seizures, dysrhythmias, hyperthermia.
- **Treatment:**
  - Supportive: Benzodiazepines, cooling measures.
  - Physostigmine:
    - Binds to acetylcholinesterase, ↑ ACh.
    - Indicated only for unstable/refractory cases (seizures and dysrhythmias are common).
    - Avoid in tricyclic antidepressant (TCA) ingestions (asystole).

Anticholinergic toxidrome:
- Mad as a hatter: Altered mental status
- Blind as a bat: Mydriasis
- Red as a beet: Flushed skin
- Hot as a hare: Hyperthermia (can't sweat)
- Dry as a bone: Dry mucous membranes and armpits

Sympathomimetic

- Agitation, mydriasis, tachycardia, hypertension, hyperthermia.
- Sympathomimetic toxidrome resembles anticholinergic except for diaphoresis (sympathetic-mediated ACh stimulation of sweat glands causes diaphoresis), and hypoactive bowel sounds (hyperactive in sympathomimetics).

Sympathomimetic = Wet
Anticholinergic = Dry

441

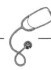

Toxins associated with mydriasis—
AAAAS
Antihistamines
Antidepressants
Anticholinergics
Atropine
Sympathomimetics

Examples of sympathomimetics—
ABC
Amphetamines
Beta agonists
Cocaine

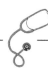

Toxins associated with tachycardia—
FAST
Free base (cocaine)
Anticholinergics/
antihistamines/
amphetamines
Sympathomimetics
Theophylline

Opiate toxidrome:
- Coma
- Respiratory depression
- Pinpoint pupils

- Multiple mechanisms of action of sympathomimetics:
  - Direct stimulation of α/β-adrenergic receptors.
  - Amphetamines stimulate release of norepinephrine (NE) into synapse.
  - Cocaine/TCAs prevent reuptake of NE from synapse.
  - MAOIs inhibit breakdown of NE.
- **Treatment:** Supportive—benzodiazepines, hydration, cooling.

Opioid

- Heroin, morphine, propoxyphene, meperidine, codeine, fentanyl
- Triad: ↓ level of consciousness, respiratory depression and pinpoint pupils (except meperidine)
- Hypothermia, bradycardia, hypotension, pulmonary edema
- **Treatment:** Naloxone (Narcan), a competitive opiate receptor antagonist
  - Dose depends on sensitivity of receptors to particular opiate
  - Caution: May precipitate agitation (withdrawal), seizures (especially tramadol), noncardiogenic pulmonary edema

Sedative-Hypnotic

- Benzodiazepines and barbiturates both work by potentiating γ-aminobutyric acid (GABA) (inhibitory neurotransmitter).
- Dose-dependent central nervous system (CNS) and respiratory depression (with barbiturates). Distinguish from ethanol (EtOH) intoxication by lack of vasodilation.
- Coingestion of alcohol, tranquilizers, or other depressants may potentiate these effects and → coma and/or apnea.
- **Treatment:** Supportive; flumazenil:
  - Competitive benzodiazepine receptor antagonist (caution—withdrawal seizures are common).
  - Benzodiazepine overdoses usually low morbidity so flumazenil rarely used.

DIAGNOSTIC ADJUNCTS

A variety of diagnostic studies and interventions are available to guide management.

"Coma Cocktail"

- Dextrose, oxygen, naloxone, thiamine
- Both a diagnostic and therapeutic intervention (hypoglycemia, hypoxia, opiates are common and easily reversible causes of CNS depression)

Acid-Base

- Blood gas, venous (VBG) or arterial (ABG), may be obtained if indicated clinically:
  - Respiratory acidosis in comatose patients suggests opiates/sedatives

- Respiratory alkalosis may be seen in sympathomimetic overdoses
- Respiratory alkalosis with metabolic acidosis is suggestive of acetylsalicylic acid (ASA)
- Serial ABG may be indicated in patients who require mechanical ventilation.
- Alkalinization of serum (TCA) and urine (ASA).

Electrolytes

- Metabolic acidosis should be classified as anion gap versus nonanion gap using serum electrolytes (anion gap metabolic acidosis may be seen in certain toxic ingestions—CAT MUDPILES).
- STAT electrolytes may be sent with ABG for potassium (useful in management of digoxin overdoses).
- **Anion gap** $= Na^+ - (Cl^- + HCO_3^-)$
- May be used in conjunction with serum osmolarity to detect toxic alcohol ingestion (with elevated osmole gap).

Spot Tests

- Classic example is ferric chloride test for salicylates (ferric chloride drops turn urine purple in presence of ASA).
- Spot tests also exist for acetaminophen, phenothiazines, barbiturates, ethanol, and certain types of mushrooms (most require high drug concentrations and have low sensitivity).

Immunoassays

- Most popular screening tool in emergency setting.
- Antibodies generated to representative antigen in each class (ie, amitriptyline for TCA, morphine for opiates, etc).
- Limited utility:
  - Time consuming: therapy should not be delayed waiting for drug screens.
  - Tests have varying sensitivities and low specificity (negative test does not rule out all types of TCA, opiates, etc).

Quantitative Tests

Useful for determining concentrations of specific toxins:

- May be useful in guiding management (acetaminophen and aspirin).
- Serial levels (assess adequacy of decontamination/elimination).
- Predicting clinical outcome.

Radiography

Certain toxins appear radiopaque on plain films.

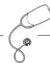

Coma cocktail—
DON'T
Dextrose (1 amp D$_{50}$)
Oxygen (supplemental)
Narcan (titrated slowly)
Thiamine (to prevent Wernicke's)
Remember, thiamine before glucose.

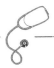

Causes of anion gap metabolic acidosis—
CAT MUDPILES
Carbon monoxide (CO)/ **C**yanide
Alcoholic ketoacidosis
Toluene
Methanol
Uremia
Diabetic ketoacidosis
Phenothiazines (Haldol)
Isoniazid (INH)
Lactic acidosis
Ethanol, ethylene glycol
Salicylates

Radiopaque substances—
CHIPS
Chlorinated substances (pesticides)
Heavy metals (lead, mercury, arsenic)
Iodine/iron
Phenothiazines
Sustained-release preparations/**S**alicylates (enteric coated)

Forced Emesis

- Rarely used anymore.
- Syrup of ipecac:
  - Plant derivative containing alkaloids (emetine and cephaeline).
  - Direct emetic effect on stomach.
  - Central effect on chemotactic trigger zone.
  - Produces emesis in over 90% of patients after single dose.
- Complications of ipecac include intractable vomiting, myocardial toxicity, and aspiration.

Gastric Lavage

Indications for lavage:
- Acute toxic ingestion.
- Patient's condition may deteriorate rapidly.
- Toxin doesn't bind to charcoal.

- Technique for orogastric lavage ("stomach pumped"):
  - Use large-bore tubes for intact pills (size 36–40 in adults, 22–24 in children).
  - Place patient in left lateral decubitus position (to minimize aspiration risk).
  - Have suction ready, measure length of tube, insert, and confirm position in stomach.
  - Lavage with fluid until aspirate is clear.
- Rarely performed secondary to complications.
- Potential indications:
  - Dangerous overdoses within 1 hour (eg, iron, TCA, etc).
  - Toxic ingestions that delay gastric emptying (ie, anticholinergics).
  - Drugs that form concretions (aspirin) take longer to clear stomach.
- Complications include aspiration pneumonia, perforation of esophagus, laryngospasm, hypoxia, and cardiac dysrhythmias.

Activated Charcoal

Substances that do not bind to charcoal—PHIALS
Pesticides
Hydrocarbons
Iron
Acids/Alkalies/Alcohols
Lithium
Solvents

- Directly binds to toxin in gut lumen.
- ↓ concentration of toxin in stomach, creating a gradient favoring flow of toxin from blood into stomach.
- Binds to toxin in bile (interrupts enterohepatic circulation).
- Multiple-dose charcoal:
  - May be beneficial with certain toxins (digoxin, phenytoin, etc).
  - Given empirically for ingestions of sustained-release products and drugs that form concretions.
- Avoid repeat doses of cathartics with charcoal.

Cathartics

- Limited role in toxic ingestions.
- May relieve constipating effects of charcoal.
- May prevent "desorption" of toxin from charcoal over time by decreasing transit time through gut.

- Sorbitol causes catharsis in < 2 hours; may cause abdominal cramping.
- Magnesium citrate causes catharsis in 4–6 hours; contraindicated in patients with renal failure.
- **Concerns:**
  - May cause significant fluid and electrolyte shifts.
  - ↓ transit time gives charcoal less time to bind.
- Current recommendations are to routinely give only single dose of cathartic with charcoal.
- **Contraindications** to cathartic use:
  - Patients with impaired gag reflex
  - Intestinal obstruction
  - Caustics

Whole Bowel Irrigation (WBI)

- A technique of flushing out the entire GI system with large volumes of fluid.
- Polyethylene glycol (Go-Lytely) is an isotonic fluid that does not cause significant bowel edema or fluid and electrolyte shifts.
- WBI minimally requires adults to drink 2 L/h of polyethylene glycol (0.5 L/h in children).
- End point of therapy is clear rectal effluent.
- Concerns:
  - Vomiting, bloating, and rectal irritation are common.
  - Polyethylene glycol may occupy charcoal binding sites.
  - It is time consuming, labor intensive, and messy.
- **Indications:**
  - Toxins that do not bind to charcoal
  - Ingestions of sustained-release products
  - Body-packers (smuggling illicit drugs in GI tract)

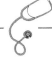

Toxins for which alkalinization may be helpful:
- Aspirin
- Phenobarbital
- Chlorpropamide

Urinary Alkalinization

- If pH of urine is raised to 7.5–8.0, "ion trapping" mechanism eliminates certain toxins.
- Hypokalemia impairs alkalinization by dumping H^+ ions in urine in exchange for K^+ (supplemental K^+ should be given intravenously [IV] with bicarbonate for alkalinization).

Hemodialysis and Hemoperfusion

Hemoperfusion: Charcoal filter in series with dialysis—most useful for theophylline.

Toxins that can be dialyzed—
I STUMBLE
Isopropyl
Salicylates
Theophylline
Uremia
Methanol
Barbiturates
Lithium
Ethylene glycol/Ethanol

Factors that accelerate acetaminophen toxicity:
- Prior induction of P450 (smokers, alcoholics, certain drugs)
- Malnutrition (↓ glutathione stores)

How to administer NAC:
- Identify patients with a toxic level of APAP (use Rumack-Matthew nomogram; *Figure 17-1*). *Note:* Nomogram was designed for use with single APAP level.
- Give loading dose of 140 mg/kg PO, followed by 70 mg/kg q4h for 17 more doses.

Acetaminophen

A 27-year-old woman with a history of depression presents approximately 6 hours after taking an estimated 30 Extra Strength Tylenol pills. EMS providers found an empty bottle of acetaminophen on the floor. She admits to trying to end her life and denies any other ingestion. Her only symptom is mild nausea. Her physical exam is unremarkable. Her vital signs are all normal and her weight is 70 kg. What should be the next step in management?

She should receive N-acetylcysteine (NAC) immediately. A rough estimate of a potential toxic dose of acetaminophen is 140 mg/kg (adults and pediatrics). Each Extra Strength Tylenol pill has 500 mg of acetaminophen. This puts her at an estimated dose of 214 mg/kg (30 × 500 mg = 15,000 mg/70 kg = 214 mg/kg), well within the toxic range. An acetaminophen level should be obtained, but care should not be delayed while awaiting the results. Charcoal is unlikely to be helpful given the delayed presentation.

- Chemical name is N-acetyl-para-aminophenol (commonly abbreviated as APAP).
- Most commonly reported potentially toxic ingestion; accounts for one third of all emergency department (ED) visits for overdose in the United States.
- Frequent coingestant.

EXPOSURE
- Tylenol, Paracetamol.
- Cold and flu preparations.
- Percocet (acetaminophen/oxycodone), Vicodin (acetaminophen/hydrocodone).

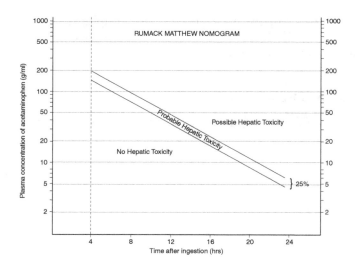

FIGURE 17-1. Rumack-Matthew nomogram.

(Reproduced, with permission, from *Management of Acetaminophen Overdose*. McNeil Consumer Products Co., 1986.)

446

- Metabolism of acetaminophen (therapeutic doses):
  - > 90% is metabolized by liver into nontoxic sulfate and glucuronide conjugates.
  - < 5% is directly excreted in urine.
  - < 5% is processed by cytochrome P450 system in liver to form N-acetyl-para-benzoquinoneimine (NAPQI).
- Metabolism of acetaminophen (in overdoses):
  - Sulfation and glucuronidation pathways become saturated.
  - P450 processes more APAP, generating more NAPQI.
  - NAPQI is a toxic intermediate of APAP.
  - NAPQI depletes glutathione stores and starts to accumulate.
  - Glutathione reduces NAPQI into nontoxic mercaptate conjugate.
  - NAPQI binds nonspecifically to intracellular proteins, causing cell dysfunction.

CLINICAL SIGNS OF TOXICITY

- Overdose is usually marked by a lack of clinical signs or symptoms in the first 24 hours.
- Toxic level of APAP at 4 hours is 150 µg/mL.
- **24–48 hours:** Begin to have right upper quadrant pain with elevation of liver function tests (LFTs) and prothrombin time (PT)/international normalized ratio (INR).
- **48–96 hours:** Severe liver dysfunction with coagulopathy, renal failure, death.
- Survivors will recover hepatic function over next 2 weeks.

MANAGEMENT

- Decontamination:
  - Activated charcoal (can be given with NAC).
  - Avoid emesis (this delays NAC administration).
  - Lavage only for coingestants.
- Administration of NAC:
  - Acts as glutathione precursor or substitute.
  - Acts as a sulfate precursor.
  - Directly reduces NAPQI back to APAP.
- After 24 hours, acts as a hepatocellular protectant.
- Administer as soon as toxic acetaminophen overdose suspected (better outcome if < 8 hours from ingestion).
- Oral dosing: 140 mg/kg × 1, followed by 17 doses at 70 mg/kg.
- IV dosing (Acetadote): Loading dose 150 mg/kg over 60 minutes, followed by 50 mg/kg over 4 hours, followed by 100 mg/kg over 16 hours.

Acetaminophen 140s:
140 mg/kg = potential toxic dose
>140 µg/mL = 4-hour level with possible hepatic toxicity
140 mg/kg = initial dose of PO NAC

Oral NAC smells and tastes like rotten eggs. Mix with cola or citrus soda over ice, cover with plastic wrap (blocks smell), and drink through a straw.

Aspirin

Acetylsalicylic acid (ASA).

EXPOSURE

- Present in over 200 oral and topical preparations (aspirin, Pepto-Bismol, Alka-Seltzer, Dristan, Ben-Gay, Tiger Balm, etc).
- Present in oil of wintergreen.

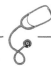

Causes of noncardiogenic pulmonary edema—MOPS
Meprobamate/**M**ountain sickness
Opioids
Phenobarbital
Salicylates

A 67-year-old woman presents with 6 days of headache and 2 days of "ringing in the ears" and fever. She is breathing deeply at a rate of 22/min. *Think: Aspirin toxicity.*

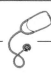

If you intubate a patient with metabolic acidosis and compensatory respiratory alkalosis, do not impede their ability to "blow off" acid. Use paralytics with extreme caution, and set the vent at a high minute ventilation. Often, ventilator is not as efficient as patient.

"Normal" ASA level does not rule out toxicity—repeat every 1–2 hours until levels decline and clinical status improves.

MECHANISM OF TOXICITY

- Absorption:
  - Normally 1–2 hours
  - 4–6 hours in overdose (delayed gastric emptying, concretion formation)
- Distribution:
  - Normally weak acid that remains ionized.
  - Acidosis in overdose makes it easier for ASA to penetrate tissues.
- Metabolism:
  - Conjugated in liver via first-order kinetics.
  - Liver enzymes saturated in overdose, zero-order kinetics.
- Elimination:
  - Small amount of free salicylate excreted in urine.
  - Maximizing urinary excretion may be beneficial in overdose. Consider for levels > 50 mg/dL.

CLINICAL SIGNS OF TOXICITY

- Respiratory:
  - Tachypnea/hyperpnea
  - Noncardiogenic pulmonary edema
- CNS:
  - Tinnitus
  - Headache
  - Cerebral edema/coma
- Other:
  - Platelet dysfunction
  - Hyperthermia

ACID-BASE DISTURBANCES

Mixed picture:

- Respiratory alkalosis: Direct stimulation of medulla (tachypnea/hyperpnea).
- Metabolic acidosis: Uncoupling of oxidative phosphorylation → to anaerobic metabolism with lactic acidosis.
- Metabolic alkalosis (less pronounced): Vomiting, diaphoresis, and tachypnea cause dehydration and volume contraction.

MANAGEMENT

- Check for presence of ASA: Ferric chloride—spot test turns urine purple if ASA is present.
- Decontamination: Activated charcoal.
- Respiratory support: Intubate if necessary but maintain hyperventilation (respiratory alkalosis buffers metabolic acidosis).
- IV fluids: Correct dehydration with glucose-containing crystalloid fluid.
- Urine alkalinization: Maintain urine pH around 8.0 to trap ionized ASA in urine. Alkalinize with bicarbonate drip.
- Extracorporeal removal: Hemoperfusion is better at removing ASA; hemodialysis is better for correcting acid-base and electrolytes (consider for ASA level > 100 mg/dL or as indicated clinically).
- Consider hemodialysis if there is: ASA level > 100 mg/dL; progressive deterioration despite aggressive care; renal impairment; or pulmonary edema.

Iron

Iron is an essential component of human red blood cells (RBCs), hemoglobin (Hgb), myoglobin, and cytochromes.

EXPOSURE

Accidental or intentional ingestion of iron-containing tablets.

Patients can die in any stage of iron toxicity.

MECHANISM OF TOXICITY

- < 10% of ingested iron is bioavailable:
  - Iron absorbed by intestinal mucosa, stored as ferritin.
  - Transported throughout body, complexed with transferrin.
  - Elimination is primarily via sloughing of intestinal mucosa (ferritin).
- Overdose:
  - Ingested iron overwhelms protein carriers, enters via passive diffusion.
  - Iron is corrosive to GI mucosa, enters circulation directly.
- Free iron in circulation → toxicity:
  - Direct corrosive effect on GI tract
  - Causes vasodilation and myocardial depression
  - Disrupts oxidative phosphorylation, which → buildup of lactic acid (metabolic acidosis)
  - Delayed hepatotoxicity

CLINICAL SIGNS OF TOXICITY

- **Stage I: 1–6 hours:** GI symptoms:
  - Abdominal pain
  - Nausea, vomiting, diarrhea
  - Hematemesis
- **Stage II: 6–24 hours:**
  - Resolution of GI symptoms
  - Early shock
- **Stage III: Variable time course:**
  - Shock.
  - Metabolic acidosis.
  - Coagulopathy.
  - Multiorgan failure may occur.
- **Stage IV: 2–5 days:** Hepatic insufficiency, may progress to failure.
- **Stage V: 4–6 weeks after ingestion:** Gastric outlet obstruction.

Toxic dose of iron:
< 20 mg/kg nontoxic
> 60 mg/kg severe toxicity
Calculate on basis of amount of elemental iron ingested
Toxic level of iron:
< 300 µg/dL nontoxic
> 500 µg/dL moderate toxicity
> 1,000 µg/dL severe toxicity

MANAGEMENT

- Obtain serum level.
- Supportive care.
- Decontamination:
  - WBI effective at clearing large GI loads.
  - No ipecac (iron already induces emesis).
  - Lavage usually ineffective (large iron pills).
  - Charcoal does not adsorb well to iron.
- Deferoxamine:
  - Chelates free iron to form ferrioxamine (water soluble, excreted in urine).
  - Ferrioxamine turns urine "vin rosé" (or rusty brown) color.
  - Dose: 5–15 mg/kg/h (not given for acute toxicity treatment).

Beta Blockers

Timmy is an 18-month-old child who is brought to the ED after ingesting some of his grandmother's medications. On further review, it appears that he took some of her propranolol and ibuprofen, but exact amounts are unknown. The parents called Poison Control and were instructed to come to the ED. He appears tired but otherwise well on physical exam, although the parents do note that he has been "lethargic and drooling." His vital signs are: temperature 36.6°C (97.9°F); pulse 65; respiratory rate 25; blood pressure 84/40. What is the most appropriate management?

He likely has sustained a significant beta blocker overdose. An acute ibuprofen overdose is not likely to be harmful. Given the bradycardia (< 90 in an 18-month-old) and hypoglycemia, he could benefit from glucagon, which has inotropic and chronotropic effects and counteracts the hypoglycemia. He will require admission and close monitoring for further symptoms (bradycardia, hypoglycemia, hypotension, etc).

EXPOSURE

Commonly prescribed for hypertension, atrial fibrillation, hyperthyroidism, etc.

MECHANISM OF TOXICITY

- Stimulation of β-adrenergic receptor causes an ↑ in intracellular cyclic adenosine monophosphate (cAMP) → phosphorylation of calcium channels (opens channels).
- ↑ calcium influx triggers release of intracellular calcium stores → excitation-contraction coupling.
- Pharmacologic differences among beta blockers:
    - Selectivity: Agents may have β_1 or β_2 selectivity, which is lost in overdose.
    - Solubility: More lipid-soluble agents are more likely to penetrate CNS.
    - Agents with intrinsic sympathomimetic activity may present atypically.
    - Membrane stabilizing: These agents may cause sodium channel blockade.

CLINICAL SIGNS OF TOXICITY

- Bradycardia and hypotension.
- Sinus node suppression.
- Slowed atrioventricular (AV) nodal conduction.
- QRS widening with agents that block Na channels.
- ↓ myocardial contractility.
- ↓ cardiac output.
- Smooth muscle relaxation, peripheral vasodilation.
- Lipophilic agents may cause sedation and/or seizures (penetrate CNS).
- β_2 receptor blockade may → bronchospasm.

β-adrenergic receptors:

β_1:
- Myocardium (↑ inotropy)
- Eye (↑ aqueous humor)
- Kidney (↑ plasma renin)

β_2:
- Smooth muscle relaxation
- Liver (glycogenolysis, gluconeogenesis)

β_3: Adipose tissue (lipolysis)

MANAGEMENT

- Supportive treatment.
- Fluid resuscitation.
- Decontamination: Gastric lavage (if within 1–2 hours) and activated charcoal.
- Glucagon bypasses beta receptor to ↑ intracellular cAMP.
- Catecholamines (dopamine/NE) for pressor support.
- Phosphodiesterase inhibitors (amrinone) block cAMP breakdown.
- Transcutaneous/transvenous pacing, intra-aortic balloon pump (IABP), bypass as indicated.

Calcium Channel Blockers

EXPOSURE

Commonly prescribed for hypertension.

MECHANISM OF TOXICITY

- Blockade of L-type calcium channels in cell membranes.
- ↓ calcium influx disrupts excitation-contraction coupling.
- Different classes of calcium channel blockers:
  - Both phenylalkylamines (verapamil) and benzothiazepines (diltiazem) cause ↓ myocardial contractility and conduction, as well as vasodilation.
  - Dihydropyridines (nifedipine, amlodipine) cause mostly peripheral vasodilation.

CLINICAL SIGNS OF TOXICITY

- Hypotension
- Bradycardia
- ↓ conduction/automaticity
- Hypoperfusion
- Lactic acidosis
- Insulin resistance, hyperglycemia/hyperkalemia

MANAGEMENT

- Supportive care.
- Fluid resuscitation.
- Decontamination with lavage (if early) and charcoal.
- Consider WBI for sustained release preparations.
- Correct acidosis.
- IV calcium:
  - ↑ gradient across calcium channel
  - Stabilizes membranes in presence of hyperkalemia
- Glucagon acts to ↑ cAMP and phosphorylate calcium channels.
- Electrical pacing and/or pressors (dopamine) as indicated.
- Refractory cases: Consider amrinone (inhibits cAMP breakdown), insulin (inotrope/chronotrope), IABP, or dialysis.

Cardiac Glycosides (Digoxin)

Commonly used in the treatment of congestive heart failure (CHF) and supraventricular tachycardias.

Causes of bradycardia --
PACED
Propranolol (beta blockers)
Anticholinesterase drugs
Clonidine/**C**alcium channel blockers
Ethanol, other alcohols
Digoxin/**D**arvon (opiates)

Toxicity from chronic digoxin use may be seen with normal levels.

Salvador Dali mustache: Scooped ST segments are seen with digoxin use at therapeutic levels *(not an indicator of toxicity).*

Pathognomic for digoxin toxicity: Bidirectional ventricular tachycardia.

Digoxin levels are meaningless once Digibind is administered.

Without Digibind therapy, mortality in digoxin overdose is:

- 100% for K > 5.5 mEq/L
- 50% for K = 5.0–5.5 mEq/L
- 0% for K < 5.0 mEq/L

Never use calcium as therapy for hyperkalemia in digoxin overdose (reports of myocardial tetany [ie, "stone heart"] have been reported).

EXPOSURE

- Digoxin
- Foxglove plant
- Oleander plant

MECHANISM OF TOXICITY

- Inhibits Na^+-K^+ ATPase pump:
  - ↑ intracellular Na^+, extracellular K^+.
  - Less Ca^{2+} is pumped out in exchange for Na^+ (↑ intracellularn Ca^{2+} → ↑ inotropy).
  - Membrane resting potential becomes less negative (as Na^+ and Ca^{2+} accumulate inside cell), → ↑ automaticity (tachydysrhythmias).
- ↑ vagal tone (→ bradydysrhythmias):
  - ↓ conduction through AV node.
  - Also → sinus bradycardia.

CLINICAL SIGNS OF TOXICITY

- Cardiac toxicity (wide range of rhythm disturbances):
  - Sinus bradycardia/block
  - Atrial fibrillation/flutter
  - AV node blocks (junctional rhythms)
  - Premature ventricular contractions, ventricular tachycardia/fibrillation
- Hyperkalemia (inhibition of Na^+-K^+ pump).
- Nausea, vomiting, and headaches are common in acute overdose.
- Visual disturbances:
  - Amblyopia
  - Photophobia
  - Yellow-green halos around light

MANAGEMENT

- Decontamination with activated charcoal for acute overdose (avoid lavage, as it may ↑ vagal tone).
- Treat bradydysrhythmias—atropine and/or pacing.
- Treat tachydysrhythmias—lidocaine, phenytoin.
- Treat hyperkalemia—indicator for digoxin toxicity as above; severe hyperkalemia: Insulin/glucose and bicarbonate.
- Treat hypokalemia—may potentiate digoxin toxicity, replace as indicated (may see toxic effects with normal digoxin levels).
- Digibind:
  - Digoxin-specific antibody fragments bind to digoxin in serum, eliminated by kidneys. Use for:
    - Ventricular dysrhythmias
    - Hemodynamically significant bradydysrhythmias
    - Hyperkalemia > 5.0 in setting of overdose
    - Digoxin level > 4 ng/mL
  - Digibind dosing:
    - Unknown ingestion (empiric): 5–10 vials
    - Known ingestion: 1.6 × amount ingested
    - Known digoxin level: [wt(kg) × level (ng/mL)/100]

GLUCOSE METABOLISM

- Serum levels maintained by balance among three mechanisms:
  - Gut absorption of ingested glucose.
  - Glycogenolysis—mobilization of liver stores.
  - Gluconeogenesis—major mechanism for glucose control in hypoglycemic states.
- Physiologic response to hypoglycemia:
  - CNS: Confusion, lethargy, seizures, coma, focal neurologic deficits
  - Autonomic response
  - Release of counterregulatory hormones (epinephrine, glucagon, etc)
  - Diaphoresis, tremors, palpitations, anxiety

EXPOSURE

- Insulin:
  - Immediate- (Lispro), short- (regular), intermediate- (NPH), and long- (Ultralente) acting formulations
  - Secreted by beta-islet cells of pancreas
  - Stimulates uptake/utilization of glucose in body
  - Insulin absorption variable in overdose
- Sulfonylureas:
  - Oral hypoglycemic agents are commonly prescribed for type 2 diabetes.
  - ↑ endogenous insulin secretion and sensitivity to insulin in peripheral tissues.
  - Long duration of hypoglycemia.
- Biguanides:
  - Oral hypoglycemic agents (eg, metformin [Glucophage])
  - ↑ peripheral sensitivity to insulin
  - Suppresses gluconeogenesis
  - Causes hypoglycemia rarely

CLINICAL SIGNS OF TOXICITY

- Hypoglycemia (glucose < 60 mg/dL)
- Anxiety, diaphoresis, hypothermia
- Delirium, coma, seizure, or focal neurologic deficit

MANAGEMENT

- Decontamination with charcoal for overdose.
- Dextrose:
  - PO solutions if patient awake
  - IV if altered mental status (see dosing in Endocrine chapter)
- Glucagon:
  - Can be given IM if patient obtunded and no IV access
  - May not help if hepatic glycogen stores are already depleted

Patients with hypoglycemia due to a long-acting oral hypoglycemic should be admitted.

HIGH-YIELD FACTS

Emergency Toxicology

Tricyclic Antidepressants (TCAs)

A 19-year-old woman with a history of an eating disorder is brought in by EMS providers. She apparently had a fight with her boyfriend and over-dosed 2 hours ago on an unknown medication. EMS found her agitated and moaning incoherently. Her vital signs are significant for a temperature of 38.1°C (100.6°F), pulse of 110, and a blood pressure of 98/50. Her physical exam reveals an agitated female moaning incoherently with dilated pupils and a dry mouth and skin. What is the most likely diagnosis?

TCA overdose. An ECG should be obtained and will reveal a QRS of >150 msec. Her physical exam findings are explained by the anticholinergic effects of TCAs. She is likely taking a TCA for her eating disorder. She should receive aggressive supportive care and sodium bicarbonate immediately. A further investigation for coingestions (eg, acetaminophen) should be undertaken.

TCAs are responsible for more drug-related deaths than any other prescription medication.

EXPOSURE

Commonly prescribed for depression, chronic pain.

MECHANISM OF TOXICITY

- Blocks reuptake of dopamine, serotonin, NE
- Binds to GABA receptor, lowering seizure threshold
- Sodium channel blockade: Wide QRS
- α-adrenergic blockade: Orthostatic hypotension
- Antihistamine effect: Sedation
- Anticholinergic effect

CLINICAL SIGNS OF TOXICITY

- Central nervous system effects:
  - Sedation
  - Seizure
  - TCAs block GABA$_A$ receptors
- Cardiac effects:
  - Arrhythmias:
    - Sinus tachycardia most common
    - Ventricular tachychardia (VT) or fibrillation (VF)
  - ↓ contractility and peripheral vasodilation
  - Hypotension
- Anticholinergic symptoms: Hyperthermia, dry skin/membranes, mydria-sis, urinary retention, altered mental status

Check an ECG on all patients with a suspected TCA OD.

DIAGNOSIS

- Abnormal electrocardiogram (ECG) (Figure 17-2):
  - ECG changes suggestive of TCA OD:
    - QRS > 100 msec
    - Abnormal QRS (deep, slurred S in I and aVL)

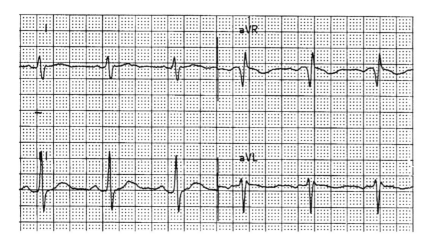

FIGURE 17-2. ECG of TCA toxicity.

(Reproduced, with permission, from Goldfrank LR et al. *Goldfrank's Toxicology*, 7th ed. New York: McGraw-Hill, 2002: 123.)

- aVR: R wave > 3 mm, R:S ratio > 0.7
- Sinus tachycardia, right axis deviation (RAD), and prolongation of PR, QRS, and QT intervals

MANAGEMENT

- Decontamination:
  - Charcoal is effective at binding TCA.
  - Lavage only effective early in course.
- Sodium bicarbonate:
  - Use if suspect TCA OD and QRS > 100 msec or VT/VF.
  - 1–2 mEq/kg rapid IV push followed by an infusion.
  - Goal of therapy is to maintain narrow QRS. Avoid excessive alkalemia (pH > 7.55).
- Treat hypotension with sodium bicarbonate, IV crystalloid, and NE (if necessary).
- Treat seizures:
  - Benzodiazepines/barbiturates.
  - Avoid phenytoin (risk of dysrhythmia).
- Treat dysrhythmias:
  - Sodium bicarbonate is first-line intervention (improves conduction/contractility and ↓ ectopy).
  - Cardioversion if unstable.

ECG and TCA:
- QRS < 100, no significant toxicity
- QRS > 100, seizures in one third of patients
- QRS > 160, ventricular dysrhythmias in one half of patients

Action of sodium bicarbonate in heart in TCA overdose is due to the *sodium* component; it alters the interaction between the drug and sodium channels.

Selective Serotonin Reuptake Inhibitors (SSRIs)

EXPOSURE

Commonly prescribed for depression, premenstrual syndrome.

MECHANISM OF TOXICITY

- Selectively inhibit reuptake of serotonin without affecting dopamine/NE.
- No direct effect on presynaptic/postsynaptic receptors (fewer side effects than TCAs).

Serotonin syndrome:
Usually results from combination of SSRI with:
- MAOI
- Cocaine
- Methylene dioxymetamphetamine (MDMA) (ecstasy)
- Lithium/tryptophan

Characterized by:
- Hyperthermia
- Tachycardia
- Rigidity
- Hyperreflexia
- Confusion/agitation

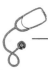

Do not use the following agents in patients on MAOIs (partial list — check all agents given to patients on MAOIs):
- Other MAOIs
- Amphetamines
- Dopamine
- Epinephrine, NE
- Meperidine
- Buspirone
- Dextromethorphan
- SSRIs
- Tyramine-containing foods
- Cocaine

- High toxic-to-therapeutic drug ratio (lower incidence of toxicity from overdose).
- Extrapyramidal symptoms (EPS): Dystonic reactions, parkinsonism, etc.
- Hyponatremia secondary to syndrome of inappropriate antidiuretic hormone secretion (SIADH).
- Seizures, QT prolongation: Rare, mostly with citalopram (Celexa).
- Serotonin syndrome:
  - Potentially life-threatening syndrome caused by ↑ serotonergic activity.
  - Clinical diagnosis:
    - Mental status changes
    - Autonomic hyperactivity (hypertension, tachycardia, hyperthermia, diaphoresis)
    - Neuromuscular hyperactivity (hyperreflexia, clonus, tremor, muscle rigidity)

MANAGEMENT

- Decontamination with activated charcoal
- Benzodiazepines/barbiturates for seizures
- Sodium bicarbonate for wide QRS
- For serotonin syndrome:
  - Supportive care, cooling.
  - Sedation with benzodiazepines.
  - Consider cyproheptadine (antihistamine with antiserotonin properties).
  - Discontinue causative medications.

Monoamine Oxidase Inhibitors (MAOIs)

EXPOSURE

Now only occasionally prescribed for depression.

MECHANISM OF TOXICITY

- MAO: Enzyme found in nerve terminals; degrades epinephrine, norepinephrine (NE), dopamine, and serotonin.
- MAOIs: Form an irreversible covalent bond with MAO in nerve terminals. ↑ the amount of biogenic amines available at nerve terminals:
  - ↑ catecholamines.
  - Synergy with SSRIs may → serotonin syndrome.
  - Tyramine-containing foods may cause sympathomimetic crisis.
  - Other drugs (cocaine, amphetamines) may contribute to or cause sympathomimetic crisis.

CLINICAL SIGNS OF TOXICITY

- Tachycardia, hyperthermia, hypertension, mydriasis, agitation.
- Eventual catecholamine depletion can cause sympatholytic crisis (hypotension, bradycardia, CNS depression).
- Serum levels of MAOI correlate poorly with toxicity.
- Onset of toxicity may be delayed up to 24 hours.

MANAGEMENT

- Supportive care.
- Gastric lavage, if acute.
- Discontinue drugs that may interact with MAOI.
- Control hypertension (phentolamine, nitroprusside).

- Treat seizures, hyperthermia, and rigidity with benzodiazepines.
- Treat ventricular dysrhythmias with lidocaine or procainamide.
- Treat hypotension with fluids and NE.

Lithium

EXPOSURE

Commonly prescribed for bipolar disorder.

MECHANISM OF TOXICITY

- Overall, not well understood.
- ↑ synthesis and turnover of serotonin.
- Downregulates number of adrenergic receptors (β and α_2).
- Inhibits adenylate cyclase (↓ cAMP).
- Inhibits inositol monophosphatase.
- Deposits in bone and other tissues, forming a reservoir of lithium.
- Competes with other molecules of similar size.
- Ninety-five percent is excreted in urine (glomerular filtration rate dependent).

CLINICAL SIGNS OF TOXICITY

- Acute toxicity:
  - Nausea, vomiting, abdominal pain.
  - Acute ingestions can tolerate higher Li+ levels without toxicity.
- Chronic toxicity: Resting tremor, hyperreflexia, seizure, coma, EPS.
- Acute or chronic:
  - Prolonged QT, flipped T waves (hypokalemia).
  - Nephrogenic diabetes insipidus.

MANAGEMENT

- Decontaminate with WBI for acute ingestions.
- Fluid resuscitation.
- Kayexalate is effective at binding lithium but requires massive doses so not done in practice.
- Hemodialysis for:
  - Lithium level > 4 (acute) or > 2.5 (chronic)
  - Significant CNS or cardiovascular toxicity
  - Renal failure
  - Heart failure

Lithium does not bind to charcoal.

Antipsychotics

EXPOSURE

- Older "typical" agents:
  - Haloperidol, chlorpromazine
  - More effective in controlling positive symptoms (hallucinations, delusions)
- Newer "atypical" agents:
  - Olanzapine, risperidone, ziprasidone.
  - More effective at controlling negative symptoms (apathy, blunted affect).

Antipsychotics: Toxicity can occur with overdose or therapeutic dose.

EPS:
- Dystonic reactions
- Akathisia (motor restlessness)

NMS:
- Hyperthermia
- Altered mental status
- Autonomic instability
- Muscular rigidity

Toxicologic causes of hyperthermia—NASA
NMS
Antihistamines
Salicylates/
Sympathomimetics/
Serotonin syndrome
Anticholinergics

MECHANISM OF TOXICITY

- Older agents block D_2 (dopaminergic) receptor, possess antihistamine, anticholinergic.
- Newer agents block 5-HT_2 (serotonergic) receptor.
- Neuroleptic malignant syndrome (NMS) caused by central dopaminergic blockade.

CLINICAL SIGNS OF TOXICITY

- EPS
- Orthostatic hypotension with tachycardia
- Sedation

MANAGEMENT

- Decontamination.
- Supportive care.
- Treat EPS symptoms with IV diphenhydramine and discontinue agent if possible.
- Treat NMS with discontinuation of agent, cooling, benzodiazepines, and dantrolene. Consider carbidopa/levodopa to ↑ dopamine activity.

ANTICONVULSANTS

Phenytoin

- First-line agent useful for all types of seizures except absence.
- Blocks voltage-sensitive and frequency-dependent sodium channels in neurons.
- Suppresses ability of neurons to fire action potentials at high frequency.
- Fosphenytoin (Cerebyx):
  - Phenytoin prodrug, soluble in aqueous solution with pH ~8.8.
  - Converted to phenytoin in blood and peripheral tissues.
  - Well tolerated both IV and IM routes (fewer side effects—faster administration possible).

EXPOSURE

Commonly prescribed for seizure disorder.

MECHANISM OF TOXICITY

In overdose, kinetics change from first-order to zero-order.

CLINICAL SIGNS OF TOXICITY

- CNS toxicity: Nystagmus, lethargy, ataxia, seizures, coma
- Local effects (IM): Crystallization, abscess, tissue necrosis
- Hypersensitivity: Systemic lupus erythematosus (SLE), toxic epidermal necrolysis, Stevens-Johnson syndrome (1–6 weeks after initiating therapy)
- Gingival hyperplasia
- Cardiovascular toxicity:
  - Almost always seen as infusion rate–related complication of IV therapy due to diluent.
  - Phenytoin diluent: Propylene glycol, ethanol solution (pH ≈12).
  - Hypotension, bradycardia, AV blocks, asystole.
  - ECG: Prolonged PR and QRS, nonspecific ST-T wave changes.

MANAGEMENT

- Use multiple-dose charcoal for oral overdose.
- Hemodialysis and hemoperfusion are ineffective.
- Supportive care; discontinue infusion for signs of toxicity.

Carbamazepine (Tegretol)

- First-line agent useful for all types of seizures except absence.
- Also used in the management of trigeminal neuralgia and bipolar disorder.
- Available only in oral formulation (no parenteral forms).

CLINICAL SIGNS OF TOXICITY

- CNS: Nystagmus, ataxia, dystonia, seizures, coma
- Cardiac: QRS widening, prolonged QT, AV blocks

The cardiovascular side effects of IV phenytoin are due to the diluent.

MANAGEMENT

- Decontamination with multiple-dose charcoal.
- Hemodialysis ineffective.
- Hemoperfusion with charcoal is effective.
- Bicarbonate for QRS widening > 100 msec.
- Benzodiazepines for seizures.

Valproic Acid

- Used for the treatment of absence, myoclonic, and tonic-clonic seizures.
- Also used as mood stabilizer for treatment of bipolar disorder.
- Metabolized extensively in liver, with several biologically active metabolites (2-N-valproic acid is active and accumulates in CNS and other tissues).

CLINICAL SIGNS OF TOXICITY

- Nausea/vomiting and abdominal pain.
- Cerebral edema from accumulation of metabolites.
- Respiratory depression, cardiac arrest.
- Metabolic derangements:
  - Hyperammonemia +/– hypocarnitinemia.
  - Metabolic acidosis.
  - Hypernatremia.
  - Hypocalcemia.
- Hepatotoxicity.

MANAGEMENT

- Supportive care.
- Decontamination with multiple-dose activated charcoal.
- Hemodialysis improves clearance; reserve for most toxic patients.
- Carnitine supplementation in hyperammonemic patients.

Blood alcohol level (BAL):
- One drink equals ~25–35 mg/dL BAL.
- Average person metabolizes 15–20 mg/dL/h.
- Chronic drinkers metabolize ~30 mg/dL/h.

General Principles

- Group of structurally similar molecules with common R–OH group.
- Level of inebriation after consumption is related to number of carbons in R group (methanol < ethanol < ethylene glycol < isopropyl alcohol).
- Calculated serum osmolarity: 2 (Na$^+$) + (BUN/2.8) + (Glucose/18).
- Osmol gap: Difference between measured and calculated serum osmolarity.
- Estimate toxic alcohol level as follows: Osmol gap = alcohol level/N (where N = molecular weight/10 [i.e., N = 3.2 for methanol, 4.6 for ethanol, etc]).
- "Normal" osmol gap is between –14 and +10; baseline gap is usually unknown.
- Patients with "normal" gap may in fact be elevated from their baseline.
- Elevated gap of 10 corresponds to methanol level of 32, ethanol level 46, etc.
- Bottom line: Elevated gap is useful; normal gap does not rule out toxic ingestion.

Ethanol

Most commonly used and abused intoxicant in the United States.

EXPOSURE

- Ethanol is frequently consumed with other intoxicants.
- Ethanol + cocaine → cocaethylene (40 times more potent than regular cocaine).

MECHANISM OF TOXICITY

- CNS depressant that cross-reacts with other depressants (benzodiazepines, barbiturates).
- Majority of ethanol is absorbed in proximal small bowel.
- Up to 10% is eliminated by lungs, urine, and sweat.
- Remainder is metabolized by liver as follows:
  - Catalyzed by alcohol dehydrogenase and aldehyde dehydrogenase (inhibited by disulfiram)
  - Microsomal alcohol oxidizing system
- Elimination follows zero-order kinetics:
  - ~15–20 mg/dL/h in normal individuals
  - ~30 mg/dL/h in chronic alcoholics

CLINICAL SIGNS OF TOXICITY

- Slurred speech.
- Nystagmus.
- Disinhibition.
- CNS depression.
- Degree of clinical intoxication correlates poorly with blood alcohol level (BAL).

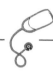

Causes of elevated osmol gap —
E-MEDIA
Ethylene glycol
Methanol
Ethanol
Diuretics (mannitol)
Isopropyl alcohol
Acetone

MANAGEMENT

Management of acute intoxication is supportive:

- Thiamine, folate, IV fluids.
- "Banana bag" consists of 1 L of D$_5$NS with 100 mg thiamine, 1 mg folate, and 1 amp of multivitamin (which turns bag yellow). Can be given for chronic alcoholics, but is not always necessary.

ALCOHOLIC KETOACIDOSIS (AKA)

- Anion gap acidosis in heavy alcohol user who has temporarily stopped drinking and eating.
- Acid-base: Frequently metabolic acidosis with respiratory alkalosis (compensatory) and metabolic alkalosis (vomiting). The pH may be normal.
- Treat with IV fluid replacement, IV glucose, and thiamine.

In AKA, most ketones are β-hydroxybutyrate and are poorly detected by lab.

Methanol

EXPOSURE

Product of wood distillation, found in:

- Antifreeze
- Windshield wiper fluids
- Paint thinners

MECHANISM OF TOXICITY

Toxicity is secondary to formic acid (Figure 17-3):

- Formic acid accumulation produces high-anion-gap metabolic acidosis.
- Formaldehyde accumulates in retina causing "snowfield vision."
- Onset of symptoms is usually delayed ~12–18 hours until metabolites form (delay is even longer if ethanol is coingested).
- Folate is a required cofactor to degrade formic acid to carbon dioxide and water.

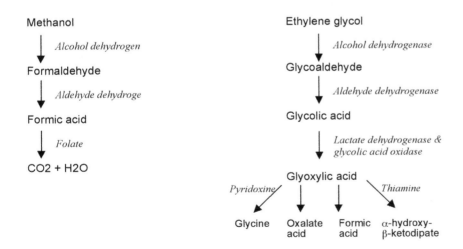

FIGURE 17-3 **Metabolism of methanol and ethylene glycol.**

Blood glucose levels need to be monitored during ethanol therapy.

CLINICAL SIGNS OF TOXICITY

- ■ CNS depression.
- ■ Visual changes (funduscopic examination demonstrates optic papillitis and edema).
- ■ Abdominal pain (direct GI mucosal irritation).
- ■ High anion gap metabolic acidosis.
- ■ Severity of acidosis is better predictor of outcome than methanol level.

MANAGEMENT

- ■ Charcoal:
  - ■ Binds poorly to all alcohols.
  - ■ Rapid GI absorption of alcohols limits utility of charcoal.
- ■ Folate: Hastens degradation of formic acid. Dose is 50 mg IV q4h; the first dose is given as activated folate (leucovorin).
- ■ Fomepizole:
  - ■ Competitive inhibitor of alcohol dehydrogenase.
  - ■ Blocks metabolism of methanol to toxic metabolites.
  - ■ Affinity for alcohol dehydrogenase 8000 times greater than methanol.
  - ■ Dose is 15 mg/kg IV, then four doses at 10 mg/kg each 12 hours apart.
- ■ Ethanol (if fomepizole unavailable):
  - ■ Affinity for alcohol dehydrogenase 20 times greater than methanol.
  - ■ BAL of ethanol should be maintained ~100–150 mg/dL.
  - ■ Methanol is cleared renally (slow) while on ethanol drip.
  - ■ Dose is 8 g/kg IV load, then continuous infusion at 11 g/h (average drinker) or 15 g/h (heavy drinker).
- ■ Dialysis:
  - ■ Indicated for large ingestions or with severe acidosis
  - ■ Indicated when methanol level > 25 mg/dL

Ethylene Glycol

A 23-year-old man is brought in by EMS with an altered mental status. He was found by his roommate at home acting funny. EMS providers believe that he is drunk. His heart rate is 105, he is breathing 24 times per minute, and his blood pressure is 138/88. He is acting grossly intoxicated with slurred speech and ataxia on exam, but his ethanol comes back negative. He was noted to have an osmol gap of 105 mOsm. His roommate arrives with what appears to be an empty bottle of antifreeze that he found in their apartment. What diagnosis should you suspect?

The intoxication alone in the presence of negative ethanol is concerning for a toxic alcohol. Combining this with the elevated osmol gap and history of antifreeze ingestion suggests ethylene glycol toxicity. An ethylene glycol level will not be immediately available. Further, tests such as detection of urine fluorescence or calcium oxalate crystals are unreliable.

Colorless, odorless, and sweet-tasting liquid.

EXPOSURE

- ■ Coolant/antifreeze
- ■ Commercial solvents

- Detergents
- Polishes
- Deicers

MECHANISM OF TOXICITY

Toxicity is secondary to toxic metabolites (Figure 17-3):

- Ethylene glycol → glycoaldehyde causes lactate formation.
- Glyoxylic acid broken down to glycine and ketoadipate (nontoxic).
- When above pathways are saturated, formic acid and oxalic acid are formed.
- Formic acid contributes to metabolic acidosis as with methanol.
- Oxalic acid crystallizes (calcium oxalate) causing renal stones and hypocalcemia.

CLINICAL SIGNS OF TOXICITY

- Early phase (1–12 hours): CNS depression, slurred speech, ataxia
- Cardiopulmonary phase (12–24 hours): Tachycardia, tachypnea, CHF, adult respiratory distress syndrome (ARDS)
- Nephrotoxic phase (24–72 hours): Oliguric renal failure, acute tubular necrosis, hypocalcemia

MANAGEMENT

- Quickly absorbed by gut and only 50% adsorbed to charcoal; charcoal has limited benefit.
- Obtain blood levels of ethanol, methanol, and ethylene glycol.
- Ethanol infusion or fomepizole to competitively inhibit toxic pathways.
- Calcium supplementation as indicated for hypocalcemia.
- Pyridoxine and thiamine supplementation to preserve nontoxic pathways.
- Dialysis as indicated clinically or for ethylene glycol level > 25 mg/dL.
- Asymptomatic patients are admitted for observation due to concern for delayed manifestation of toxicity.

Isopropanol

Clear liquid with bitter burning taste and characteristic odor.

EXPOSURE

- Rubbing alcohol
- Disinfectants
- Skin and hair products

MECHANISM OF TOXICITY

- Twice as potent as ethanol in causing CNS depression, with longer half-life.
- Metabolism of isopropanol follows first-order (concentration-dependent) kinetics.

CLINICAL SIGNS OF TOXICITY

- Hallmark of isopropanol ingestion is ketosis without significant acidosis:
  - Acetic acid and formic acid formation contribute to mild acidosis.
  - Acetone formation causes ketonemia/ketonuria in absence of hyperglycemia.

Ethylene glycol is often consumed as an ethanol substitute or in suicide attempts.

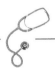

Funduscopy in ethylene glycol poisoning is normal; this distinguishes it from methanol poisoning.

Hallmark of ethylene glycol toxicity: Calcium oxalate crystals in urine (50% present).

How to calculate osmolarity:
$2 \times Na + BUN/2 + Glucose/18 + ETOH/4.6$
If there is a difference between the measured (lab) and calculated osmolarity, consider toxic alcohols.

HIGH-YIELD FACTS

Emergency Toxicology

- Marked CNS depression (greater than ethanol).
- Hypotension secondary to peripheral vasodilatation.
- Hemorrhagic gastritis from direct mucosal irritation.

MANAGEMENT

- Rapidly absorbed and binds poorly to charcoal.
- Supportive treatment for coma/respiratory depression.
- IV fluids (pressors if necessary) for hypotension.
- H₂ blockers, nasogastric tube, and transfusion as indicated for hemorrhagic gastritis.
- Dialysis for refractory hypotension or peak level > 400 mg/dL.
- Asymptomatic patients can be discharged after 6–8 hours.

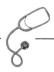

The hallmark of isopropanol ingestion is ketosis and elevated osmolal gap without significant acidosis.

DRUGS OF ABUSE

Cocaine

Naturally occurring alkaloid extract of *Erythroxylon coca* (South American plant).

EXPOSURE

- Cocaine hydrochloride: Absorbed across all membranes (usually snorted or injected)
- Cocaine alkaloid (crack): Stable to pyrolysis (may be inhaled), rapid onset/short duration

MECHANISM OF TOXICITY

- Mechanisms of action:
  - Blocks presynaptic reuptake of biogenic amine transmitters: Dopamine, serotonin, NE
  - Local anesthetic effect by blocking fast sodium channels
- Initial euphoria secondary to release of biogenic amines, subsequent dysphoria secondary to depletion of neurotransmitters (dopamine)

CLINICAL SIGNS OF TOXICITY

- Euphoria followed by dysphoria.
- Hypertension.
- Tachycardia, dysrhythmias.
- Chest pain (coronary vasoconstriction).
- Seizures, infarction, hemorrhage (cerebral vasoconstriction).
- Cocaine psychosis.
- Rhabdomyolysis.
- Hyperthermia.
- QRS widening (sodium channel blockade) and QT prolongation (potassium channel blockade).
- Adulterants and direct toxicity cause pulmonary edema, hemorrhage, and barotrauma (patients try Valsalva to ↑ drug effect).
- Mesenteric vasospasm (common in body-stuffers).
- Uterine vasospasm causes abortions, abruption, prematurity, intrauterine growth retardation.
- Cocaine wash-out syndrome.

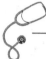

Causes of toxin-induced seizures —
OTIS CAMPBELL
Organophosphates/**O**ral hypoglycemics
Tricyclic antidepressants
INH/**I**nsulin
Sympathomimetics
Camphor/**C**ocaine
Amphetamines
Methylxanthines
PCP/**P**henol/**P**ropranolol
Benzodiazepine withdrawal
Ethanol withdrawal
Lithium/**L**indane
Lidocaine/**L**ead

Beta blockers are traditionally considered contraindicated in cocaine toxicity due to concern that unopposed alpha stimulation could ↑ blood pressure.

MANAGEMENT

- Initial supportive therapy includes sedation and cooling measures.
- Decontamination (charcoal and/or WBI) for body packers; endoscopy is contraindicated due to high incidence of bags rupturing.
- Benzodiazepines are effective in controlling tachycardia, hypertension, and seizures.
- Aggressive fluid resuscitation to maintain urine output.
- Aspirin/nitrates/morphine for myocardial ischemia.
- Bicarbonate for patients with widened QRS or rhabdomyolysis.
- Nitroprusside or phentolamine for control of severe hypertension (beta blockers contraindicated, unopposed alpha stimulation may ↑ blood pressure).

Opioids

EXPOSURE

Naturally occurring or synthetic derivatives of poppy plant:

- Morphine
- Codeine
- Fentanyl
- Heroin
- Methadone
- Others

MECHANISM OF TOXICITY

- There are three main opioid receptors: OP1 (formerly δ), OP2 (formerly κ), and OP3 (formerly μ).
- Stimulation of OP3 receptors produces analgesia, cough suppression, euphoria, and repiration depression.

CLINICAL SIGNS OF TOXICITY

- CNS depression.
- Hypothermia, bradycardia, hypotension.
- Miosis (not for every drug in the class).
- Histamine release may contribute to hypotension.
- Respiratory depression.
- Noncardiogenic pulmonary edema.
- ↓ GI motility—obstipation/constipation.

MANAGEMENT

- Respiratory support using bag-valve mask or endotracheal intubation (respiratory depression is the major cause of mortality with opiates).
- Charcoal and WBI for body-packers.
- Naloxone (Narcan):
  - Pure antagonist at all three opiate receptors.
  - Use incremental doses and titrate to response.
  - Small initial doses (≤ 0.4 mg) less likely to precipitate withdrawal.
  - Patients given naloxone should be observed until effects of naloxone have worn off (> 2 hours) to ensure they do not have prolonged opioid effects.
  - Obtain acetaminophen level for any combined opioid preparations.

Causes of miosis—
COPS
Cholinergics/**C**lonidine
Opiates/**O**rganophosphates
Phenothiazines/
Pilocarpine/**P**ontine bleed
Sedative—hypnotics

Meperidine:
- Dilated pupils
- Can cause seizures
- Is renally excreted
- Can precipitate serotonin syndrome in combination with MAOIs

Toxic causes of hypertension —
CT SCAN
Cocaine
Theophylline
Sympathomimetics
Caffeine
Amphetamines/
Anticholinergics
Nicotine

Amphetamines

EXPOSURE

- Long history of use and abuse as stimulants and nasal decongestants
- Currently used in the management of narcolepsy, attention-deficit/hyperactivity disorder, and short-term weight reduction
- Methamphetamine (crystal, ice): High-potency stimulant effect
- MDMA (Ecstasy, X, Adam): Serotonin affects, intensifies emotions
- Ephedrine: Amphetamine-like structure, used to ward off drowsiness

MECHANISM OF TOXICITY

- Release of catecholamines (dopamine and NE) from presynaptic nerve terminals
- Blocks reuptake of catecholamines (presynaptic)
- At higher doses, causes release of serotonin

CLINICAL SIGNS OF TOXICITY

- Hyperadrenergic: Tachycardia, hypertension, myocardial infarction, dysrhythmias
- CNS effects: Agitation, seizures, coma, ischemia/hemorrhage, psychosis (hallucinations, etc) with serotonergic amphetamines
- ↑ metabolism: Hyperthermia, dehydration, rhabdomyolysis

MANAGEMENT

- Decontamination using activated charcoal for oral ingestions
- Benzodiazepines for sedation and anticonvulsant
- External cooling and aggressive rehydration for hyperthermia
- Phentolamine or nitrates for control of severe hypertension

Sedative-Hypnotics

A 27-year-old man is brought to the ED by EMS. He was at a rave when friends noticed he was acting very bizarre and then became unresponsive. EMS providers found him unresponsive and intubated him with no medications. He is being ventilated at about 20 breaths per minute, and his vital signs are stable. Approximately 45 minutes after his arrival, you hear him yelling from the room with his endotracheal tube in his hand (he extubated himself). You find him awake, alert, and wishing to go home. What was the cause of his symptoms?

Given the background of his coming from a rave party, polysubstance abuse is likely. A profoundly altered mental status that rapidly improves is common with GHB use. He is likely to do well at this point if there are no other concerning coingestions.

A diverse group of drugs that cause sedation and hypnosis, used for:

- Insomnia
- Anxiety
- Seizures
- Alcohol withdrawal
- Anesthesia

- Benzodiazepines
- Barbiturates
- GHB (γ-hydroxybutyrate)
- Others

MECHANISM OF TOXICITY

- Benzodiazepines/barbiturates both work by potentiating GABA:
  - GABA is the primary inhibitory neurotransmitter in the CNS.
  - $GABA_A$ receptor in cell membrane controls chloride ion flow.
  - Receptor has separate binding sites for benzodiazepines and barbiturates.
- GHB:
  - GHB is an endogenous metabolite of GABA.
  - Available by prescription, used to treat cataplexy associated with narcolepsy.
  - Used as a "date-rape drug" secondary to euphoria, aphrodisiac, and amnesia.

CLINICAL SIGNS OF TOXICITY

- Sleepiness and sedation
- Muscle relaxation
- May induce general anesthesia
- May be associated with respiratory depression
- Tolerance may develop rapidly
- Benzodiazepine overdose:
  - Isolated benzodiazepine overdose is rarely associated with death.
  - May potentiate other CNS depressants (ethanol, opioids, etc).
  - Cardiorespiratory depression usually seen only with parenteral administration.
- Barbiturate overdose:
  - Barbiturate overdose has a significant incidence of morbidity/mortality.
  - Confusion/lethargy progresses to coma with hypothermia, cardiovascular collapse, and respiratory arrest.

MANAGEMENT

- Control airway, breathing, and circulation (ABCs).
- Volume replacement and pressors as required for hemodynamic stability.
- Consider lavage (agents cause ↓ gut motility) and charcoal.
- Alkalinization of urine promotes elimination of phenobarbital.
- Hemodialysis/hemoperfusion has limited utility in removing drug.
- Antidote:
  - Flumazenil is competitive antagonist at benzodiazepine receptor site.
  - Most appropriate for reversing benzodiazepines administered IV by physicians (procedural sedation).
  - Should not be used in overdose setting, as it may precipitate seizures.

Causes of hypothermia—
COOLS
CO
Opiates
Oral hypoglycemics
Liquor (alcohols)
Sedative-hypnotics

Sedative-hypnotics are frequently used in suicide attempts, especially in combination with alcohol. Patients should not receive regular prescriptions from the ED.

Flumazenil is of limited use in benzodiazepine overdose due to the risk of seizures.

HIGH-YIELD FACTS

Emergency Toxicology

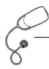

HIGH-YIELD FACTS

Emergency Toxicology

Hydrocarbons with low viscosity and low surface tension are more likely to be aspirated. Halogenated hydrocarbons are associated with myocardial sensitization.

A 3-year-old boy presents with cough and tachypnea after being found in the kitchen. He smells like pine cleaner. *Think: Aspiration of hydrocarbon with pulmonary toxicity.*

A 15-year-old boy presents after being found by his mother in the garage passed out with a rag soaked in paint stripper. *Think: Inhalation of halogenated hydrocarbon with cardiac toxicity.*

Hydrocarbons

Compounds consisting primarily of carbon and hydrogen.

EXPOSURE

- Household products:
  - Polishes
  - Pine oils
  - Glues
- Petroleum distillates:
  - Kerosene
  - Gasoline
- Abused solvents (inhalants):
  - Nail polish remover
  - Paints, paint stripper
  - Typewriter correction fluid

MECHANISM OF TOXICITY

- The number of carbons determines physical state:
  - 1–4 = gas, low viscosity
  - 5–19 = liquid, low viscosity
  - 20–60 = solids, high viscosity
- Structures:
  - Aliphatics: Saturated straight/branched chain hydrocarbons
  - Aromatic: Unsaturated, contain at least one benzene ring
  - Alkene: Contain at least one carbon-carbon double bond
  - Cycloparaffins: Saturated hydrocarbons in closed rings
  - Halogenated: Chloride-containing hydrocarbons

CLINICAL SIGNS OF TOXICITY

- Pulmonary toxicity:
  - Most common organ system affected.
  - Due to aspiration with direct toxic effects and disruption of surfactant.
  - Associated with cough, rales, bronchospasm, tachypnea, pulmonary edema.
  - Forty to 88% will have pneumonitis on chest film.
- CNS toxicity: Seizures and/or coma.
- GI toxicity:
  - Ulcers
  - Hematemesis
- Cardiac toxicity:
  - Myocardial sensitization and dysrhythmias.
  - More common with halogenated hydrocarbons.
- Dermatologic toxicity:
  - Dermatitis
  - Full-thickness burns reported

MANAGEMENT

- Control ABCs.
- Intubation, mechanical ventilation with positive end-expiratory pressure for respiratory distress.

- Avoid catecholamines if possible (myocardial sensitization).
- Gastric emptying is controversial:
  - May ↑ risk of aspiration.
  - Consider if ingestion is > 30 mL.
  - Consider if hydrocarbon is associated with systemic toxicity.

Caustics

Acidic or alkaline substances capable of causing damage on contact with body surfaces.

ACIDS

EXPOSURE

- Drain cleaners
- Disinfectants
- Rust removers
- Photography solutions

MECHANISM OF TOXICITY

- Acids cause coagulation necrosis.
- Dehydration of superficial tissues produces an eschar that limits tissue damage.
- Systemic absorption of strong acids causes acidosis, hemolysis, and renal failure.
- Acid exposure is associated with a higher mortality than alkali despite less local tissue destruction.

CLINICAL SIGNS OF TOXICITY

- Hematemesis, melena
- Abdominal pain
- Gastric perforation with peritonitis
- Gastric outlet obstruction
- Dermal burns

MANAGEMENT

- Supportive care (control ABCs).
- Decontamination contraindicated (risk of emesis, perforation, and impairing endoscopy with charcoal).
- Obtain upright chest film to look for free air.
- Endoscopy of gastric mucosa.
- Surgical intervention if indicated.

ALKALIS

EXPOSURE

- Industrial cleaners
- Industrial bleach (sodium hypochlorite)
- Batteries
- Clinitest tablets

Associated with systemic toxicity—CHAMPS
Camphor
Halogenated hydrocarbons
Aromatic hydrocarbons
Hydrocarbons associated with **M**etals
Hydrocarbons associated with **P**esticides
Suicidal ingestions

Most common caustic exposure: Household bleach (sodium hypochlorite)

ACids cause **C**oagulation; a**L**kalies cause **L**iquefaction.

Dermal exposure to hydrofluoric acid, found in rust removers, can result in systemic absorption, hypocalcemia, hypomagnesemia, and death. Treat with supportive care, calcium gluconate paste to dermal burn, and possibly IV/IA calcium.

MECHANISM OF TOXICITY

- Cause liquefaction necrosis.
- Lipids saponified, proteins denatured, causing deep local tissue injury.
- Alkali exposure is associated with a lower mortality than acid despite more local tissue destruction.

CLINICAL SIGNS OF TOXICITY

- Orofacial burns
- Drooling, odynophagia
- Stridor, dyspnea
- Esophageal perforation, chest pain, mediastinitis
- Dermal burns

MANAGEMENT

- Supportive care (control ABCs).
- Upright chest film to look for free air, button batteries.
- Decontamination contraindicated (risk of emesis, perforation, and impairing endoscopy with charcoal).
- Orofacial burns, drooling, vomiting, stridor, or inability to drink sips of water, admit for endoscopy within 12–24 hours.
- Eye exposure: For both acid and alkali exposures to the cornea, irrigate with normal saline (2–10 L) until the pH is 7.5. Alkaline eye exposures may result in continued local tissue destruction and always require ophthalmology consultation.
- Endoscopic removal of ingested batteries is required for batteries lodged within the esophagus. Once they are below the lower esophageal sphincter, they will likely pass without incident.
- Surgical intervention if indicated.

Why endoscope?
- Safe 12–24 hours after exposure
- May identify surgical candidates
- Grades injuries and predicts risk of strictures
- Patients who develop strictures are far more likely to develop neoplasm at stricture site than those without exposure.

Common alkalies:
- Sodium hydroxide
- Lithium hydroxide
- Ammonium hydroxide
- Sodium hypochlorite

Organophosphate chemical warfare agents:
- GA: Tabun
- GB: Sarin
- GD: Soman
- VX

PESTICIDES

Organophosphates

EXPOSURE

- Pesticides
- Animal care
- Household products
- Chemical warfare

MECHANISM OF TOXICITY

- Irreversibly binds to cholinesterase, inactivating it by phosphorylation.
- Acetylcholinesterase in RBC/CNS, pseudocholinesterase in serum.
- Phosphorylation ("aging") takes place between 24 and 48 hours post-exposure for most pesticides. Nerve agents age more quickly. Once aging is complete, enzyme must be resynthesized (takes weeks).
- Accumulation of ACh in synapse causes cholinergic crisis.

- Muscarinic effects: "SLUDGE" symptoms
- Nicotinic effects:
  - Diaphoresis
  - Hypertension
  - Tachycardia
- Neuromuscular effects:
  - Fasciculations
  - Muscle weakness
- CNS effects:
  - Anxiety
  - Tremor
  - Confusion
  - Seizures
  - Coma
- Long-term effects:
  - Delayed neurotoxicity
  - Delayed polyneuropathy
  - Transient paralysis 24–96 hours after exposure

MANAGEMENT

- Supportive care (including airway).
- Atropine reverses CNS and muscarinic effects (may require multiple large doses).
- Pralidoxime (2-PAM) regenerates acetylcholinesterase (must be given before 24–36 hours, before "aging" is complete).

Carbamates

Structurally related to organophosphates, carbamates also work by inhibiting cholinesterase.

EXPOSURE

- Insecticides
- Wartime pretreatment (carbamate pyridostigmine given in Gulf War)
- Myasthenic agents

MECHANISM OF TOXICITY

Inhibit cholinesterase via carbamoylation, a transient and reversible process.

CLINICAL SIGNS OF TOXICITY

- Similar to organophosphates: "SLUDGE," nicotinic and neuromuscular effects.
- CNS effects not prominent.
- All effects transient (24 hours).

MANAGEMENT

- Supportive care as with organophosphates
- Atropine for reversal of muscarinic symptoms
- 2-PAM usually not necessary (carbamate inhibition is transient)

Organophosphates inactivate acetylcholinesterase, causing cholinergic crisis.

Causes of diaphoretic skin —
SOAP
Sympathomimetics
Organophosphates
Aspirin (salicylates)
PCP

HIGH-YIELD FACTS

Emergency Toxicology

Methemoglobin

EXPOSURE

- Environmental: Nitrites (well water, food, chemicals/dyes)
- Medications: Local anesthetics (eg, benzocaine spray), dapsone, Pyridium, nitroglycerin
- Hereditary: Deficiency of reducing enzymes or abnormal Hgb

MECHANISM OF TOXICITY

- **Oxidation of Hgb:** Normal Hgb has Fe^{2+} group (able to bind oxygen). Oxidant stress causes $Fe^{2+} \rightarrow Fe^{3+}$ (methemoglobin).
- **Inability to transport oxygen:**
  - Ferric ion (Fe^{3+}) in methemoglobin is unable to bind oxygen.
  - Methemoglobin shifts oxygen dissociation curve to left (impairs release).
  - With severe oxidant stress, methemoglobin begins to accumulate.

CLINICAL SIGNS OF TOXICITY

- **General signs:**
  - Cyanosis with normal pO_2 that doesn't respond to supplemental oxygen
  - "Chocolate-brown" color of blood (compare with normal blood color)
  - Confirmation of methemoglobin level by co-oximetry
- **Mild:**
  - Methemoglobin level < 20%
  - Cyanosis present
- **Moderate:**
  - Methemoglobin level 20–50%
  - Cyanosis, dyspnea, headache, fatigue
- **Severe:**
  - Methemoglobin level 50–70%
  - Seizures/coma, myocardial ischemia, acidosis
- **Death:** Methemoglobin level > 70%

MANAGEMENT

- Supportive care
- Antidote therapy: Methylene blue:
  - Indicated for patients with moderate to severe symptoms or level > 20%.
  - An electron carrier that allows methemoglobin $\rightarrow$ Hgb.
  - Utilizes NADPH pathway to reduce itself back to methylene blue.
  - Can't use in patients with glucose-6-phosphate dehydrogenase deficiency (can't generate NADPH).
  - Pulse oximetry will drop transiently due to bluish discoloration of blood.
- Exchange transfusions and hyperbaric oxygen for refractory cases

Measurement of O_2 in methemoglobinemia:
- Pulse oximetry trends toward 85% (measures color).
- pO_2 from ABG measures dissolved oxygen and may be normal. Calculated O_2 saturation will also be normal.
- Accurate measurement by co-oximetry

Carbon Monoxide (CO)

A 33-year-old pregnant woman and her 35-year-old husband arrive at the ED with the complaint of a headache. It is December and they have recently moved into an older home. Both she and her husband have normal vital signs and normal physical exam findings. Neither of them smoke and both have CO-Hgb levels of 22%. What should be the next step in management? Given her pregnancy, she meets criteria for Hyperbaric O_2 (HBO). She may need to be transferred to a center that can perform this. He does not meet criteria for HBO, but should be treated with 100% oxygen by nonrebreather mask.

CO is responsible for the most deaths due to poisoning in the United States.

EXPOSURE

- **Combustion:** Fires, vehicle exhaust, home generators.
- **Metabolism:** Methylene chloride (paint remover) is metabolized to CO in the liver.

MECHANISM OF TOXICITY

- Binds to Hgb with ~250 times greater affinity than oxygen
- Shifts oxygen-Hgb dissociation curve to left (↓ release of O_2)
- Binds to myoglobin in heart and skeletal muscle
- Binds to and inactivates cytochrome oxidase
- Associated with CNS ischemic reperfusion injury

Fetal Hgb binds to CO with even greater affinity than adult Hgb.

CLINICAL SIGNS OF TOXICITY

- **Mild:** Headache, nausea, vomiting
- **Moderate:**
  - Chest pain, confusion, dyspnea
  - Tachycardia, tachypnea, ataxia
- **Severe:**
  - Palpitations, disorientation
  - Seizures, coma, hypotension, myocardial ischemia, dysrhythmias, pulmonary edema, ARDS, rhabdomyolysis, renal failure, multiorgan failure, disseminated intravascular coagulation

A couple and their son present to the ED with flulike symptoms and mild confusion 1 day after using a home generator in the garage. *Think: CO poisoning.*
- Multiple victims
- Initial flulike symptoms
- Exposure to products of combustion

MANAGEMENT

Elimination.

- CO dissociates from Hgb at different rates depending on F_{IO_2}:
  - Room air (21% O_2): ~4 hours
  - 100% O_2 (1 ATM): ~90 minutes
  - 100% O_2 (3 ATM): ~23 minutes
- Hyperbaric O_2 (HBO):
  - Enhances pulmonary elimination of CO as above.
  - Displaces CO from myoglobin and cytochromes in peripheral tissues.
  - ↓ reperfusion injury.
  - May ↓ delayed neurologic sequelae in some patients.
  - Indications for HBO:
    - Evidence of end-organ ischemia (syncope, coma, seizure, focal neurologic deficits, myocardial infarction, ventricular dysrhythmias)

- CO-Hgb level > 25% (> 20% in pregnancy, children)
- Severe metabolic acidosis
- Unable to oxygenate (pulmonary edema)
- No improvement with 100% O_2

Cyanide

Among the most potent and potentially lethal toxins.

EXPOSURE

- **Inhalation:** Smoke from fires involving chemically treated wool, silk, rubber, polyurethane.
- **Ingestion or cutaneous exposure:**
  - Accidental or intentional ingestion of chemical baths used in photography, jewelry making, and electroplating
  - Food and drug tampering (poisoning)
  - Ingestion of plants or fruits containing cyanogenic compounds
- **Iatrogenic:** Nitroprusside contains cyanide.

MECHANISM OF TOXICITY

- Inhibits cytochrome oxidase at cytochrome aa₃ of the electron transport chain
- Causes cellular hypoxia and lactic acidosis
- Blocks production of adenosine triphosphate

CLINICAL SIGNS OF TOXICITY

- CNS dysfunction: Headache, seizures, coma
- Cardiovascular dysfunction: Bradycardia, ↓ inotropy, hypotension
- Pulmonary edema
- Hemorrhagic gastritis

MANAGEMENT

- Supportive care (manage airway, fluids)
- Decontamination
- Antidote therapy:
  - Administration of nitrites generates methemoglobin.
  - Methemoglobin draws cyanide groups from cytochrome oxidase.
  - Thiosulfate transfers sulfur group to cyanomethemoglobin.
  - Thiocyanate (relatively harmless) is excreted in urine.
- Cyanide antidote (Lilly antidote kit):
  - Amyl nitrite pearls—crush and inhale.
  - Sodium nitrite—give IV over 20 minutes.
  - Sodium thiosulfate—IV (after nitrites).
  - Monitor excessive methemoglobin production during antidotal therapy.

Treat coexistent CO poisoning in fires (further compromises O_2 supply).

"Classic" signs of cyanide toxicity such as bitter almond odor and cherry-red skin color are unreliable.

Environmental Emergencies

DEFINITION

Impaired gas exchange at altitude.

ALTITUDE CLASSIFICATION

- High altitude: 5000–11,500 feet
- Very high altitude: 11,500–18,000 feet
- Extreme altitude: > 18,000 feet

SIGNS AND SYMPTOMS

- **High altitude:**
  - ↓ exercise performance
  - ↑ ventilation at rest
- **Very high altitude:**
  - Maximal SaO < 90%, PaO_2 < 60 mm Hg
  - Stress and sleep hypoxemia
- **Extreme altitude:**
  - Severe hypoxemia and hypocapnia
  - Acclimatization impossible

HIGH-ALTITUDE ACCLIMATIZATION

DEFINITION

Adjustment of the body to lower ambient oxygen concentrations.

PHYSIOLOGY

- Carotid body hypoxemia stimulates ↑ in ventilation, which → ↓ $PaCO_2$ and ↑ PaO_2.
- Without adequate O_2, hyperventilation → acute respiratory alkalosis.
- Renal response is to excrete more bicarbonate, returning the pH to normal.
- ↑ erythropoietin within 2 hours of ascent gives rise to an ↑ red cell mass in days to weeks, hence a minimal and subclinical ↓ O_2-carrying capacity.

ACUTE MOUNTAIN SICKNESS (AMS)

DEFINITION

Syndrome of several constitutional complaints related to hypobaric hypoxemia and its physiologic consequences.

SIGNS AND SYMPTOMS

- At 24 hours: Hangover (lassitude, anorexia, headache, nausea, vomiting).
- Then oliguria, peripheral edema, retinal hemorrhages.
- Finally, high-altitude pulmonary edema (HAPE), high-altitude cerebral edema (HACE), death.

> **Late effects:** Chronic mountain polycythemia:
> - Headache
> - Sleep difficulty
> - Mental slowness
> - Impaired circulation

> **Associated high-altitude symptoms:**
> - Snow blindness (ultraviolet keratitis)
> - Pharyngitis
> - Retinopathy

HIGH-YIELD FACTS

Environmental Emergencies

RISK FACTORS

- Children
- Rapid ascent
- Higher sleeping altitudes
- Chronic obstructive pulmonary disease
- ↓ vital capacity
- Cold
- Heavy exertion
- Sickle cell disease

Patients with sickle cell disease require supplemental oxygen for high-altitude exposures.

TREATMENT (SEE TABLE 18-1)

- Descent
- Oxygen
- Acetazolamide

TABLE 18-1. Medications Used for High-Altitude Illness

DRUG	MECHANISM OF ACTION	INDICATIONS
Acetazolamide	■ ↓ the formation of bicarbonate by inhibiting the enzyme carbonic anhydrase ■ Diuretic action counters the fluid retention of AMS ■ ↓ bicarbonate absorption in the kidney, resulting in a metabolic acidosis that stimulates hyperventilation (to blow off excess CO_2) ■ This compensatory hyperventilation is normally turned off as soon as the pH reaches close to 7.4 ■ By maintaining a constant forced bicarbonate diuresis, acetazolamide causes the central chemoreceptors to continually reset, permitting the hyperventilation to continue, thereby countering the altitude-induced hypoxemia	■ Abrupt ascent to > 10,000 feet ■ Nocturnal dyspnea ■ AMS ■ History of altitude illness (used as prophylaxis)
Dexamethasone	■ ↓ vasogenic edema ■ ↓ intracranial pressure ■ Antiemetic ■ Mood elevator	HACE
Oxygen	Low-flow oxygen improves sleeping problems by ameliorating the normal hypoxemia that occurs during sleep	■ AMS ■ HAPE ■ HACE
HBO	■ Improves hypoxemia for all altitude illness ■ In nitrogen narcosis, raises ambient pressure and PaO_2 in order to convert nitrogen bubbles back to solution and restore O_2 to deprived areas while the body eliminates the problem gas	■ AMS ■ HAPE ■ HACE ■ Nitrogen narcosis
Nifedipine	↓ pulmonary artery pressure	HAPE when descent or oxygen is unavailable
Morphine, furosemide	Reduce pulmonary blood flow and ↓ hydrostatic force, resulting in less fluid available for extravasation	HAPE

478

- HBO chamber
- Nonsteroidal anti-inflammatory drugs (NSAIDs) for headache
- Prochlorperazine for nausea and vomiting
- Other helpful tips:
  - Avoidance of alcohol and overexertion
  - High-carbohydrate diet

Definitive treatment for all high-altitude syndromes is descent; when not possible, descent may be simulated with a Gamow bag (a portable hyperbaric oxygen [HBO] chamber).

HIGH-ALTITUDE PULMONARY EDEMA (HAPE)

DEFINITION

Noncardiogenic pulmonary edema seen at altitude associated with ↓ vasoconstriction, ↑ pulmonary hypertension, and capillary leak.

SIGNS AND SYMPTOMS

- Dry to productive cough
- Tachypnea
- Tachycardia
- Peripheral cyanosis
- Fatigue
- Orthopnea
- Rales

Best prevention for AMS is graded ascent with enough time at each altitude step for acclimatization.

TREATMENT (SEE TABLE 18-1)

- Immediate descent to lower altitude.
- Oxygen to keep SaO > 90%.
- Hyperbaric oxygen (HBO) if descent is not possible.
- Continuous positive airway pressure.
- Consider nifedipine if descent or HBO is not available.
- Minimize exertion.
- Keep warm (cold stress elevates pulmonary artery pressures).
- Consider morphine/furosemide.

Early diagnosis of HAPE is key, because it is reversible in the early stages. Patients need not develop any signs of AMS before developing HAPE. Early presentation may be just a dry cough.

HIGH-ALTITUDE CEREBRAL EDEMA (HACE)

DEFINITION

Progressive neurologic deterioration in someone with AMS.

SIGNS AND SYMPTOMS

- Altered mental status
- Ataxia
- Cranial nerve palsy
- Seizure
- Strokelike symptoms
- Coma (usually not permanent)
- Headache
- Nausea, vomiting

TREATMENT (SEE TABLE 18-1)

- Immediate descent to lower altitude
- Oxygen to keep SaO > 90%
- Dexamethasone
- Loop diuretic
- HBO chamber

HIGH-PRESSURE DYSBARISM

Descent Barotrauma

DEFINITION

Barotrauma associated with descent or dive in body spaces that cannot equalize pressure; also known as the "squeeze."

SIGNS AND SYMPTOMS

- Middle ear squeeze (barotitis media):
  - Eustachian tube dysfunction
  - Ear fullness or pain
  - Nausea and vertigo
  - Hemotympanum
- External ear squeeze:
  - Due to occlusion of external ear canal with cerumen
  - Bloody otorrhea
  - Petechiae in canal
- Inner ear squeeze:
  - Rare
  - Associated with rapid descent
  - Tinnitus, vertigo, hearing loss
  - Nausea, vomiting
- Sinus squeeze:
  - Sinus pain or pressure
  - Usually frontal and maxillary
  - Can have epistaxis
  - Associated with preexisting sinus inflammation or blockage
- Lung squeeze:
  - Occurs in divers who hold their breath going down
  - Hemoptysis
  - Shortness of breath
  - Pulmonary edema
- Equipment squeeze:
  - Conjunctival/scleral/periorbital petechiae under face mask
  - Petechiae on skin under suit

TREATMENT

- All types of squeeze:
  - Cease dive.
  - Equilibrate spaces in advance (remove foreign body, use decongestants).

Boyle's Law
$P \propto K/V$
As pressure ↑, volume ↓.
P = pressure
K = temperature in degrees Kelvin
V = volume

- Give antibiotics for:
  - Frontal or sphenoid sinus squeeze
  - Otitis externa
  - Tympanic membrane rupture
- Inner ear fistula requires surgical repair.

Ascent Barotrauma

DEFINITION

Barotrauma caused by expansion of gas on ascent in body spaces that cannot equilibrate.

SIGNS AND SYMPTOMS

- Reverse ear squeeze:
  - Tympanic membrane rupture
  - Ear pain
  - Bloody otorrhea
  - Occurs with rapid ascent
- Pulmonary barotrauma:
  - Dissection of air into pulmonary tissue with failure to exhale during ascent
  - Associated with:
    - Pneumomediastinum
    - Pneumopericardium
    - Local subcutaneous emphysema
    - Pulmonary interstitial emphysema
    - Pneumothorax

TREATMENT

- All types of ascent barotrauma: Rest, decongestants
- Reverse ear squeeze: Ear, nose, and throat consult
- Pulmonary barotrauma:
  - Oxygen.
  - Observation.
  - Most resolve without intervention.

Dysbaric Air Embolism (DAE)

DEFINITION

Arterial air embolism associated with ruptured alveoli; enters left heart through pulmonary veins and may occlude an area of systemic circulation.

SIGNS AND SYMPTOMS

- Coronary artery emboli:
  - Chest pain
  - Dysrhythmias
- Central nervous system (CNS) emboli:
  - Focal neurologic deficit
  - Aphasia
  - Seizure

Most types of descent barotrauma resolve with ascent and rest.

Risk factor for reverse ear squeeze is upper respiratory tract congestion/infection.

DAE: Occurs within 10 minutes of surfacing. Not related to depth of dive. Can occur at less than 30 feet of depth.

Environmental Emergencies

A 24-year-old male diver syncopizes upon ascent to the surface. *Think: DAE.*

- Dizziness
- Headache
- Confusion
- Visual field loss

TREATMENT

- HBO.
- Avoid air transport (ascent).

Decompression Sickness

A 38-year-old man presents to the emergency department (ED) with left arm weakness and back pain that began during a flight home from a diving vacation in Mexico. The flight was diverted so that he could receive medical care for a possible stroke. He has no medical problems and has been in his usual state of health. His last dive was approximately 10 hours ago and was uneventful. His vital signs are stable. What is the diagnosis and the next step in therapy?

This is a case of decompression sickness. He is very young to be having a stroke, but other concerns such as an aortic dissection always need to be considered. He should receive HBO therapy immediately. This is not available at all centers, so he may require transfer to another center, preferably by ground rather than air. Current recommendations are to avoid flying within 24 hours of diving.

Decompression sickness: Also known as "the bends." Related to the depth of dive and time at depth. Need to be at least 30 feet.

DEFINITION

Illness due to nitrogen bubbles in the blood, which form on decompression (ascent).

SIGNS AND SYMPTOMS

Type 1: Skin, Lymphatic, Musculoskeletal "Bends"
- *Skin:* Pruritus, redness, mottling
- *Lymphatic:* Lymphedema
- *Musculoskeletal:* Periarticular joint pain

Type 2: Cardiovascular, Respiratory, CNS "Bends"
- *Cardiovascular:* Tachycardia, acute coronary syndrome
- *Respiratory:* Dyspnea, cough, pulmonary edema, pneumothorax, hemoptysis
- *CNS:* Focal neurologic deficit, back pain, urinary retention, incontinence

TREATMENT

- Transport immediately to HBO chamber.
- Supine position.
- Intravenous (IV) fluids.
- 100% O_2.
- Avoid air evacuation.
- Steroids controversial.

Nitrogen Narcosis

DEFINITION

- The partial pressure of nitrogen in inspired tank air is ↑ at depth and as it accumulates in the tissues; the inert gas exerts an anesthetic effect on the diver.
- Becomes a problem at 70- to 100-foot dives.

SIGNS AND SYMPTOMS

- Euphoria, disinhibition, overconfidence, poor judgment
- Slow reflexes
- Fine sensory discrimination loss
- At greater depths: Hallucinations, coma, death

TREATMENT

Ascend at a reasonable rate with assistance.

NEAR DROWNING/IMMERSION SYNDROME

DEFINITION

- *Drowning:* Death from an immersion.
- *Near drowning:* Survival after an immersion.

PATHOPHYSIOLOGY

- Mechanism of injury is suffocation from aspiration and associated laryngospasm.
- Fresh water (lakes, rivers, pools, baths): Hypotonic liquid disrupts surfactant and causes intrapulmonary shunting and fluid retention.
- Sea water (oceans and some lakes): Hypertonic liquid draws intravascular fluid into alveoli and causes intrapulmonary shunting.

SIGNS AND SYMPTOMS

- Vary significantly:
  - Mild cough and shortness of breath.
  - Full cardiac arrest due to pneumonia/pneumonitis.
- Once stable, hospital course can also vary, depending on:
  - Aspiration (usually contaminated water).
  - Physiologic reserve of victim.

TREATMENT

- Rapid and cautious rescue.
- C-spine immobilization.
- Control airway, breathing, and circulation (ABCs).
- Rewarm as needed (see section on hypothermia).
- Treat associated injuries.
- Obtain chest x-ray, arterial blood gas, finger-stick glucose, electrolytes, toxicology screen, C-spine x-rays.
- No role for empiric steroids or antibiotics.

High-risk groups for drowning:
- Children < age 4
- Teens (poor judgment)
- Elderly (tubs)
- Alcohol and drug users

"Secondary drowning" is death after initial stabilization.

Risk factors for near drowning:
- Hypoglycemia
- Head trauma
- Seizure

PROGNOSIS

- Cerebral anoxic injury begins within a few minutes of no oxygen.
- Some authorities believe resuscitation should not be initiated if immersion > 10 minutes.
- Scattered case reports of survival without neurologic deficit in up to 24% of children requiring cardiopulmonary resuscitation (CPR).

MARINE LIFE TRAUMA AND ENVENOMATION

The emergency physician must be familiar with the fauna of ocean and lake environments in order to diagnose and treat injuries and illnesses inflicted by them.

Type of Injury

- Marine life can be grossly divided into those that have stingers to cause injury and those that have nematocysts.
- A **nematocyst** is a microscopic "spring-loaded" venom gland, discharged by physical contact or osmotic gradient.
  - The gland found on tentacles contracts when touched, striking victim repetitively, leaving whiplike scars.
  - Gland remains active after the animal dies or tentacle rips off.

Stingers

- Stingrays
- Starfish
- Scorpion fish
- Sea urchins
- Catfish
- Lionfish
- Cone shells

TREATMENT OF STINGER INJURY

- Immerse wound in nonscalding hot water (45°C [113°F]) for 90 minutes (or until pain is gone) to break down venom.
- X-ray to find and remove stings.
- Aggressive cleaning, antibiotics.

Nematocysts

- Portuguese man-of-war
- Corals
- Fire corals
- Anemones
- Sea wasps
- Jellyfish

TREATMENT OF NEMATOCYST INJURY

- ABCs.
- Inactivate nematocysts by immersing them in vinegar (5% acetic acid).

They're not dead until they're warm and dead (see hypothermia).

The main difference in treatment between a stinger and nematocyst injury is that you use water for a stinger and vinegar for a nematocyst.

- Do not use tap water (causes venom discharge by osmotic gradient).
- Immobilize limb.
- IV access and fluids.
- Antivenin: 1 ampule diluted 1:10 IV (20,000 U/ampule).
- Antihistamines/epinephrine/steroids for anaphylaxis.
- Shave off remaining nematocysts.
- Pain control.
- Tetanus prophylaxis.

Shark Attacks

- Generally, sharks attack humans only when they can't see well enough to tell them apart from seals and sea lions.
- Great white, mako, hammerhead, blue, bull, reef, and tiger sharks make up the majority of species reported to attack.
- If attacked, a force of ~18 tons per square inch and razor-sharp teeth digging into a limb or torso can quickly be a fatal blow, especially if the victim doesn't immediately receive medical attention.

Sharks: < 100 attacks per year worldwide with < 10% mortality.

Blue-Ringed Octopus Envenomation

- Found off Australian coast.
- Bites when handled and antagonized.
- Beak injects venom containing tetrodotoxin (TTX), a paralyzing neurotoxin that blocks voltage-gated Na^+ channels.
- **Signs and symptoms:** Paresthesias, diffuse flaccid paralysis, respiratory failure, local erythema.

TTX also found in puffer fish flesh.

Gila Monster and Mexican Beaded Lizard

- Normally timid, bite those who handle them.
- Venom: Phospholipase-A, hyaluronidase, arginine esterase, and a kallikrein-like hypotensive enzyme secreted by glands in lower jaw.
- Animal sometimes continues to bite/chew; the longer it holds on, the more venom gets in.

SIGNS AND SYMPTOMS

- Crush and puncture wounds; may have teeth in wound
- Burning pain, radiates up extremity, lasts 8 hours, edema and cyanosis
- Rare systemic effects: Weakness, fainting, hypotension, sweating

TREATMENT

- Remove animal (if still attached).
- Remove teeth, clean copiously and aggressively, broad-spectrum antibiotics, tetanus.
- Observation for systemic effects.

Amphibians

- Colorado River toad, Columbian poison-dart frogs, and several species of newt and salamander secrete toxins in their skin and internal organs:
  - Batrachotoxin: Opens Na^+ channels irreversibly

- Tetrodotoxin: Blocks Na+ channels irreversibly
- Bufotalin: Cardiac toxin, acts like digitalis
- Samandarine: Opens CNS Na+ channels irreversibly
- **Treatment:** Supportive

A medical control call comes in from an EMS crew providing care to a patient that is more than 30 minutes away from a hospital. He was bitten 1 hour ago by a rattlesnake. He has swelling around the bite site and appears very anxious. The crew is seeking directions on what they should do in route to your hospital, which is the closest. What should you tell them?

They should provide supportive care and drive safely but quickly to the nearest ED, in this case your own. Interventions such as cutting and suction or tourniquets should not be used, as they will only increase the patient's morbidity. Since you know the patient is coming and will require antivenom, it would be appropriate to order 4–6 vials of antivenom (FabAV) and consider mixing (takes > 20 minutes) prior to the patient's arrival.

Crotalidae Family (Pit Vipers)

Includes rattlesnakes, massasauga, copperheads, and water moccasins (see Table 18-2).

SIGNS AND SYMPTOMS

- **Local** (see Table 18-3):
  - Burning pain (severity related to amount of venom)
  - Edema spreading proximally
  - Local petechiae, bullae, and skin necrosis
- **Systemic:**
  - Nausea
  - Fever
  - Metallic taste
  - Weakness
  - Sweating
  - Perioral paresthesias
  - Hypotension

TABLE 18-2. **Characteristics of Poisonous versus Nonpoisonous Snakes**

POISONOUS	NONPOISONOUS
Triangle-shaped head	Rounded head
Elliptical pupil	Round pupil
Pit between eye and nostril	Absence of pit
Fangs	Absence of fangs

TABLE 18-3. Snake Bite Grading System

GRADE	PIT VIPER	CORAL SNAKE
0	▪ Fang marks ▪ No pain ▪ No systemic symptoms ▪ Don't give antivenin	▪ No envenomation ▪ Minimal fang scratches or punctures ▪ Minimal local swelling ▪ No systemic symptoms in 24 hours ▪ Give 3 vials antivenin
I	▪ Fang marks ▪ Mild pain/edema ▪ No systemic symptoms ▪ Give antivenom	▪ Fang scratches or punctures ▪ Minimal local swelling ▪ Systemic symptoms present, but no respiratory paralysis ▪ Give 3 vials antivenin
II	▪ Fang marks ▪ Severe pain ▪ Moderate edema ▪ Mild systemic symptoms ▪ Give antivenom	▪ Severe envenomation ▪ Respiratory paralysis occurs within 36 hours ▪ Give 5–10 vials antivenin
III	▪ Fang marks ▪ Severe pain/edema ▪ Severe symptoms (hypotension, dyspnea) ▪ Evidence of systemic coagulopathy ▪ Give antivenom	

- Fasciculations
- Compartment syndrome (rare)
- Pulmonary edema
- Anaphylaxis
- Shock, intravascular coagulation, hemorrhage, and death

TREATMENT

Avoid harmful interventions (cutting, sucking, tourniquets, etc). All sympomatic patients should be treated with antivenom:

- Antivenom Crotalidae polyvalent (ACP):
  - No longer made
  - From horse serum
- Polyvalent Crotalidae ovine immune Fab (FabAV):
  - From sheep
  - Less adverse reactions than ACP
  - Dosing:
    - 4–6 vials (4–6 g) IV immediately.
    - Repeat dose in 1 hour if no response.
    - Once symptoms controlled, smaller doses (2 g) can be given every 6 hours.
    - Dosing is the same in children (same amount of venom as in adults).
- Poison Control (1-800-222-1222) is a reference if unsure.

HIGH-YIELD FACTS

Environmental Emergencies

Elapidae Family (Coral Snakes)

- Includes the corals, cobras, kraits, and mambas.
- Venom is a neurotoxin.

SIGNS AND SYMPTOMS

- Painless bite site
- Weak/numb within 90 minutes
- Euphoria
- Drowsiness
- Tremors
- Salivation
- Slurred speech
- Diplopia
- Flaccid paralysis
- Respiratory failure

TREATMENT

Antivenin for all coral snake bites (regardless of symptoms).

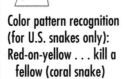

Color pattern recognition
(for U.S. snakes only):
Red-on-yellow . . . kill a
fellow (coral snake)
Red-on-black . . . venom
lack

SPIDERS

Brown Recluse Spider

Loxosceles reclusa.

DEFINITION

Identified by violin design on its back (Figure 18-1).

EXPOSURE

- Found in midwestern, mid-Atlantic, and southern states.
- Inhabits warm, dry places—typically woodpiles, cellars, and abandoned buildings.
- Venom: Proteases, alkaline phosphatase, lipase, complement-system substances.

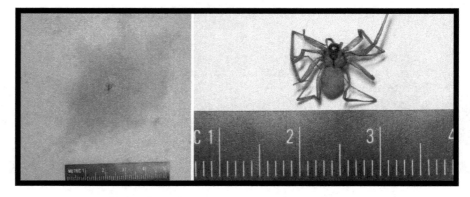

FIGURE 18-1. Brown recluse spider.

(Reproduced, with permission, from Laack TA, Stead LG, Wolfe ME. Images in emergency medicine. *Loxosceles reclusa* bite, *Ann Emerg Med* 50: 368–370, 2007.)

HIGH-YIELD FACTS

Environmental Emergencies

SIGNS AND SYMPTOMS

- Necrosis at bite site due to local hemolysis and thrombosis associated with ischemia.
- Mild red lesion, may be bluish/ischemic.
- Varying degrees of pain, blistering, necrosis within 3–4 days.
- May take weeks to heal.
- Systemic symptoms:
  - Fever
  - Chills
  - Nausea
  - Myalgias, arthralgias
  - Hemolysis, petechiae
  - Seizure
- Renal failure
- Death

Loxoscelism is a reaction to *Loxosceles* spider venom proportional to amount of venom exposure.

TREATMENT

- Monitor ABCs.
- Daily wound care.
- Analgesia.
- Tetanus prophylaxis.
- Antibiotics if wound becomes infected.

Brown recluse spider bites are often overdiagnosed, even in areas that do not have these spiders.

Black Widow Spider

Latrodectus mactans.

DEFINITION

- Identified by red-orange hourglass on abdomen.
- Female two times size of male, has design, is only one that can envenomate humans.

EXPOSURE

- Found throughout the continental United States.
- Inhabits warm, dry, protected places, typically woodpiles, cellars, barns, under rocks, etc.
- Venom: Neurotoxic protein causing acetylcholine and norepinephrine release at synapses.

SIGNS AND SYMPTOMS

- Local pinprick sensation, red, swollen
- Then slow progression of painful muscle spasm of large groups
- Lasts a few hours, resolves spontaneously
- Systemic signs:
  - Hypertension
  - Coma
  - Shock
  - Respiratory failure
  - Death (more often in children)

Abdominal muscle spasm of black widow spider bite may mimic peritonitis.

TREATMENT

- Pain control and muscle relaxants (narcotics and benzodiazepines).
- Tetanus, local wound care.
- Antivenin available for severe reactions (1–2 vials IV over 30 minutes).

SCORPION

Bark scorpion (*Centruroides exilicauda*).

DEFINITION

Has venom gland and stinger in last segment of tail.

EXPOSURE

- Found in Arizona, California, Nevada, and Texas.
- Bark scorpion inhabits areas around trees.
- Other species usually under rocks, logs, floors, boots.
- Victims usually children and campers/hikers.
- Venom activates Na^+ channels, damaging parasympathetic, somatic, and sympathetic nerves.
- Other proteins may cause hemolysis, hemorrhage, and local tissue destruction.

SIGNS AND SYMPTOMS

Severe and immediate pain (erythema and swelling are species dependent). Then tachycardia, ↑ secretions, fasciculations, nausea, vomiting, blurred vision, dysphagia, roving eye movements, opisthotonos, respiratory failure, syncope, death (rare).

TREATMENT

- ABCs
- Sedation with benzodiazepines
- Tetanus prophylaxis, local wound care
- Antivenin: Previously available in Arizona; now available only in Mexico

Patients who should get antivenin:
- Extremes of age
- Pregnant
- Underlying medical conditions (check for hypersensitivity/allergy with skin test prior to administration)

A 14-year-old boy is rushed to the ED by his mother. He is complaining of a tightness in his throat and difficulty breathing that began suddenly after he was stung by a wasp. He has not had any problems with allergies in the past, he has no medical problems, and he takes no medications. His vital signs are significant for a heart rate of 120 beats per minute, respiratory rate of 24 breaths per minute, oxygen saturation of 98%, and a blood pressure of 80/40. He is ill in appearance but able to speak in full sentences. He is warm to the touch. His weight is 65 kg. What is the appropriate treatment for this patient?

He has anaphylaxis from a Hymenoptera sting. This is a type of distributive shock and should be treated with IV fluids and vasopressors (epinephrine). The epinephrine dose can be given IM. The dose for children is 0.01 mg/kg, but this would be 0.65 mg in this child. A more appropriate dose is the starting dose for adults, 0.3 mg of 1:1000 epinephrine (the same dose as an EpiPen).

DEFINITION

- The order Hymenoptera includes the insects with most severe sting-related injuries.
- Winged Hymenoptera:
  - Apids: Honeybees, bumblebees.
  - Vespids: Wasps, hornets, yellow jackets.
  - "Africanized" honeybees: Much more aggressive but venom contains same substances.
  - Yellow jackets cause most allergic reactions.
- Wingless Hymenoptera:
  - Formicids: fire ants.
  - *Soleneopsis invicta*—"unvanquished ant," Brazilian import to the United States in 1930s.

EXPOSURE

- Venom: Mostly proteins and peptides (phospholipase-A, hyaluronidase, histamine, serotonin, bradykinin, dopamine), also lipids and carbohydrates.
- Systemically, toxicity from venom or anaphylaxis can occur within minutes.

SIGNS AND SYMPTOMS

- Apids and vespids:
  - Most commonly local: Burning pain, erythema, edema at sting site, lasting ~24 hours.
  - Local/systemic delayed reaction up to 1.5–2 weeks later.
  - Toxicity: Vomiting, diarrhea, fever, drowsiness, syncope, seizure, muscle spasm, and rarely neuritis, nephritis, vasculitis.
  - Anaphylaxis is possible.
- Formicids:
  - Immediate intense burning pain locally.
  - Becomes sterile pustule in 6 hours.

Apids sting only once—stinger detaches in skin, bee then dies.
Vespids can sting again and again—stinger has no retroserrate barbs.

- With multiple stings in sensitized individuals, nausea, sweating, dizziness, and anaphylaxis can occur.
- No cross-reactivity with that of bees.

TREATMENT

- ABCs:
  - Airway can be compromised early (ask about prior bee stings).
  - For any systemic signs (anaphylaxis).
- Visual representation of anaphylaxis criteria:
  - Epinephrine (1:1,000): 0.3–0.5 mg IM in adults, 0.01 mg/kg in children.
  - Antihistamine (eg, 50 mg diphenhydramine IV).
  - Steroid (eg, 125 mg methylprednisolone IV).
  - β_2 agonist for wheezing (eg, albuterol nebulizer treatment).
  - Admit and observe.
- Local wound care:
  - Remove stingers
  - Local cleaning
  - Pain medications

1:1000 epinephrine 1 mg = 1 mL (concentrated for IM/SQ).
1:10,000 epinephrine 1 mg = 10 mL (for IV use).
EpiPen contains 0.3 mg of 1:1000 epinephrine.

TERRESTRIAL ANIMAL TRAUMA

Dog Bites

- 80–90% of reported animal bites
- Usually lacerations, crush injury, punctures, and avulsions
- Wounds are infection and tetanus prone, bacteria from animal oral flora (not human skin):
  - Aerobes: *Streptococcus, Staphylococcus aureus, Pasteurella multocida* (20–30%), *Staphylococcus intermedius, Eikenella corrodens.*
  - Anaerobes: *Bacteroides* spp., *Actinomyces* spp., *Fusobacterium* spp., *Peptostreptococcus* spp.

TREATMENT

- ABCs as appropriate.
- Local wound care: Aggressive irrigation, debridement; repair lacerations, but may consider loose suturing or leave open for delayed primary closure of hand lacerations.
- If stray and cannot be observed, initiate rabies immunization.
- Tetanus prophylaxis.
- Prophylactic antibiotics for the immunocompromised and frail (amoxicillin/clavulanic acid for outpatient, ampicillin/sulbactam inpatient) (see Table 18-4).

Cat and dog bite infection rules of thumb:

- Infection in < 24 hours: *P multocida.* Rx: penicillin, if penicillin allergic, tetracycline, or erythromycin
- Infection in > 24 hours: *Staph or Strep* Rx: Dicloxacillin or cephalexin
- Prophylaxis: amoxicillin-clavulanate

Cat Bites

- 5–18% of reported animal bites in United States
- More likely to contain *P multocida* in wound

TABLE 18-4. Closure and Prophylaxis for Bites

ANIMAL BITE	CLOSE?	MAIN OFFENDING ORGANISM	ANTIBIOTICS?
Dog	Yes, except if crush injury or bite to hand	*Capnocytophaga canimorsus*	Yes, if severe
Cat	No	*Pasteurella multocida*	Yes
Rodent	No	Multiple	No
Monkey	No	Herpesvirus	Acyclovir for high-risk bites
Human	Yes, except if closed-fist injury	*Eikenella corrodens*	Yes

SIGNS AND SYMPTOMS

- Punctures (57–86%)
- Abrasions (9–25%)
- Lacerations (5–17%)

TREATMENT

See dog bites.

Humans

- Behavior at times animal-like.
- Clenched-fist injuries (CFIs) from punches in the face have high incidence of poor wound healing and complications.
- Bites to areas other than the hand have similar rates of infection as non-bite lacerations.
- Human oral flora is polymicrobial:
    - Aerobes: *Streptococcus viridans*, *S aureus*, *Haemophilus* spp., *E corrodens*.
    - Anaerobes: *Bacteroides* spp., *Fusobacterium* spp., *Peptostreptococcus* spp.

TREATMENT

- CFIs: Copious irrigation, debridement, tetanus, penicillin, and second-generation cephalosporin for *Staphylococcus* coverage. Diabetics should get an aminoglycoside.
- Immobilize, daily dressing changes, elevate extremity.

E corrodens: A gram-negative rod of the normal human oral flora, distinguished by being susceptible to penicillin but resistant to penicillinase-resistant penicillins, clindamycin, metronidazole, cephalosporins.

HIGH-YIELD FACTS

Environmental Emergencies

> A 65-year-old woman is brought in to the ED by ambulance after being rescued from a house fire. She smells strongly of smoke and has extensive burns over her face. She is moaning in pain, coughing, and is noted to have carbonaceous sputum and burnt material in her mouth. Her vital signs are significant for a respiratory rate of 25 breaths per minute, oxygen saturation of 92%, and a heart rate of 105 beats per minute. What should be your first priority in treatment?
>
> She is at high risk for a significant inhalation injury and appears to already be in some respiratory distress (↑ respiratory rate, altered mental status, hypoxia). A rapid sequence intubation (RSI) should be performed. Once she is intubated, a secondary survey for other injuries and the extent of her burns can be performed. Priority also needs to be given to maintain adequate pain control and sedation. She should be transferred to a burn center. Her predicted mortality is high (age and inhalation injury).

DESCRIPTION OF DEPTH

- **First degree:** Superficial burn, epidermis only, mild to moderate erythema, heals without scar.
- **Second degree:**
  - Superficial partial thickness, epidermis and part of dermis (follicles and glands spared), blisters and erythema, very painful, heals with or without scar in 2–3 weeks.
  - Deep partial thickness, epidermis and deeper dermal layers (follicles and glands), blisters, erythema, some charring, painful, heals in 3–4 weeks with some scarring.
- **Third degree:** Full thickness, epidermis, dermis, subcutaneous fat; pale, charred, painless, leathery; surgical skin grafts necessary for healing; moderate to severe scarring.
- **Fourth degree:** Skin, fat, muscle, bone involvement; severe, life-threatening injury.

DESCRIPTION OF SIZE

- Estimate size with rule of nines (Figure 18-2).
- Size of patient's palm roughly 1% of their total body surface area (TBSA).

CATEGORIZATION

- **Minor burns:**
  - < 15% TBSA for ages 10–50.
  - < 10% TBSA for ages < 10 or > 50.
  - < 2% TBSA full thickness, any age, no other injury.
- **Moderate burns:**
  - 15–25% TBSA second degree for ages 10–50
  - 10–20% TBSA second degree for ages < 10 or > 50
  - 2–10% TBSA full thickness, any age
  - No perineal, facial, foot, hand, or circumferential limb burns

Typical cause of burns:
First degree: Sunburn
Second degree: Hot liquids
Third degree: Hot liquids, steam, hot oil, flame
Fourth degree: Flame, hot oil, steam

Poor-risk burn patients: Age > 60, burn > 40% TBSA, inhalation injury.

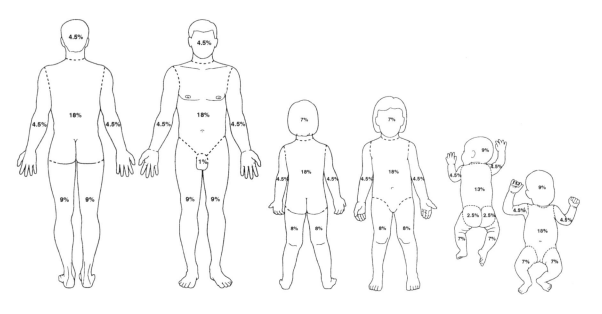

FIGURE 18-2. Rule of nines for adults, children, and infants.

(Reproduced, with permission, from Stead L. BRS: *Emergency Medicine*. Philadelphia, PA: Lippincott Williams & Wilkins, 2000: 558.)

- **Major burns:**
  - > 25% TBSA second degree for ages 10–50.
  - > 20% TBSA second degree for ages < 10 or > 50.
  - > 10% TBSA full thickness, any age.
  - Hand, foot, perineal, circumferential limb, major joint, electrical burns.
  - Associated inhalation injury or other trauma in elderly, infants, poor-risk patients.

TREATMENT

- Prehospital: Transport to nearest burn-capable hospital, preferably within 30 minutes.
- ED: Ask age, medical history, tetanus status, what burned, was there an explosion/blast injury, were there toxic substances, enclosed space?
- Fiberoptically evaluate airway for edema and injury, or intubate and protect the airway prior to respiratory failure in high risk injuries.
- Humidified 100% O_2.
- Fluid resuscitation according to **Parkland formula.**
- Beware of overaggressive fluid resuscitation → excessive pulmonary and peripheral edema.
- Foley catheter to monitor urine output (maintain 1 cc/kg/h).
- Primary and secondary surveys: Treat all associated injuries appropriately.
- Management of the burn wound:
  - Within 30 minutes: "Put out the fire"—cool water.
  - Always cover with clean, sterile, saline-soaked dressings to small areas.
- Protect against hypothermia: Cover with sterile sheets.

Parkland formula: 4 × weight (kg) × % TBSA burned = mL IV fluids over 24 hours; one-half over first 8 hours from time of burn, and remaining one-half over next 16 hours. Ringer's lactate is fluid of choice.

High risk for airway injury and need for endotracheal intubation in burn victims:

- Known smoke inhalation in enclosed space
- Respiratory distress (cough, stridor, wheezing)
- Hypoxia or hypercapnia
- Hoarse voice
- Singed facial hairs/ facial burns
- Carbonaceous sputum

Children have ↑ TBSA relative to their weight, ↑ evaporative water loss, and therefore ↑ fluid requirements.

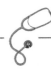

Any chemical burn to the eye needs immediate irrigation. Test ocular pH before and after irrigation; goal is 7.3–7.7, ideally 7.45.

HF is found in glass etching, dyes, high-octane gas, and germicides.

Phenol is found in dyes, deodorants, agriculture, and disinfectants.

- Escharotomy for full-thickness or circumferential burns.
- Analgesia with morphine.
- Blisters: Best left intact until consulting service can evaluate (skin is protective); incise and drain sterilely all those not on palms and soles if delayed transfer or consultation.
- No role for prophylactic antibiotics.
- Antibiotic skin cream/ointment application only if delay of transfer to burn unit or delay in arrival of consulting service for many hours; silver sulfadiazine or bacitracin.
- Tetanus prophylaxis.

CRITERIA FOR TRANSFER TO BURN UNIT

- > 10% TBSA in ages < 10 or > 50
- > 20% TBSA in ages 10–50
- Significant burns to face, eyes, ears, hands, feet, genitalia, perineum, or major joints
- > 5% TBSA third-degree burn
- Electrical and chemical burns
- Inhalational injury
- Children

CHEMICAL BURNS

General

- Determine what chemical is by history and physical examination.
- Remove patient from agent, then remove agent from patient.
- If wet agent, dilute with water.
- If dry agent, wipe off first.
- Remove clothing.
- Assess size and depth of burn.

Hydrofluoric Acid (HF)

Penetrates tissues like alkalies and releases flouride ion, which immobilizes intracellular Ca^{2+} and Mg^{2+}, poisoning enzymes.

TREATMENT

- Dilute with water for 30 minutes.
- Detoxify: Local intramuscular/subcutaneous/transdermal, IV, or intra-arterial 5–10% calcium gluconate solution.

Phenol (Carbolic Acid)

Causes local coagulation necrosis, protein denaturation, and systemic life-threatening complications.

TREATMENT

- Dilute with water.
- Isopropyl alcohol ↓ local absorption and necrosis.

Lime (Calcium Oxide)

- Desiccates
- Converted to alkali by water (calcium hydroxide)

TREATMENT

Brush off, then dilute.

Lime is found in agriculture and cement.

Lyes (KOH, NaOH, Ca(OH)$_2$, LiOH)

- Strong alkalies burn more deeply and longer, → liquefaction necrosis.
- High tissue absorption.
- If swallowed, aggressively manage airway and have surgical intervention available. Dilute aggressively.

TREATMENT

Dilute with water.

Metals (Industrial, Molten)

Water can cause severe exothermic reaction.

TREATMENT

- Cover hot metal fragments with mineral oil.
- Brush off or excise fragments.

Hydrocarbons

- Tar causes deep thermal burns.
- Dissolve tar, don't peel it off (takes skin too).

Tar is found in gasoline and hot tars.

TREATMENT

- Dilute gasoline with water.
- Aggressively cool tar.
- Use Neosporin (polysorbate) to remove tar.

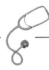

Do not try to remove tar with acetone. It will make the tar stick to the skin even more and continue burning.

ELECTRICAL BURNS

PHYSICS OF ELECTRICITY

- I = current (amps), R = resistance (ohms), E = energy (joules), V = voltage (volts).
- As current flows through a resistor (tissue), energy is deposited as heat.
- Current flows through path of least resistance.
- High voltage: ≥ 1,000 V (> 600 V clinically).
- U.S. household circuits = 110 V (220 V entering home).
- Tasers = 50,000 V, 10–15 pulses per second.

Ohm's law: $V = I \times R$
Joule's law:
$E = I^2 \times R \times \text{time}$

SIGNS AND SYMPTOMS

- On scene: Look for source, entrance/exit wounds, extent of cutaneous injury (may reflect internal).

- Underlying internal damage far exceeds skin burns (rule of nines does not apply).
- Blood vessels, nerves, and muscle damaged most ($\rightarrow$ compromised vasculature, vasospasm, rhabdomyolysis, paralysis, neuropathies).
- Children biting electric cords: Risk of delayed hemorrhage from labial artery at mouth edges.
- Delayed cataracts with ocular involvement.

TREATMENT

- Scene safety.
- ABCs, support respirations.
- Advanced cardiac life support (ACLS) protocol as appropriate.
- IV access and fluids—20 cc/kg bolus.
- Treat thermal burns.
- Tetanus prophylaxis.
- Admit if poor risk, pregnant, high voltage, or systemic injury.

Lightning Injury

 A 29-year-old man is found lying in a big open field, not breathing and pulseless. His clothes are tattered, he has no shoes, and he has blood in his ear canals. He is awake but confused. You notice fernlike burns on his skin. What is the most likely explanation for these findings?

He has most likely suffered a lightning injury. This can create a classic fernlike pattern on the skin and is associated with ruptured tympanic membranes.

PHYSICS OF LIGHTNING

- Ten million to 2 billion V.
- Unidirectional impulse of current.
- Temperature 14,432–90,032°F.
- Hot, humid days.
- Strikes metal or tall objects.
- Electricity flows over the body (flashover) as well as through, causing pathognomonic fern-shaped mark on the skin caused by electron showering.

DEFINITIONS

- Direct strike: Lightning versus person
- Contact strike: Lightning versus object person is touching
- Side flash: Lightning versus object near person, then flash from object
- Ground current: Lightning versus ground near person, then up person's foot
- Stride potential/step voltage: Lightning versus ground near person, then up one foot and down the other; temporarily cold, numb, paretic, pulseless legs

SIGNS AND SYMPTOMS

- Fernlike pattern to skin (cutaneous streaking; Figure 18-3)
- Ruptured tympanic membranes
- Often unconscious
- Cardiac arrhythmias

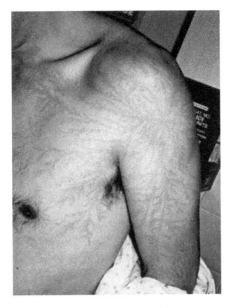

FIGURE 18-3. Characteristic cutaneous streaking pattern of lightning injury.

(Reproduced, with permission, from Tintinalli JE, Kelen GD, Stapczynski JS. *Emergency Medicine: A Comprehensive Study Guide*, 5th ed. New York: McGraw-Hill, 2000: 1300.)

TREATMENT

- ABCs, secure airway.
- ACLS protocol as appropriate.
- Reverse triage if multiple injured: Care for "dead" first—they recover if supported.
- Immobilize C-spine.
- Tetanus prophylaxis.
- Electrocardiogram (ECG) and cardiac monitor.
- Urinalysis, complete blood count, creatine kinase (CK) and CK-MB, lytes, blood urea nitrogen (BUN)/creatinine.
- Treat any bony fractures; admit for observation.

HEAT ILLNESS

Heat Transfer

- Radiation:
  - 65% of normal body cooling
  - Heat transfer from electromagnetic waves
- Convection:
  - 10–15% of normal body cooling
  - Heat transfer from cooler water vapor in air current
- Conduction:
  - 2% of normal body cooling
  - Heat transfer from direct physical contact
- Evaporation:
  - 15–25% of normal body cooling
  - Heat transfer from evaporated sweat/breath

Associated heat-related symptoms:

- Heat syncope (postural hypotension)
- Prickly heat (maculopapular rash under clothed areas)
- Heat tetany (carpopedal spasm, hyperventilation)
- Heat cramps (muscle cramping due to electrolyte loss)

Heat Exhaustion

DEFINITION

Syndrome of vague constitutional symptoms associated with salt and water depletion, and heat exposure or heavy exertion.

SIGNS AND SYMPTOMS

- Dizziness or fatigue with normal mental status
- Nausea/vomiting
- Headache
- Positional hypotension/syncope
- Mildly elevated temperature
- Diaphoresis
- Heat-related illnesses: Prickly heat, heat cramps, or heat tetany

TREATMENT

- Remove from heat.
- Rest.
- IV hydration with normal saline, oral hydration with sports drinks.
- Check and correct electrolytes.
- Observe for resolution of symptoms.

Heat Stroke

DEFINITION

Rapid rise in core temperature ($> 40.5°C$ [$104.9°F$]) associated with:

- Altered mental status
- Symptoms of heat exhaustion
- Anhidrosis
- Loss of temperature regulation

SIGNS AND SYMPTOMS

- CNS abnormalities:
  - Ataxia
  - Combativeness
  - Hallucination
  - Seizure
  - Posturing
  - Hemiplegia
  - Coma
- Renal failure:
  - $\downarrow Ca^{2+}$
  - Hypo- or hypernatremia
  - $\downarrow PO_4^-$
  - Hypo- or hyperkalemia
- Coagulation:
  - $\uparrow$ bleeding times
  - Consumptive coagulopathy and disseminated intravascular coagulation
- Liver failure:
  - Abnormal liver function tests.
  - $\uparrow$ creatine phosphokinase (CPK) and rhabdomyolysis.
- Hypotension
- Death

TREATMENT

- Rule out other causes of fever and altered mental status (sepsis, thyrotoxicosis, meningitis, neuroleptic malignant syndrome [NMS], etc).
- Remove from heat sources.
- Control ABCs, O_2; monitor rectal temperature.
- Use cooling techniques (see below); avoid rebound hypothermia.
- Correct electrolyte abnormalities.
- Check complete blood count, urinalysis, CPK, prothrombin time, partial thromboplastin time, BUN/creatinine, and ECG.
- Benzodiazepines for shivering.

Antipyretics (ibuprofen, acetaminophen) are not helpful in heatstroke.

COOLING TECHNIQUES

- **Evaporation:**
  - Water mist and blowing fans
  - Heat dissipated by evaporation
  - Rapid
  - Most practical in the ED
- **Immersion:**
  - Tub of water and ice
  - Heat dissipated by conduction
  - Impractical
  - Can't monitor patient
- **Ice packing:**
  - Ice bags to groin and axillae
  - Heat dissipated by conduction
  - Easy
  - Slow
  - Poorly tolerated
- **Cool lavage:**
  - **Gastric:**
    - Via nasogastric tube
    - Heat dissipated by conduction
    - Invasive
    - Slow
    - Poorly tolerated
  - **Peritoneal:**
    - Via peritoneal catheter
    - Heat dissipated by conduction
    - Invasive
    - Very rapid
    - Questionable sterility

MALIGNANT HYPERTHERMIA

DEFINITION

Autosomal dominant pseudocholinesterase deficiency.

SIGNS AND SYMPTOMS

- Hyperthermia.
- Rhabdomyolysis.

Malignant hyperthermia is associated with halothane and succinylcholine administration.

- Muscle rigidity.
- Not related to exogenous heat sources.
- Pathophysiology is distinct from NMS.

TREATMENT

- Dantrolene 2–3 mg/kg IV q6h
- No more succinylcholine

NEUROLEPTIC MALIGNANT SYNDROME (NMS)

- See Toxicology chapter for more details.
- Reaction to antipsychotic agents.
- **Symptoms:**
  - Hyperthermia.
  - Also associated with "lead pipe rigidity," altered mental status, and autonomic dysfunction (labile blood pressure, dysrhythmias).

COLD INJURIES

Chilblains

DEFINITION

- Local injury from dry cold at nonfreezing temperatures
- Most commonly affects extremities and ears

SIGNS AND SYMPTOMS

- Local edema
- Nodules or blisters
- Erythema or cyanosis
- Rarely ulcers or bullae

TREATMENT

- Reversible with gentle rewarming
- Moisturizer
- Avoidance of the cold

Trench Foot

DEFINITION

- Nonfreezing injury from wet cold
- Due to prolonged immersion in standing water
- Causes direct soft-tissue injury and nerve damage

SIGNS AND SYMPTOMS

- Numbness/tingling, permanent numbness possible
- Pallor, mottling
- Lack of pulses

TREATMENT

- Rest, elevation, local skin care
- Avoidance of the cold

Frostbite

DEFINITION

- Freezing injury when skin temperatures fall below 0°C (32°F) from body trying to maintain normal core temperature (prefreeze state).
- Ice crystals form in extracellular space (freeze state).
- Tissue loss.
- Most commonly occurs on extremities and face.

Frostnip: Mild reversible, superficial frostbite.

SIGNS AND SYMPTOMS

- Throbbing, shooting pain in joints
- Numbness, tingling
- Edema
- Blisters (clear or hemorrhagic)
- Eschars (develop over a few days)

TREATMENT

- Active rewarming in warm water (40–42.2°C [104–108°F]).
- Tetanus, analgesia.
- Aspirate clear blisters.
- Limb elevation.
- Topical aloe vera.
- Treat for associated hypothermia (see below).

Hypothermia

A 56-year-old homeless man is brought into the ED after being found by law enforcement drunk on a park bench. It is a cool, rainy fall day. His clinical exam is consistent with alcohol intoxication. His vital signs are stable, but the nurse reports that she cannot get a temperature on the patient. What should you do next?

This patient is hypothermic, which often makes obtaining a temperature difficult. A rectal or bladder temperature (via a urethral catheter) should be obtained. In this case, the rectal temperature is 31°C (87.8°F), consistent with moderate hypothermia. This patient should have his wet clothing removed, and he should receive active rewarming measures (warming with blankets, IV fluids, bladder irrigation, etc).

DEFINITION

- Core temperature < 35°C (< 95°F)
- Usually due to prolonged overwhelming cold exposure; can occur in any season

At risk for hypothermia:
- Extremes of age
- Alcohol users
- Homeless
- Altered mental status (including psychiatric disorders)
- Trauma victims
- Underlying chronic illness
- Hypoglycemia
- Sepsis

Tympanic membrane temperature measurements are not reliable below 34.4°C (94°F). *Get a rectal temperature!*

SIGNS AND SYMPTOMS

Mild Hypothermia: 32–35°C (90–95°F)
- Shivering
- Excitation
- Tachypnea
- Tachycardia
- Apathy
- Poor judgment
- Dysarthria
- Ataxia

Moderate Hypothermia: 28–32°C (82–90°F)
- Shivering ceases
- Stupor
- Bradycardia
- Dysrhythmias (often atrial fibrillation)
- Dilated pupils

Severe Hypothermia: < 28°C (< 82°F)
- Coma
- Hypotension
- ↓ cardiac output
- Areflexia
- ↓ respiratory rate
- Dysrhythmias (often ventricular fibrillation, agonal, or asystole)
- May appear dead

TREATMENT

- **All patients:**
  - Remove wet clothing.
  - Get rectal temperature.
  - Get ECG (Figure 18-4).
  - Look for and treat concomitant illness (alcohol, hypoglycemia, trauma).

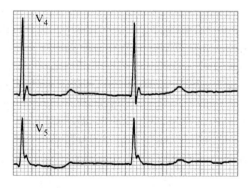

FIGURE 18-4. Osborn (J) wave of hypothermia.

- **Mild hypothermia:** Passive rewarming with blankets.
- **Moderate and severe hypothermia:**
  - Active rewarming.
  - Handle with care: Sudden manipulation can precipitate cardiac dysrhythmias.
  - Cardiac monitoring.
- **Cardiac dysrhythmias:**
- Treat cardiac dysrhythmias as per ACLS protocol.
- Remember, the best treatment for cardiac dysrhythmias in hypothermia is rewarming.
- Severely hypothermic patients who appear dead can have normal or near-normal neurologic outcomes: **Continue resuscitation until warm!**

Methods of active rewarming (in order of invasiveness):
- Warmed blankets
- Mechanical warming blanket
- Warmed IV fluids
- Warmed bladder irrigation
- Warmed gastric lavage
- Warmed peritoneal irrigation
- Warmed cardiopulmonary bypass
- Warmed pleural cavity with chest tube lavage

"Nobody is dead until they are warm and dead."

Environmental Emergencies

HIGH-YIELD FACTS

Environmental Emergencies

Ethics, Medicolegal Issues, and Evidence-Based Medicine

The **"duty to warn"** was established by the Tarasoff case. In this case, a physician caring for a patient who made homicidal statements about another person was found liable for her death because he failed to protect or warn her, or to report the situation to police.

- **Beneficence:** To act in the best interest of one's patient.
- **Nonmaleficence:** Do no harm—this includes protecting one's patient from personnel not qualified to deliver appropriate care due to lack of training, experience, or impairment.
- **Privacy and confidentiality:** Physicians have a duty to protect the confidentiality of patient information. Disclosure of sensitive information is appropriate only when such disclosure is necessary to carry out a stronger conflicting duty, such as a duty to protect an identifiable third party from serious harm or to comply with a just law.
- **Autonomy:** The ability to function independently and to make decisions about one's care free from the undue influence or bias of others.
    - All patients are considered autonomous if they have capacity, defined as the ability to understand the situation and the consequences of their action.
    - Physicians have a duty to respect the health care preferences of their patients, whenever possible. However, some patient preferences cannot be honored (eg, suicide, unnecessary testing, etc).
- **Justice:** The principle of equal and fair allocation of benefit.
    - Provision of emergency medical treatment should not be based on gender, age, race, socioeconomic status, or cultural background.
    - No patient should ever be abused, demeaned, or given substandard care.

Consent for Treatment

A 35-year-old man presents with the worst headache of his life. You are concerned about the possibility of a subarachnoid hemorrhage. His head computed tomography (CT) does not reveal a bleed. You discuss a lumbar puncture and the patient refuses. What do you do?

Under the principle of autonomy, patients have the right to refuse care as long as they have the capacity to understand the risks and benefits or consequences of their decisions. If there is a question of impaired decision-making capacity, efforts need to be made to protect the patient until this can be further assessed. For example, an obviously intoxicated patient may not refuse care if it is life threatening and time sensitive. If the care can be delayed until the patient is sober, that is an alternative possibility.

A 65-year-old man is sent to the emergency department (ED) from dialysis because he refused dialysis. After talking with your patient, you realize that he is depressed and does not want to live. He is therefore refusing dialysis. His vital signs are stable without respiratory compromise. His potassium is normal. What is the next step?

The patient is depressed and suicidal and may lack the capacity to refuse dialysis. At this point, he does not need emergent dialysis, and therefore he should not be forced to have dialysis immediately. He should undergo emergent psychiatric evaluation in the ED and should be placed on a psychiatric hold.

Consent for treatment should be obtained when the patient is capable of providing such consent.

- The informed consent process should include a description of the proposed treatment, the risks and benefits of treatment, alternatives to treatment, and the potential outcomes of the treatment options.
- Implied consent is inferred when a patient is unable to give consent, the condition is life threatening without emergent treatment, and it is assumed the patient would want the treatment if he or she were able to give consent.

Discharge Against Medical Advice

Patients who have capacity may refuse care. Oral or written instructions from a patient to family members and health care professionals about health care decisions.

Privacy and Confidentiality

- Patient information is privileged and confidential. Information may not be released to other parties without patient's consent. Such other parties include family members, employers, and police.
- The **Health Insurance Portability and Accountability Act (HIPAA) of 1996** protects and governs such disclosures.
- There are specific exemptions and requirements under the law that may mandate disclosure such as gunshot wounds and child abuse.

Emergency Medical Treatment and Labor Act (EMTALA)

- A federal law that requires anyone coming to an ED receive a medical screening exam to determine if a medical emergency exists, and further if an emergency exists, it needs to be stabilized and treated, regardless of their insurance status or ability to pay.
- EMTALA was passed as part of Consolidated Omnibus Budget Reconciliation Act (COBRA) in 1986.
- Governs the interfacility transfer of patients and was design to prevent dumping of uninsured patients.

EMTALA was passed to ensure appropriate emergency care to all patients, regardless of their ability to pay.

Patients should participate in these decisions unless they are unable (lack capacity). In such situations, other options may be available.

Advance Directives

- Oral or written instructions from a patient to family members and health care professionals about health care decisions.
- May include living wills; designation of a health care proxy; specific instructions about which therapies to accept or decline, such as intubation, surgery, medical treatments, and Do Not Resuscitate (DNR) orders.

- A DNR order applies only to advanced cardiac life support resuscitation and may not include intubation and ventilation unless specifically addressed.
- Comfort Measures Only (CMO) or comfort care refers to therapies designed only to make the patient comfortable but not necessarily sustain life.

Medical Decision Surrogates

Also known as a **health care proxy**; appointed by the patient. Surrogates should make decisions based on the patient's preferences and not on their own wishes.

PHYSICIAN IMPAIRMENT

Physicians have a duty to report an impaired or incompetent colleague to the chief of staff or appropriate regulatory agency. Many states have mechanisms in place whereby anonymous reporting can be done. Physicians who conscientiously fulfill this responsibility should be protected from adverse political, legal, or financial consequences. Action toward the impaired physician may include internal discipline and/or remedial training. It does not necessarily mean the physician will lose his or her license to practice medicine.

MEDICAL RECORD DOCUMENTATION GUIDELINES

General Principles

- Medical record should be legible and complete.
- Rationale for ordering laboratory and other ancillary tests should be documented.
- Patient's emergency department course, including response to any treatment, should be documented.
- Documentation in record should support Current Procedural Terminology and ICD-9-CM codes submitted on insurance form and billing statement.

Key Elements of Chart

- Reason for encounter (chief complaint)
- History, physical exam (including addressing of any abnormal vital signs)
- Assessment, clinical impression, or diagnosis
- Care plan
- Date and legible identity of observer

LEGAL CONCEPTS

- **Battery:** Unwanted touching
- **Malpractice:** Four elements:
  - Duty to care for the patient

- Breach of duty by not meeting the standard of care.
- Causation: The breach was the proximate cause of injury.
- Harm: Damages were incurred.

Cost Containment

The practice of conscientiously limiting medical expenses without compromising the medical care of the patient. The factor most directly in the control of the physician is the judicious use of laboratory and radiographic tests.

Child Abuse

All human services professionals, including physicians, are required by all 50 states to report known or *suspected* child abuse. There is no penalty for the reporting of cases that turn out not to be cases of abuse.

Communicable Diseases

Many infectious diseases that are transmissible are reportable to both the federal and state authorities. The process and list of diseases varies from state to state. The list includes:

- Acquired immune deficiency syndrome (AIDS)
- Anthrax
- Botulism
- Brucellosis
- Chancroid
- *Chlamydia trachomatis*, genital infections
- Cholera
- Coccidioidomycosis
- Cryptosporidiosis
- Diphtheria
- Encephalitides
- *Escherichia coli* O157
- Gonorrhea
- *Haemophilus influenzae*, invasive
- Hansen disease (leprosy)
- Hantavirus pulmonary syndrome
- Hepatitis
- Legionellosis
- Lyme disease
- Malaria
- Measles
- Meningococcal disease
- Mumps
- Pertussis
- Plague

- Poliomyelitis
- Psittacosis
- Rabies, animal and human
- Rocky Mountain spotted fever
- Rubella
- Salmonellosis
- Shigellosis
- *Streptococcus pneumoniae*, invasive drug-resistant disease
- Syphilis
- Tetanus
- Toxic shock syndrome
- Trichinosis
- Tuberculosis
- Typhoid fever
- Yellow fever

Public Health Issues

Many states have laws regarding other public health issues where public safety is involved or to protect a vulnerable individual such as:

- Gunshot wounds
- Elder neglect and abuse
- Domestic violence
- Driving with certain medical conditions: seizure, syncope

PRINCIPLES OF EVIDENCE-BASED MEDICINE

Evidence-based medicine is the practice of incorporating the best available evidence from the medical literature for a diagnostic test or treatment into daily patient care. It is an active process that requires five steps:

1. Identify a clinical problem.
2. Formulate a question.
3. Search for the best evidence.
4. Appraise the evidence.
5. Apply the information to the clinical problem.

A thorough search of the medical literature requires a computer or Internet search of MEDLINE, through OVID, Grateful Med, or Pub Med. All relevant articles should be considered. The best evidence is most often provided by meta-analysis or randomized clinical trials.

Sensitivity

- (People with disease who tested positive)/(All people with disease) true positive (TP)/(TP + false negative [FN])
- Low rate of false negatives gives high value.

Specificity

- (People without disease who tested negative)/(All people without disease) true negative (TN)/(TN + false positive [FP]).
- Low rate of false positives gives high value.

It is important to note that many well-established practices are not in fact proven by high-quality evidence, but rather consensus.

SpinS out:
High **specificity** rules **in**, high **sensitivity** rules **out** disease.

The more sensitive a test, the less likely the test is to fail to detect a positive result.

The more specific a test, the less likely the test is to fail to detect negative result.

Positive Predictive Value

> A 19-year-old woman presents with pleuritic chest pain. She is on birth control pills. A D-dimer is ordered. How do you interpet the result?
>
> D-dimer is a highly sensitive test for pulmonary embolus (PE), but has a low specificity. In a relatively low prevalence population, the test has high negative predictive value, but low positive predictive value. So if the test is negative (high negative predictive values), she most likely does not have a PE. If the test is positive (low positive predictive value), the patient may or may not have a PE. A confirmatory test is needed, such as a CT of the chest. A D-dimer may be a good screening test in low-risk patients because it is very sensitive; it should not be used too broadly, however, as it has a large number of false-positive results.

Tests with high predictive values are likely to be correct; this is impacted by sensitivity and specificity of the test as well as the prevalence of the disease.

- (People with disease who tested positive)/(All people who tested positive) TP/(TP + FP)
- All positive variables

Negative Predictive Value

- (People without disease who tested negative)/(All people who tested negative)
- TN/(TN + FN)
- All negative variables

Likelihood Ratio (LR)

A high positive LR ↑ the pretest likelihood that a patient has a disease.

- Measures the fixed relationship between the chance of given test result in a patient with the disorder and the chance of the same test result in a patient without the disorder.
- LR for a positive test result = Sensitivity/(1 − specificity)
- LR for a negative test result = (1 − sensitivity)/Specificity

Number Needed to Treat

Measures the number of patients with a given disease that a clinician would need to treat with the tested therapy in order to see one beneficial event or prevent one adverse event.

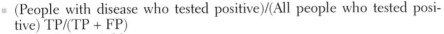

SOURCES OF MEDICAL EVIDENCE

Meta-analysis

Evaluates the data of many trials that address the same question and attempts to combine the information: These studies are best used when the clinical problem is infrequent and large randomized trials cannot be done.

Randomized Controlled Clinical Trial (RCT)

The selected population is randomized to receive either the treatment in question or a placebo, and the outcome is measured. The ideal RCT is triple-blinded, meaning that the treating physician, the patient, and the investigators do not know which treatment has been given until the analysis is complete. These studies can establish cause and effect.

Cohort Study

The selected population is identified as being exposed or not exposed and is monitored for subsequent effects. These studies are used when the exposure cannot be assigned for logistical or ethical reasons.

Case Control Study

Populations with and without a given outcome are selected, and historical (retrospective) data are collected on exposure to a given agent or treatment.

Consensus

A panel of experts in the field who make recommendations about treatments given limited or unclear evidence.

Awards and Opportunities for Students Interested in Emergency Medicine

The Emergency Medicine Residents' Association (EMRA) is the largest emergency medicine organization for residents and medical students interested in emergency medicine as a career choice. A number of publications are offered as part of membership, which are listed on their web site: www.emra.org.

For medical students, EMRA has a Medical Student Committee (MSC) that:

- Educates medical students about the specialty of emergency medicine and its importance to the practice of medicine in this country.
- Provides information to those students interested in emergency medicine regarding career options and emergency medicine training programs.
- Develops a network of physician advisors for third- and fourth-year medical students who may not have access to role models in emergency medicine.
- Establishes a peer network for medical students aspiring to careers in emergency medicine and allows them the opportunity to assume leadership roles in organized emergency medicine.
- Provides American College of Emergency Physicians (ACEP) and Society for Academic Emergency Medicine (SAEM) with a resource for dissemination of materials and information to medical students and training institutions.

Dr. Alexandra Greene Medical Student Award

The EMRA Medical Student Award has been named in honor of Dr. Alexandra Greene. The award is given to recognize the great talent, hard work, and true compassion embodied by Dr. Greene, and to pass her memory on to students who might carry on her work.

Award Criteria: The Dr. Alexandra Greene EMRA Medical Student Award recognizes a student who displays a significant dedication to emergency medicine. More important, this student goes out of his or her way for patients and colleagues. This student demonstrates compassion and professionalism even when faced with difficult situations and stresses.

Application Process: Single letter of support, the nominee's curriculum vitae (CV), and application form.

Eligibility: Medical student member of EMRA.

Selection Criteria: Leadership and service to students.

Award: Plaque and $500.

EMRA Research Grant

Purpose of Award: To provide research funding to physicians in training (residents or medical students) interested in completing a research project during residency/medical school. This grant promotes the involvement of emergency medicine trainees in research that supports the specialty of emergency medicine and its training.

Application Process: Submit cover letter, grant proposal form (using the EMRA research project proposal form), and CV(s) of primary author(s) to

CLASSIFIED

EMRA. Preferred method of submission is by e-mail to gachilles@emra.org. You may also submit materials by mail or fax.

Eligibility: Grants will be available to any EMRA medical student or resident member, or any emergency medicine interest group whose principal applicant is an EMRA student or resident member.

Selection Criteria: The proposed project must be consistent with EMRA's purposes and objectives. The EMRA Research Committee will review grant applications, and projects will be selected based on the perceived importance and possible impact of the research, as described on the research project proposal form.

Award: One award of $500 each spring.

Application Deadline: March 15.

EMRA Travel Scholarship to SAEM

Purpose: To assist a resident or student member of EMRA in the costs associated with attendance of the SAEM annual meeting.

Application Process: Letter of intent explaining need and purpose of attendance (no greater than one page), single letter of support, current CV, and application form.

Eligibility: Resident or student member of EMRA (international members included).

Selection Criteria: Up to three applicants may be chosen based on financial need and academic pursuit.

Award: $500.

Application Deadline: March 15.

About SAEM: The SAEM annual meeting brings together academic emergency medicine physicians from many regions to a single location. Thus, these meetings provide an opportunity for organizations other than SAEM to access the academic emergency medicine community. Visit www.saem.org for more information.

EMRA Travel Scholarship to Scientific Assembly

Purpose: To assist a resident or student member of EMRA in the costs associated with attendance of this national event.

Application Process: Letter of intent explaining need and purpose of attendance (no greater than one page), single letter of support, current CV, and application form.

Eligibility: Resident or student member of EMRA (international members included).

Selection Criteria: Up to three applicants may be chosen based on financial need and academic pursuit.

Award: $500.

Application Deadline: August 15.

517

About Scientific Assembly: Scientific Assembly is the largest gathering of emergency physicians in the country, as thousands of medical professionals from across the nation and more than 30 countries meet to learn the latest medical advances and debate the medical and policy issues of vital interest to them and their patients. For more information, visit www.acep.org/sa.

EMRA Local Action Grants

Purpose of Award: To promote the involvement of emergency medicine residents in community service and other activities that support the specialty of emergency medicine.

Application Process: Submit cover letter, grant proposal form (using the EMRA local action grant template), and CV(s) of primary author(s) to EMRA. Preferred method of submission is by email to gachilles@emra.org. You may also submit materials by mail or fax. Application and cover letter may be submitted using the general award application form.

Eligibility: Grants will be available to any EMRA member (medical students, residents, fellows) or any emergency medicine interest group whose principal applicant is an EMRA member.

Selection Criteria: The proposed project must be consistent with EMRA's purposes and objectives. Grants will be awarded in support of projects relating to: improving community health through education, direct services or preventive programs (eg, developing a local bicycle helmet education program); supporting the specialty of emergency medicine through community awareness, advocacy of local and state medical societies, or involvement with local and state government (eg, development of a state "Emergency Medicine Day"); improving opportunities for resident education and interaction on the residency, state, or regional level (eg, travel honorariums for speakers, development of a regional EM resident conference).

Award: One award not to exceed $1000 each spring and fall.

Application Deadline: March 15 for spring award, August 15 for fall award.

AMERICAN COLLEGE OF EMERGENCY PHYSICIANS AWARDS

The American College of Emergency Physicians (ACEP) is a national medical specialty society representing emergency medicine, with more than 28,000 members. It administers two awards specifically for medical students: (1) the National Outstanding Medical Student Award, and (2) the Medical Student Professionalism and Service Award.

Please contact Academic Affairs at academicaffairs@acep.org or 800-798-1822, ext. 3143 for more information.

National Outstanding Medical Student Award

This award is intended to recognize students who excel in compassionate care of patients, professional behavior, and service to the community and/or specialty. Up to 10 awards per year are given.

Award recognition includes:

- A plaque from ACEP.
- Free 1-year membership in ACEP.
- Free registration to ACEP's annual meeting.
- Convocation at ACEP's annual meeting.
- Publication of winners' names in ACEP News or other college publications.
- Notification of the award recipients to state chapters.

SELECTION PROCESS

ACEP is asking the chair of emergency medicine, the emergency medicine program director, or the medical student clerkship director to select one medical student who is emergency medicine bound, to complete the application that addresses:

- Humanism, professionalism, and clinical judgment as attested to by the nominating individual.
- Scholarly achievement: Grades, academic rank, the U.S. Medical Licensing Exam (USMLE) scores for allopathic residencies or the Comprehensive Medical Licensing Exams (COMLEX) scores for osteopathic residencies, and honors (AOA, etc.).
- CV-driven listing of activities with annotated description of each of the following:
  - Leadership and service to medical organizations: Focus on professional service and advocacy (service to the College with emphasis on the College's priority objectives, or local emergency medicine interest group [EMIG]).
  - Community service.
  - Research and publications.

Application Deadline: February 15.

Medical Student Professionalism and Service Award

This award is intended to recognize students who excel in compassionate care of patients, professional behavior, and service to the community and/or specialty.

Award recognition includes:

- A certificate from ACEP and a reception for award winners at ACEP's annual Scientific Assembly. Any monetary award is to be decided at the local level.
- Award recipients will be announced in an ACEP publication and on the ACEP web site.
- Announcement may also be made at your medical school's awards or graduation ceremony.

SELECTION PROCESS

ACEP is asking the chair of emergency medicine, the emergency medicine program director, or the medical student clerkship director, to select one medical student who is emergency medicine bound, using the following criteria:

- The student gives outstanding care to patients in a manner that exemplifies professionalism and a humanistic approach to patients, their families, and fellow health care workers.

- The student has evidence of active service to medical organizations and the community that demonstrates a substantial commitment of time and effort, with evidence of leadership.
- Grades and board scores are not a requisite for this award.

Application Deadline: October 30.

Emergency Medicine Medical Student Interest Group Educational Grants

The Society for Academic Emergency Medicine recognizes the valuable role of emergency medicine medical student interest groups (EMIGs) for medical students, and award grants to support these groups' educational activities. Established or developing EMIGs, located at medical schools with or without emergency medicine residencies, are eligible to apply.

The goals of the SAEM Education Grant for EMIGs are to:

- Promote growth of emergency medicine education at the medical student level.
- Identify new educational methodologies advancing undergraduate education in emergency medicine.
- Support educational endeavors of an EMIG.

Given these broad goals, there are few limitations on the nature of eligible proposals. Proposals should focus on educational activities or projects related to undergraduate education in emergency medicine. Grant monies may be used for supplies, consultation, and seed money. Faculty salary support is excluded.

Applications will be reviewed by a subcommittee of the SAEM Undergraduate Education Committee. There are usually five to seven $500 grants awarded annually.

SAEM Medical Student Excellence in Emergency Medicine Award

This award is offered annually to each medical school in the United States and Canada. It is awarded to the senior medical student at each school who best exemplifies the qualities of an excellent emergency physician, as manifested by excellent clinical, interpersonal, and manual skills, and a dedication to continued professional development leading to outstanding performance on emergency medicine rotations. The award, presented at graduation, conveys a 1-year membership in SAEM, which includes subscriptions the SAEM monthly journal, *Academic Emergency Medicine*, the SAEM Newsletter, and an award certificate.

Announcements describing the program and applications are sent to the dean's office at each medical school in February. Coordinators of emergency medicine student rotations then select an appropriate student based on the student's intramural and extramural performance in emergency medicine. Each school must submit the name of its recipient no later than June 1. The list of winners is published in a summer issue of the SAEM Newsletter.

Over 110 medical schools currently participate in this award. Contact SAEM at saem@saem.org if your school would like to participate.

SAEM Medical Student Emergency Medicine Symposium

Each year during the SAEM annual meeting, an emergency medicine medical student forum is held. This session is designed to help the medical student understand the residency and career options that exist in emergency medicine, develop an optimal senior-year schedule, evaluate residency programs, and navigate the residency application process. The medical student also learns to recognize and begin management of common and potentially life-threatening problems that present to the emergency department. A medical student/resident visual diagnosis photography contest is also held at the SAEM annual meeting. Small prizes are awarded, and winners are acknowledged in the SAEM Newsletter.

SAEM/EMF Medical Student EM Research Grants

SAEM and the Emergency Medicine Foundation (EMF) sponsor annual grants of up to a maximum of $2400 over 3 months for medical students. Applications can be obtained from EMF. The deadline is in January every year.

AMERICAN ACADEMY OF EMERGENCY MEDICINE (AAEM) AWARDS

At the time of this writing, there are no AAEM awards offered specifically for medical students per se. However, AAEM (www.aaem.org) has a residents and students association (RSA) that offers an e-mail contact list, a "medical student forum" feature in their monthly newsletter, and a great web-based residency tool called emselect.com. EM Select is a tool developed by medical students for medical students with the goal of making the application process easier to manage. The tool allows you to search through the EM residency database, create a customized list, make notes on the list, and compare your programs side by side in order to make a rank list.

ROYAL SOCIETY OF MEDICINE (UNITED KINGDOM) AWARDS

Emergency Medicine Section Students' Prize

Submission Deadline: The deadline for this academic year has now passed; next year's deadline will be advertised when available.

Meeting Date: TBA.

Prize: £500 and a 1-year membership to the RSM.

Open To: Medical students.

This prize is to contribute toward the cost of an elective abroad, with the intention of gaining experience in the practice of emergency medicine. It is open to medical students.

Applicants should provide details of the proposed elective abroad in no more than 1000 words. They should also provide a current CV. After returning from the elective, the winner will be invited to give a presentation at one of the meetings of the Section of A&E Medicine.

Web site: www.rsm.ac.uk/academ/awards/.

E-mail: emergency@rsm.ac.uk.

CLASSIFIED

AMA Foundation Awards

PHYSICIANS OF TOMORROW SCHOLARSHIPS

Purpose: The AMA Foundation has made it a priority to assist medical students in handling the rising cost of medical education. The Physicians of Tomorrow Scholarships were created in 2004 to provide financial assistance to medical students facing spiraling medical school debt. On average, medical students in the United States graduate with a debt load of nearly $155,000. A large debt burden may deter many from practicing in underserved areas of the country, in medical education and research, or in primary care medicine. To date, over $500,000 has been granted to exceptional medical students across the nation.

Eligibility: These $10,000 scholarships reward current third-year medical students or individuals who are approaching their final year of medical school. Multiple scholarships, funded by various organizations, will be awarded. The number of recipients is determined after all applications have been received. Typically, 8–12 recipients in total are selected. Each medical school can nominate one person for each of the three different scholarship opportunities (three nominees in total). All three scholarship categories take into consideration academic excellence and financial need.

Each $10,000 scholarship is based on different eligibility requirements.

- Physicians of Tomorrow Scholarship: Selection is based on academic excellence and financial need.
- Physicians of Tomorrow Scholarship, supported by the Audio-Digest Foundation: Selection is based on a commitment to "the communication of science." Communication of science may be defined as activities such as mentoring and/or teaching.
- Physicians of Tomorrow Scholarship, supported by the Johnson F. Hammond, MD, Fund: Selection is based on a commitment to a career in medical journalism.

Contact your medical school if you are interested in being nominated for the Physicians of Tomorrow Scholarships.

Deadline: Late May.

AMA SEED GRANT RESEARCH PROGRAM

An increasing number of young physician scientists are experiencing difficulty finding the resources and support to do research. Consequently, fewer physicians are choosing careers in research, which is a terrible loss to medicine.

To address this trend, the AMA Foundation established the Seed Grant Research Program in 2000 to encourage medical students, physician residents, and fellows to enter the research field. The program provides $2500 grants to help them conduct small basic science or applied or clinical research projects. These funds will round out new project budgets, rather than sustain current initiatives.

http://www.intjem.com

The *International Journal of Emergency Medicine (IJEM)* is directed toward physicians and medical personnel undergoing training or working within the field of emergency medicine. It focuses on the practice of emergency medicine in a variety of settings, from urban emergency departments to rural clinics, including humanitarian and disaster situations. The content is diverse and features case reports, with discussion on evidence-based practice, clinical images with spot diagnosis, systematic reviews, brief research reports, quality improvement, and innovations.

IJEM is an open-access journal that provides free access to its articles to anyone, anywhere, at any time, without the need of a subscription. *IJEM* is indexed in PubMed, PubMed Central, Medline, Google Scholar, EMBASE, and SCOPUS.

MENTORSHIP

IJEM offers medical students the opportunity to publish interesting case reports and clinical images, as well as opportunities to be mentored as reviewers and board members. Please direct inquires to IJEM2008@gmail.com.

BEST MEDICAL STUDENT PAPER

IJEM awards the best medical student paper for manuscripts submitted where a medical student had significant involvement in the paper/project. An announcement is sent to medical schools informing them of this opportunity.

WEB SITE RESOURCES

http://cdc.org

Presents a wealth of information, including clinical guidelines, up-to-date info on most major diseases, and an excellent search engine with links to other governmental agencies.

http://ncemi.org

Web site of the National Center for Emergency Medicine Informatics. Presented as a daily newspaper page with question of the day, ECG, x-ray photo, and cartoon of the week. Summarizes important abstracts in EM. Has several excellent links to other EM sites. Has many clever medical calculators and facts and formulae.

http://emedicine.com

This web site has online textbooks in emergency medicine and most other primary specialties for use free of charge. These textbooks have four levels of peer review and are continually updated. Opportunities for authorship in one of the many textbooks are available.

CLASSIFIED

http://emcrit.org

This is a user friendly web site dedicated to emergency medicine and emergency critical care. It has lectures, a blog, podcasts, and appendices, all neatly categorized and updated. An interesting section entitled "EM practice and philosophy" covers a group of eclectic topics, including shift work, kaizens, and training errors.

www.hopkins-abxguide.org

This guide from Johns Hopkins University provides current information about using antibiotics for the diagnosis and treatment of infectious diseases. There are multiple ways to search, and this application is available on both Apple iPhone and Blackberry.

Index

sinus tachycardia, 178–179
supraventricular tachycardia (SVT), 181–182
Wolff-Parkinson-White (WPW) syndrome, 182–183

E

Echinococcus, 231
Eclampsia, 132, 321–322
Ectopic pregnancy (EP), 315–317
Eczema, 399
Eikenella corrodens, 187, 492, 493
Elbow dislocation, 353
    posterior, 350
Electrocardiograms (ECGs), 40–43
    axis, 41–42
    cardiac catheterization or thrombolysis, criteria for, 43
    intervals, 42
    lead placement, 41
    morphology, 42
    Q waves, 43
    rate, 41
    rhythm, 41
    ST segments, 43
    U waves, 43
Electrolytes, 31–39, 443
    calcium, 31
        hypercalcemia, 31–32
        hypocalcemia, 32
        ionized, 31
    potassium, 32–35
        hyperkalemia, 34–35
        hypokalemia, 33–34
    sodium, 35–38
        balance, 36
        hypernatremia, 38
        hyponatremia, 36–37
Emergency medicine clerkship, how to succeed in, 1–10
Emesis, forced, 444
Emphysema, 159–160
Encephalitis, 125–126
    causes of, 125
End-stage renal disease (ESRD), 247–248
Endocarditis, acute bacterial (ABE), 187–188
Endometriosis, 305–306
Endometritis, 327
Endotracheal intubation, 17–18
Entamoeba histolytica, 126
Enterobacter, 126, 266
Enterobacter aerogenes, 231

Enterococcus, 406
Environmental/occupational toxins, 472
    carbon monoxide (CO), 473–474
    cyanide, 474
    methemoglobin, 472
Epididymitis, 257–258
Epidural hematoma, 64, 65
Epiglottitis, 142–143, 144
Epistaxis, 135–137
    anterior, 135–136
    posterior, 136–137
Erysipelas, 388
Erythema multiforme (EM), 400–401
Erythema nodosum, 403–404
Escape rhythms, 184–185
    junctional ectopy, 184
    torsades de pointes, 184–185
    ventricular ectopy, 184
    ventricular tachycardia, 185
Escherichia coli, 126, 230, 231, 257, 266, 307, 336
    O157:H7, 284, 285
Esophageal cancer, 216
Esophagitis, 216
Esophagus, 213–216
    Boerhaave syndrome, 216
    foreign body (FB) ingestion, 214–215
    gastroesophageal reflux disease (GERD), 215–216
    varices, 213–214
Estrogens, 313
Ethanol toxicity, 460–461
Ethics. *See* Medical ethics, principles of
Ethylene glycol toxicity, 462–463
Evidence-based medicine, principles of, 512–513
    likelihood ratio (LR), 513
    negative predictive value, 513
    number needed to treat, 513
    positive predictive value, 513
    sensitivity, 512
    specificity, 512
Extension teardrop fracture, 75
Extremity trauma, 91
Extremity x-rays, 45

F

Facial x-rays, 45
Felon, 332–333
Femoral shaft fracture, 359

Fire ant stings, 491–492
Fitz-Hugh–Curtis syndrome, 310
Flexion teardrop fracture, 74–75, 76
Flexor tenosynovitis, 333–334
Focused abdominal sonogram for trauma (FAST), 48, 59, 85–87
    abnormal, 86
    normal, 85
Foley catheter, 55–56
Foreign body airway obstruction, 15–16, 164
    complete, signs of, 16
    Heimlich maneuver (abdominal thrusts), 16
    partial, management of, 16
    risk factors, 15–16
Fournier's gangrene, 258
Fresh frozen plasma (FFP), 292
Frostbite, 503
Frostnip, 503
Fungal infections, cutaneous, 393–394
    candida, 393
    tinea infection, 394
Fusobacterium, 492, 493

G

Galeazzi fracture, 354
Gallbladder, 231–232
    cholangitis, 231
    cholelithiasis and cholecystitis, 232
Gallstone composition, 232
Ganglion cyst, 340
Gardnerella vaginalis, 302
Gas gangrene, 335–336
Gastric intubation, 56
Gastric lavage, 444
Gastric outlet obstruction, 220
Gastritis, acute, 217–218
Gastroesophageal reflux disease (GERD), 215–216
Genitourinary (GU) trauma, 89–91
    bladder rupture, 90
    renal contusion, 90
    renal laceration, 90
    renal fracture ("shattered kidney"), 91
    ureteral injury, 90
Ghon complex, 161
Gila monster and Mexican beaded lizard, 485

Hyperparathyroidism, 373
Hypertension (HTN), 205–206
  hypertensive emergency, 205–206
  hypertensive urgency, 205
  pregnancy-induced, 321–322
    preeclampsia/eclampsia, 321–322
Hyperthermia, malignant, 501–502
Hyperthyroidism, causes of, 376
Hypocalcemia, 32
Hypoglycemia, 372–373
Hypoglycemic toxicity, 453
Hypokalemia, 33–34
Hyponatremia, 36–37
Hypoparathyroidism, 373–374
Hypotension and shock, 24
  causes, 24–25
Hypothermia, 378, 503–505
Hypothyroidism, causes of, 377
Hypovolemic shock, 58

I

Idiopathic thrombocytopenic purpura (ITP), 282–283
Iliopsoas sign, 236
Immersion syndrome, 483–484
Immunogenic cutaneous disorders, 397–405
  angioedema, 397–398
  bullous pemphigoid, 398–399
  eczema, 399
  erythema multiforme (EM), 400–401
  erythema nodosum, 403–404
  Henoch-Schönlein purpura (HSP), 404
  psoriasis, 400
  Stevens-Johnson syndrome (SJS), 401–402
  systemic lupus erythematosus (SLE), 404–405
  toxic epidermal necrolysis (TEN), 402–403
  urticaria, 398
Impetigo, 387–388
Inflammatory bowel disease (IBD), 221–223
  extraintestinal manifestations of, 222
Internuclear ophthalmoplegia, 119
Intracerebral hemorrhage, 115

Intracranial lesions, 63–65
  diffuse, 63
    cerebral concussion, 63
    diffuse axonal injury (DAI), 63
  focal, 64–65
    cerebral contusion, 64
    epidural hematoma, 64, 65
    subdural hematoma, 64, 66
Intracranial pressure, measures to lower, 66
Intraosseous access, 418–419
Intravenous catheters, 56
Intravenous fluid, 56
Intussusception, 225–226
Iron toxicity, 449
Isopropanol, 463–464

J

Janeway lesions, 188
Jarisch-Herxheimer reaction, 270
Jefferson fracture, 73, 75
Joint fluid analysis, 417
Jones fracture, 358
Junctional ectopy, 184

K

Kanavel criteria, 334
Kaposi's sarcoma, 407–408
Kawasaki disease, 193
Kernig sign, 124
Kidney stones, 249–252
Kingella kingae, 187
Klebsiella, 126, 152, 266
Klebsiella pneumoniae, 150
Koebner phenomenon, 400
KOH preparation, 384

L

Labor and delivery. *See* Pregnancy
Laboratory tests, diagnostic, 31
Labyrinthitis, 122
Large intestine, 235–240
  appendicitis, 236–237
  diverticular disease, 238–239
  lower GI bleed, 239–240
  obstruction, 235–236
  Ogilvie syndrome, 238
  volvulus, 237
Laryngeal mask airway (LMA), 17
Left anterior fascicular block (LAFB), 175
Left bundle branch block (LBBB), 176

Left posterior fascicular block (LPFB), 175
Legal concepts, 510–511
Legg-Calvé-Perthes disease, 360–362
Legionella, 152
Legionella pneumophila, 150
Levine sign, 169
Lice (pediculosis), 394
Life-sustaining treatment, 509–510
  advance directives, 509
  medical decision surrogates, 510
Lightning injury, 498–499
Lisfranc fracture, 358
Listeria, 126
Lithium toxicity, 457
Liver, 227–231
  hepatic abscess, 231
  hepatic encephalopathy, 229
  hepatitis, 227–229
  hepatorenal syndrome (HRS), 229–230
  spontaneous bacterial peritonitis (SBP), 230–231
Local anesthesia, 415
Low back pain, 341–344
  cauda equina syndrome, 343–344
  epidural abscess, 342–343
  leading causes of, 341
  lumbar disk herniation, 341
  vertebral compression fracture, 342
Low-pressure dysbarism, 477
Lower extremity trauma, 357–360
  ankle fracture and dislocation, 360
  Baker cyst, 358
  calcaneal fracture, 358
  femoral shaft fracture, 359
  hip dislocation, 359
  hip fracture, 358–359
  Jones fracture, 358
  Lisfranc fracture, 358
  Maisonneuve fracture, 358
  pelvis fracture 357–358
  tibial fracture, proximal, 360
Lower GI bleed, 239–240
Ludwig's angina, 140–141
Lumbar disk herniation, 341
Lumbar spine fractures and dislocations, 77
  burst fracture, 77
  compression (wedge) fracture, 77

CPSIA information can be obtained
at www.ICGtesting.com
Printed in the USA
JSHW052127300623
43978JS00004B/260